Avian Influenza in Human

Chen Qiu • Yu-xin Shi • Pu-xuan Lu
Editors

Avian Influenza in Human

PMPH PEOPLE'S MEDICAL PUBLISHING HOUSE

Springer

Editors
Chen Qiu
Department of Respiratory Diseases
Shenzhen People's Hospital
Shenzhen
Guangdong
China

Yu-xin Shi
Department of Radiology
Shanghai Public Health Clinical Center
Shanghai
China

Pu-xuan Lu
Department of Medical Imaging
Shenzhen Center for Chronic Disease Control
Shenzhen
Guangdong
China

ISBN 978-981-16-1431-6 ISBN 978-981-16-1429-3 (eBook)
https://doi.org/10.1007/978-981-16-1429-3

Jointly published with People's Medical Publishing House, PR of China

This Springer imprint is published by the registered company Springer Nature Singapore Pte Ltd.
The registered company address is: 152 Beach Road, #21-01/04 Gateway East, Singapore 189721, Singapore

Preface

Avian influenza is an acute respiratory infectious disease caused by some of the strains of the avian influenza virus (AIV) belonging to the genus Influenza A (type A). According to the antigenicity of outer membrane hemagglutinin (HA) and neuraminidase (NA), avian influenza virus can be divided into 18 H subtypes (H1–H18) and 11 N subtypes (N1–N11). Theoretically, there are 198 avian influenza virus subtypes. However, more than a dozen subtypes of avian influenza virus have been found to infect humans. Most of these human avian influenza subtypes of human infection occurred in China for the first time in the world, including H7N9, H5N1, H10N8, H5N6, H9N2 and H7N4. The disease has become a global public health problem with rapid onset and high mortality, which has seriously affected social stability and economic development.

In the process of fighting human avian influenza, which originated and distributed in China all over the world, Chinese medical science and technology workers have continuously analyzed and studied the cases of human avian influenza and the practical application of new technologies. The imaging features, imaging diagnosis, differential diagnosis, and curative effect evaluation of human avian influenza pneumonia were studied and explored. Hundreds of scientific papers have been published and a series of scientific research achievements have been made. In order to summarize and popularize our research results in time, and to provide the theoretical basis and practical guidance for effective prevention, early diagnosis, and timely treatment of human avian influenza, thereby achieving accurate diagnosis, improving cure rate, and reducing mortality, we specially organized relevant national and international experts to compile the book Avian Influenza in Human for the benefit of the reader.

The book is written by medical science and technological workers who are directly involved in the prevention, diagnosis, treatment, and related basic research and clinical treatment of human avian influenza. The book is divided into 16 chapters, which comprehensively and systematically introduces the etiology and epidemiology of human avian influenza, pathogenesis and pathological changes, laboratory test, clinical diagnosis and treatment principles, and other basic and clinical related contents. At the same time, the epidemic history, main clinical symptoms and signs, imaging findings, imaging dynamic changes, and prognosis of human avian influenza cases that occurred in China for the first time in the world are also described in detail.

More than 300 precious case images and pathological pictures in this book add important reading value to this book. Especially, the image and pathological picture of the first case of human avian influenza have very important application and guiding value. This book is the first monograph at home and abroad with the introduction of the first human avian influenza case in the world as the main line; through the study of this book, readers can learn about their own specific prevention, diagnosis, and treatment with new methods and new technologies. It is of great reference value and guiding significance to the medical institutions and hospitals at home and abroad, as well as the relevant medical personnel, such as the Department of Infectious Diseases, the Respiratory Medicine, the Imaging Section, the Laboratory and the Pathology

Department, the health management workers, and the medical students. *Avian Influenza in Human* has guiding and reference significance for the prevention, diagnosis, and treatment of emerging infectious diseases such as coronavirus disease (COVID-19).

China Chen Qiu
China Yu-xin Shi
China Pu-xuan Lu

Contents

List of Contributors

Editors

Chen Qiu Department of Respiratory Diseases, Shenzhen People's Hospital, The Second Clinical Medical College of Jinan University, The First Affiliated Hospital of Southern University of Science and Technology, Shenzhen, Guangdong, China

Yu-xin Shi Department of Radiology, Shanghai Public Health Clinical Center, Shanghai, China

Pu-xuan Lu Department of Medical Imaging, Shenzhen Center for Chronic Disease Control, Shenzhen, Guangdong, China

Associate Editors

Shi-pin Wu Department of Infectious Diseases, Shenzhen People's Hospital, The Second Clinical Medical College of Jinan University, The First Affiliated Hospital of Southern University of Science and Technology, Shenzhen, Guangdong, China

Gui-lin Yang Department of Infectious Diseases, Shenzhen People's Hospital (The Second Clinical Medical College, Jinan University, The First Affiliated Hospital, Southern University of Science and Technology), Shenzhen, Guangdong, China

Jin-ping Wu Department of Radiology, Third People's Hospital of Changzhou, Changzhou, Jiangsu, China

Yu-lin He Department of Radiology, The First Affiliated Hospital of Nanchang University, Nanchang, Jiangxi, China

Bu-dong Chen Department of Radiology, Beijing Ditan Hospital, Capital Medical University, Beijing, China

Yi-bo Lu Department of Radiology, The Fourth People's Hospital of Nanning, Nanning, China

Editorial Board Members

Jun Chen Department of Infectious Disease and Immunology, Shanghai Public Health Clinical Center, Shanghai, China

Ying-ying Deng Department of Radiology, Yantian District People's Hospital, Shenzhen, Guangdong, China

Feng Feng Department of Radiology, Nantong Tumor Hospital Affiliated to Nantong University, Nantong, China

Yan-ling Feng Department of Pathology, Shanghai Public Health Clinical Center, Shanghai, China

Wen-zhong Hou Department of Radiology, Meizhou People's Hospital, Meizhou, Guangdong Province, China

Xiao-yan Huang The First Affiliated Hospital of Guangzhou Medical University, Guangzhou, China

Hua Huang Department of Radiology, The Third People's Hospital of Shenzhen, Shenzhen, China

Wei Huang Bacteriology & Antibacterial Resistance Surveillance Laboratory, Shenzhen Institute of Respiratory Diseases, Shenzhen People's Hospital, The Second Clinical Medical College of Jinan University, The First Affiliated Hospital of Southern University of Science and Technology, Shenzhen, Guangdong, China

Qiu-yan Jin Department of Radiology, The Third People's Hospital of Changzhou, Changzhou, Jiangsu, China

Xiao-hua Le Department of Pathology, The Third People's Hospital of Shenzhen, Shenzhen, Guangdong, China

Bin Li Department of Radiology, The First Affiliated Hospital of Nanchang University, Nanchang, China

Jia-fu Lin Department of Infection, Affiliated Hospital of North Sichuan Medical College, Nanchong, China

Hong-zhou Lu Department of Infectious Disease and Immunology, Shanghai Public Health Clinical Center, Shanghai, China

Yong-yi Lu Department of Health Studies, American University, Washington, DC, USA

Sheng-xiu Lv Department of Medical Imaging, Chongqing Public Health Medical Center, Chongqing, China

Wan-shui Shan Department of Clinical Laboratory, The Third People's Hospital of Shenzhen, Shenzhen, Guangdong, China

Fei Shi Emergency Department, Institute of Shenzhen Respiratory Diseases, Shenzhen People's Hospital, The Second Clinical Medical College of Jinan University, The First Affiliated Hospital of Southern University of Science and Technology, Shenzhen, Guangdong, China

Wei-ya Shi Department of Radiology, Shanghai Public Health Clinical Center, Shanghai, China

Xiu-dong Shi Department of Radiology, Shanghai Public Health Clinical Center, Shanghai, China

Zhi-gang Song Department of Biosafety, Shanghai Public Health Clinical Center, Shanghai, China

Dong-na Su Department of Infectious Diseases, Shenzhen People's Hospital, The Second Clinical Medical College of Jinan University, The First Affiliated Hospital of Southern University of Science and Technology, Shenzhen, Guangdong, China

Yong Sun The Second Affiliated Hospital of Kunming Medical University, Kunming, China

Gui-xia Wang Department of Infection, Affiliated Hospital of North Sichuan Medical College, Nanchong, China

Ling-wei Wang Department of Respiratory and Critical Care Medicine, Shenzhen People's Hospital, The Second Clinical Medical College of Jinan University, The First Affiliated Hospital of Southern University of Science and Technology, Shenzhen, Guangdong, China

Yu-zhe Wang Department of Radiology, Shanghai Fifth People's Hospital, Fudan University, Shanghai, China

Ru-ming Xie Department of Radiology, Beijing Ditan Hospital, Capital Medical University, Beijing, China

Chuan-jun Xu The Second Hospital of Nanjing, Nanjing University of Chinese Medicine, Nanjing, China

He-ping Xu Department of Radiology, The Children's Hospital of Hunan Province, Changsha, Hunan, China

Qin-qin Yan Department of Radiology, Shanghai Public Health Clinical Center, Shanghai, China

Shu-yi Yang Department of Radiology, Shanghai Public Health Clinical Center, Shanghai, China

Yong-xiang Yi The Second Hospital of Nanjing, Nanjing University of Chinese Medicine, Nanjing, China

Hua-bin Yin Department of Radiology, Shanghai Fifth People's Hospital, Fudan University, Shanghai, China

Qing-si Zeng The First Affiliated Hospital of Guangzhou Medical University, Guangzhou, China

Yue Zeng Department of Infection, Affiliated Hospital of North Sichuan Medical College, Nanchong, Sichuan, China

Qian-qian Zhang Magnetic Resonance Room, Zhoukou Central Hospital, Zhoukou, Henan Province, China

Guang-ping Zheng Department of Radiology, The Third People's Hospital of Shenzhen, Shenzhen, China

Qiu-ting Zheng Department of Medical Imaging, Shenzhen Center for Chronic Disease Control, Shenzhen, China

Kai Zhou Shenzhen Institute of Respiratory Diseases, Shenzhen People's Hospital, The Second Clinical Medical College of Jinan University, The First Affiliated Hospital of Southern University of Science and Technology, Shenzhen, Guangdong, China

Su Zhou Intervention Section, Shanghai Public Health Clinical Center, Shanghai, China

Zhao-qin Zhu Department of Clinical Laboratory, Shanghai Public Health Clinical Center, Shanghai, China

About the Editors

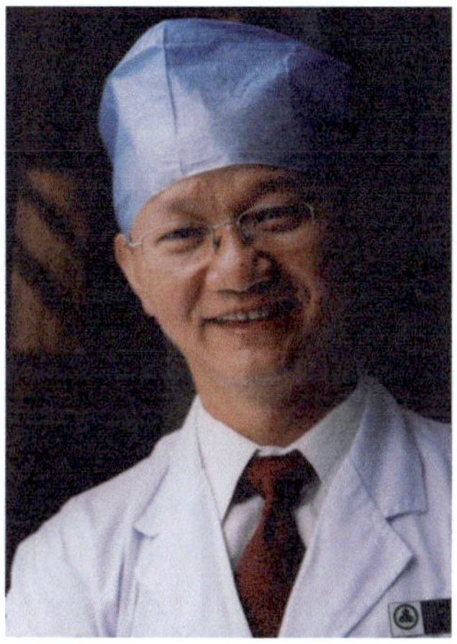

Chen Qiu is a leader in the discipline of respiratory and critical medicine, Shenzhen People's Hospital. Professor Qiu is also the director at the Institute of Shenzhen Respiratory Disease and the director of the National Drug Clinical Trial Institute.

His academic titles include committee member, Asthma Group at the Respiratory Branch of Chinese Medical Society; review expert, Medicine Branch of National Natural Science Funding Commission, China; review expert, Education Development Center for Degree and Postgraduate at the Ministry of Education, China; review expert, Provincial Science and Technology Planning Project, Guangdong, China; associate director, Provincial Hospital Association of Guangdong, China; deputy chair, Respiratory Branch of Provincial Medical Society of Guangdong, China; deputy chair, Respiratory Physician Branch of Provincial Physician Association of Guangdong, China; deputy chair, Expert Committee for Respiratory Medication of Provincial Pharmacy Society of Guangdong, China; deputy chair, Respiratory Disease Control and Prevention Branch of Provincial Preventive Medicine Society of Guangdong, China; deputy chair, Respiratory Rehabilitation Branch of Provincial Thoracic Disease Society of Guangdong, China; and chair, Respiratory Branch of Shenzhen Medical Society.

Professor Qiu is the editorial committee member of the *Chinese Journal of Tuberculosis and Respiration*, Chinese edition of *Chest*, Chinese edition of the *Lancet* (*Respiratory Medicine*), and *Journal of Guangdong Medicine*; standing editorial committee member of Medicine Review and Modern Hospital; and associate editor of *Electronic Journal of Emerging Infectious Disease*. He has edited and translated three academic treatises, finished five academic treatises as associate editor, and contributed to four academic treatises.

He also directed six projects funded by the National Natural Science Foundation of China and the Provincial Natural Science Foundation of Guangdong, China. He owns seven patents for invention and six patents for utility models.

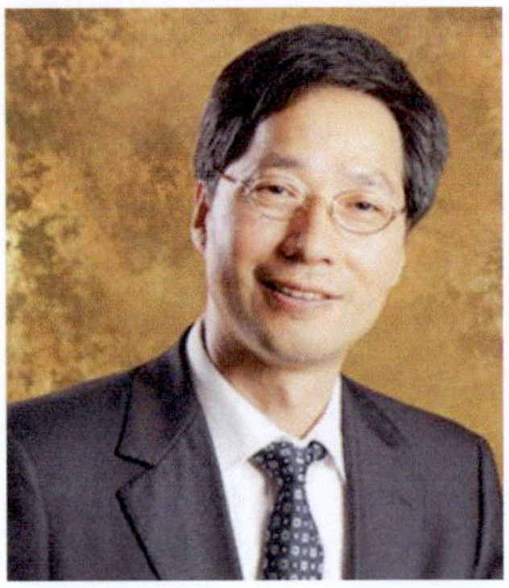

Yu-xin Shi was born in Jiangsu, January 1964, and graduated from Nantong Medical College majoring in medicine in 1986. He obtained doctoral degree of radiology and nuclear medicine in Zhongshan Hospital affiliated to Shanghai Medical University in 1995.

He is mainly engaged in the imaging research of infectious diseases, especially the radiology of AIDS-associated opportunistic infections and emerging infectious diseases. Now, he is vice-chairman of Infectious Disease Committee of the Chinese Society of Radiology, vice-chairman of Tuberculosis Diagnostic Radiology Committee of the Chinese Medical Association, vice-chairman of Infection and Inflammation Committee of China Research Hospital Society, vice-chairman of Infection Radiology of China Association of STDs and AIDS, and vice-chairman of Radiology Quality Control Group of Infectious Diseases Management of China Hospital Association. Besides, he is member of the Cardiothoracic Committee of the Chinese Society of Radiology, Hospital Architectural System Research of China Hospital Association, and Radiology Society of Shanghai Medical Association.

He has received funding from more than ten organizations, such as the National Natural Science Foundation of China, National Institute of Health of the United States, and government of Shanghai and Jiangsu Province. He has received nine times science and technology awards of provincial and ministerial level. He has published in total more than 110 papers in SCI and national core journals and edited and coedited 14 monographs, translations, and textbooks at all levels. He had trained more than 20 postgraduates. Besides, he served as an evaluation expert of the Chinese Medical Award, deputy editor of *New Infectious Diseases*, invited reviewer expert of the *Chinese Journal of Radiology* and *Shanghai Medical Radiology*, and editor of *Radiology of Infectious Diseases* and *Journal of Nantong University*.

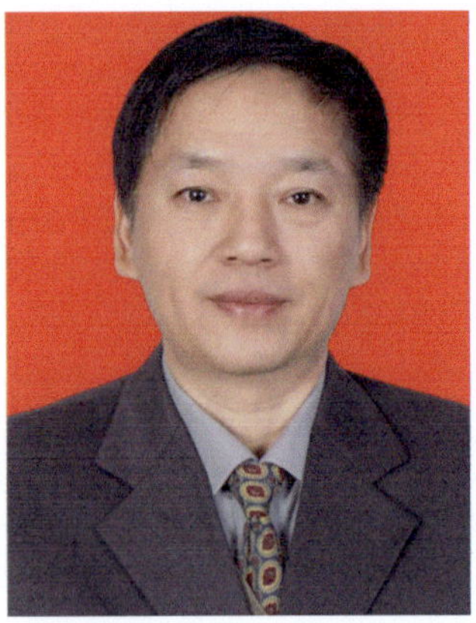

Pu-xuan Lu is a professor and graduate supervisor of Guangdong Medical University and the radiology department director of Shenzhen Center for Chronic Disease Control.

His academic titles include chief editor of *Electronic Journal of Emerging Infectious Disease*; deputy chair, Radiology of Infectious Disease Group at the Radiology Branch of Chinese Medical Society; deputy chair, Radiology of Infectious Disease Group at Chinese Radiology Society; deputy chair, Radiology Branch of Chinese Sexually Transmitted Disease and HIV/AIDS Society; deputy chair, Beijing Diagnostic Imaging Technology Innovation Alliance; deputy chair, Radiology Branch of Provincial Health Management Society of Guangdong, China; and editorial committee member of the *Journal of Radiology of Infectious Disease*.

His research fields include diagnostic imaging and differential diagnosis of emerging infectious diseases, such as SARS, MERS, AIDS, human-infected avian influenza, tuberculosis, hepatitis, and other infectious diseases as well as clinical and basic sciences of emerging infectious diseases.

Professor Lu has edited or coedited more than ten academic treatises. *Diagnostic Imaging of Emerging Infectious Diseases* has been published by Springer in November 2015, which obtained national key award for book output in May 2017 by the General Administration of News and Publishing, China. In the last 5 years, he has directed and finished five national and provincial as well as international collaborative research projects. Pu-xuan Lu has published more than 180 papers. 36 of these papers were published in SCI-indexed journals. He received 12 awards from the Chinese Medical Society, Chinese Preventive Medicine Society, Guangdong provincial government, and Shenzhen city government.

Outline of Human Avian Influenza

1

Chen Qiu, Gui-lin Yang, and Pu-xuan Lu

1.1 Introduction of Human Avian Influenza

Avian influenza, abbreviated as avian flu, is an infectious disease caused by the avian influenza virus and is commonly known as fowl plague or European fowl plague. Infection with avian influenza virus may occur in domestic fowls such as chickens, turkeys, ducks, and quails as well as wild birds, manifesting various forms from asymptomatic virus carrier to mild respiratory disease or even acute fatal disease.

Influenza virus that infects birds is called avian influenza virus (AIV), which belongs to the genera influenza virus of Orthomyxoviridae A. Now AIV can be categorized into 18 H subtypes (H1–18) and 11 N subtypes (N1–11), based on different antigenicity of hemagglutinin (HA) and neuraminidase (NA) on the outer membrane [1]. Besides infecting birds, AIV also infects human beings, pigs, horses, minks, and marine mammals. AIV can be categorized into highly, moderately, and low/non-pathogenic ones based on its virulence against chickens.

Human avian influenza is an acute respiratory infectious disease caused by the avian influenza virus (AIV) infecting human beings. The avian influenza viruses that have been confirmed to infect human beings include subtypes of H3N2, H5N1, H5N6, H7N1, H7N2, H7N3, H7N4, H7N7, H9N2, H7N9, and H10N8. Among them, the highly pathogenic subtype H5N1 and the new avian influenza virus H7N9 subtype in March 2013, were of particular interests, which not only caused human casualties but also damaged badly poultry industry. Human avian influenzas caused by infection with subtypes of H5N1, H7N9, and H5N6 manifest severe diseases with high mortality and are called highly pathogenic avian influenza (HPAI) [2–4]. Since the first outbreak of human avian influenza of subtype H5N1 in Hong Kong in 1997, 622 cases of human avian influenza with highly pathogenic H5N1 have been reported in the world up to March 2013, including 371 deaths. The patients have been distributed among 15 countries, wherein 45 have been observed in China with 30 deaths. As of March 2, 2018, 1567 cases of laboratory-confirmed cases of human avian influenza infected with H7N9 have been reported in total via International Health Regulations, including 615 deaths with an accumulative mortality of 39.2%. Twenty-one cases of human avian influenza infected with H9N2 have been reported in China's mainland, as of January 2017, including one death. Two cases of severe human avian influenza with H5N6 have been reported during 2014 including one death, and this influenza has replaced H5N1 and become the main pathogenic strain of avian influenza viruses in southern China [5–7].

The main infection source of AIV is the bird infected with or carrying avian influenzas, such as chickens, duck, and gooses, and wild birds play an important role in the natural transmission of AIV. Besides its transmission through the respiratory tract, this disease may also spread through close contact with secretion and excretion of birds, materials, and water polluted by the virus, and direct contact with viral strains. There is currently no definite evidence of human-to-human transmission.

The main clinical manifestations of human avian influenza in the early stage seems similar to those of a common

The original version of the chapter has been revised. A correction to this chapter can be found at https://doi.org/10.1007/978-981-16-1429-3_17

C. Qiu (✉)
Department of Respiratory Diseases, Shenzhen People's Hospital, The Second Clinical Medical College of Jinan University, The First Affiliated Hospital of Southern University of Science and Technology, Shenzhen, Guangdong, China

G.-l. Yang
Department of Infectious Diseases, Shenzhen People's Hospital (The Second Clinical Medical College, Jinan University, The First Affiliated Hospital, Southern University of Science and Technology), Shenzhen, Guangdong, China

Pu-x. Lu
Department of Medical Imaging, Shenzhen Center for Chronic Disease Control, Shenzhen, Guangdong, China

C. Qiu et al. (eds.), *Avian Influenza in Human*, https://doi.org/10.1007/978-981-16-1429-3_1

cold, manifesting mainly fever with the temperature persistently above 39 °C in most cases and possibly accompanied with runny nose, stuffy nose, cough, sore throat, headache, muscle aches, and general malaise. Some of the patients may have gastrointestinal symptoms such as nausea, abdominal pain, and watery diarrhea. Patients with severe disease may have unabating high fever and rapidly progressive disease, manifesting as obvious pneumonia. After a human is infected with avian influenza virus, a storm of cytokines can be induced, such as interferon-inducible protein 10 (IP-10), monocyte chemoattractant protein 1 (MCP-1), interleukin 6 (IL-6), interleukin 8(IL-8), etc., which may cause systemic inflammation as well as acute respiratory distress syndrome (ARDS), shock and multiple organ dysfunction syndrome (MODS). Pathological examination shows acute exudative inflammatory changes in both lungs, including diffuse alveolar injury and formation of the hyaline membrane. Multiple complications may occur, such as acute lung injury (ALI), ARDS, pulmonary hemorrhage, pleural effusion, multiple organ failure, DIC, shock, and Reye syndrome. It may cause secondary bacterial infection and septicemia, with a mortality rate of more than 39%.

1.2 Epidemics of Human Avian Influenza and Its Control

Now, bird-carrying viruses are considered to be the main source of human infection with avian influenza. It is particularly important to reduce and control the transmission of the avian influenza virus among birds, especially fowls. Along with the improvement of social and economic developing level in China, it is urgently needed to accelerate the transformation and upgrading of traditional poultry breeding and circulation into a modernized production mode. The conversion from decentralized breeding to centralized and large-scale cultivation, slaughtering, and scientific transportation will improve biosafety level in the cultivation and transportation of poultry and livestock, thereby reducing the populational exposure to birds that are alive or have died from illness. Meanwhile, health education should be performed continuously to advocate and cultivate personal respiratory hygiene and prevention habits, including washing hands frequently, keeping the environment clean, and processing and cooking food properly. It is necessary to strengthen the health education and protection for the high-risk population with infection of AIV and medical staff.

In addition, influenza in animals and human beings will be monitored properly. Infection of animals or epidemics will be found in time, as well as the status of viral circulation in the environment, so that measures will be carried out to eliminate infection source and block viral transmission among birds, such as animal immunization, culling, and closing market. Human avian influenza patients should be found and diagnosed as soon as possible, and isolation and treatment should be provided for patients timely, effectively, and reasonably. Epidemiological investigation and virologic monitoring of the disease should be performed properly, with constant improvement in scientific understanding of avian influenza and timely discovery of clustered cases and virus variation, so that corresponding interventions and response measures can be taken further.

Besides the implementation of scientific control, serious preparation should be done in response to pandemic influenza.

1. To control infection source of avian influenza virus in the market of live poultry. 80% of patients have the history of direct or indirect contact with poultry and are suspected to be correlated with infection source and environmental pollution, such as sewage and poultry feces. Investigations show that incidence of infection can be reduced through the closing market of live poultry, but these measures have little effect in the areas with lower level of education. Risk of infection can also be lowered by culling infected poultry and immunizing those vulnerable to infection.
2. To strengthen management in public areas. Public places densely populated with great mobility are the main places for the spread of respiratory infectious diseases. We will strengthen disinfection management, implement disinfection measures, improve health supervision and monitor the management system. Once an infected patient is found, a report should be submitted immediately to the corresponding authority, and the patient should be escorted to designated medical institution for isolation, and further diagnosis and treatment.
3. To standardize administrative systems in hospitals. It is inevitable for physicians especially nurses to have close contact with patient. They might be exposed to the patients' excrements, which increases the risk of infection. Self-disinfection must be done well by medical practitioners when entering or leaving quarantine areas. They must wear caps, masks, and insolation gowns as prescribed to avoid bringing viruses out of the quarantine areas. Hospitals are obliged to set up special clinics and wards to separate patients from those with suspected infection, which reduces the risk of mutual infection. In addition, it is important to arrange food, accommodation, and family visit for quarantined personnel.
4. Publicity and education of knowledge about controlling human avian influenza. It is necessary for corresponding authorities to organize actively the publicity of knowledge about infectious diseases. This can help more people know their harms, self-protective measures, and raise people's awareness of the avian influenza virus, which is of great importance to prevent its transmission. Measures

play an important role in cutting off the routes of infection, which also includes indoor ventilation, frequent hand washing, enhancement of nutrition, and outdoor activities.

5. To discover and cure patients. Antiviral therapy should be launched as soon as possible, such as oseltamivir, peramivir, and zanamivir.

1.3 Avian Influenza Virus

I. Pathogenic Characteristics

Avian influenza is caused by type A of influenza virus of Orthomyxoviridae. It can be categorized into four serum types A, B, C, and D, based on its difference in the antigenicity of nucleoprotein (NP) and matrix protein (MP). NP and MP exist in strains of each type, i.e., NP and MP have specificity. Avian influenza can also be categorized into different subtypes, according to different antigenicity of hemagglutinin (HA) and neuraminidase (NA). At least 18 kinds of HAs of influenza virus type A have been identified up to now, named H1–H18 respectively: there are at least 11 kinds of NAs identified and named as N1–N11 respectively. At present, there are up to a thousand of avian influenza viruses isolated.

II. Molecular Basis for Virulent Variation of AIV

Variation occurs very easily in AIV, [8] and antigenic change may take place due to antigenic drift, thereby generating easily biological variants with stronger pathogenicity. When more than one kind of AIV can infect different hosts, the virus will undergo genetic recombination, i.e., antigenic shift, which may induce gene recombination of HA and NA from different types of virus to generate novel viral types. In type A influenza virus, the antigenic shift is induced mainly by point mutation of HA and/or NA genes, with the HA gene having the highest mutation rate up to 2×10^3 for every nucleotide during each replication cycle.

(I) Genome Structure

Avian influenza virus belongs to type A of influenza virus of Orthomyxoviridae. Type A avian influenza virus mostly seems in spheres in a diameter of 80–120 nm with an outer capsule and an interior nucleocapsid in a diameter of 70 nm. The nucleocapsid consists of RNA, nucleoprotein, and three polymerases. The capsule can be divided into three layers: inner membrane protein, lipid, and glycoprotein. The nucleic acid of the avian influenza virus is segmented with a single negative-strand RNA with a length of about 14,000 nucleotide acids. The genome is characterized by the "discontinuity" of its sequence, which is divided into eight segments. These eight segments of RNA encode respectively ten proteins correlated to structures and functions of the viruses, with segment 1 and 2 encoding polymerase PB1 and PB2, segment 3 encoding PA protein that is also related to the activity of polymerase, segment 4 encoding hemagglutinin HA, segment 5 encoding nucleocapsid protein (NP), segment 6 encoding neuraminidase (NA), segment 7 encoding matrix protein M1 and M2 that act as scaffold proteins and correlate with viral morphology, and segment 8 encoding nonstructural proteins NS1 and NS2 that possibly participate in the transcription of the viral genome. The segmentation of the influenza virus makes genetic recombination happen easily during its replication, which leads to antigenic variation and even the emergence of novel virulent strains.

(II) Variance of Pathogenicity or Virulence

It has been found recently that H9N2 with low pathogenicity manifests moderate pathogenicity after infecting human being. There is a close relationship between the amino acid composition at the HA cleavage site and virulence of the virus, i.e., there are multiple alkaline amino acids at the HA cleavage site in highly pathogenic strains, which is the differential feature of highly pathogenic AIV and almost all H5 and H7 have this specific structure. All highly pathogenic avian influenzas in history have been caused by H5 and H7, but not all H5 and H7 are highly virulent.

(III) Specific Change of Hosts of AIV

Researches show that type A influenza virus (H5N1) has been evolving continuously since 1997, with continuous alteration of antigenicity and genetic recombination. Range of hosts for avian influenza keeps expanding, and the virus becomes capable of infecting animals of the cat family. Its pathogenicity increases in infected mice and ferrets in the laboratory, and may induce systemic infection in these animals. The continuous evolution of H5N1 results in expansion of the range of hosts, enhancement of pathogenicity and of stability, and genetic and antigenic changes, thereby causing eventually endless emergence of cases of human infection.

1.4 The Latest Detection Technology for Influenza Viruses

The diagnosis of avian influenza can be confirmed, based on clinical manifestations, adjuvant examination, and results of laboratory tests, especially isolated avian influenza virus from avian respiratory excretions, or positiveness of nucleic acid of avian influenza virus, or positive conversion of the specific antibody of avian influenza virus in double serum samples or its rise for more than four times [9, 10].

1. Diagnostic criteria for infection of influenza virus: the golden criteria for determining infection of avian influenza virus is the isolation and cultivation of the virus. Methods: (1) rapid detection of influenza virus: rapid detection kit for influenza A/B virus will be used for detecting influenza virus, and colloidal gold immunochromatography is used to determine core antigen of influenza virus; (2) MDCK cell cultivation: the collected throat swabs are used to inoculate MDCK cells for virus isolation, and the isolated virus strains undergo serological detection or identification of nucleotide sequence.
2. Molecular biological technology, characterized in specificity, simplicity, and sensitivity, has developed rapidly during recent years and many methods have been applied to the detection of the influenza virus.
   (1) Reverse Transcription-Polymerase Chain Reaction

   Reverse Transcription-Polymerase Chain Reaction (RT-PCR) is one of the detections in molecular biology commonly used today. This approach allows the detection of influenza virus in genetic level, with a high sensitivity, a high specificity, and simple manipulation, capable of accomplishing the detection within hours and realizing simultaneously genotyping of HA and NA of influenza virus.

   (2) Real-Time Quantitative PCR

   Compared with common RT-PCR, real-time fluorescent quantitative RT-PCR (Real-time RT-PCR) is characterized in easy operation, less time consumption, high sensitivity, high specificity, and intuitionistic results. Moreover, its reaction products do not require subsequent treatment, which reduce the risks of laboratory pollution to a certain degree. Therefore, real-time fluorescent quantitative RT-PCR is commonly used in monitoring influenza throughout the country now.

   (3) Loop-Mediated Isothermal Amplification (LAMP)

   Loop-mediated isothermal amplification (LAMP), a gene amplification method invented by Notomi et al. in 2000 and characterized in less time consumption, high sensitivity, and low cost, is suitable for detecting and diagnosing influenza virus in the early stage in basic units and on the spot. Both its sensitivity and detection rate are superior to those of traditional RT-PCR.

   (4) Gene Chip

   Gene chip, also called DNA Microarray, is to solidify cDNA or specific oligonucleotide probe of the viral gene on the chips in the form of large-scale matrix. Its working principle is consistent with that of hybridization of nucleic acid molecules, and it is a new technology allowing high-throughput detection and capable of realizing concurrently rapid detection of subtypes of H5, H7, and H9 of avian influenza viruses.
3. Conventional sequencing and a new generation of DNA sequencing method. The new generation of sequencing methods developed in recent years includes Roche's 454 genome sequencer and Illumina's genome analyzer. The most prominent feature of these sequencing technologies is the high-throughput detection, and one reaction can determine hundreds of thousands to hundreds of millions of base sequences. The new generation of sequencing method can not only detect multiple subtypes of AIV strains, but also determine the whole genome sequence of the virus. Gene chip and the new generation of sequencing method, both featuring high-throughput, speediness, and high automation, achieve a precise detection on the level of single nucleotide acids. In contrast to the prerequisite of prior understanding of nucleotide acid sequence of genomes of cells or virus to be determined when a detecting probe is designed, the new generation of sequencing does not have this limitation. Therefore, in monitoring the advent of a new AIV mutation, the new generation of sequencing method may have a greater advantage than gene chip. Although the advantages of these two methods are obvious, they have not been adopted extensively because they need expensive apparatus and analysis software. The new generation of sequencing method is anticipated to become probably an important approach for detecting AIV subtypes and sequencing the whole genome in near future, along with renewal and development of detection technology and gradual decrease of detection cost.

The development of researches on AIV detection in the future should be oriented to speediness, specificity, sensitivity, precision, high-throughput, low cost, portability, and availability for field operation. The key to prevent and control the influenza pandemic lies in early detection, rapid response, and appropriate preventive measures adopted in time. The adherence to prolonged monitoring, correlation analysis on sequences of mutated AIV strains, and their epidemiological investigation will provide a solid scientific basis for predicting the occurrence trend of avian influenza and mastering its changing patterns.

In recent years, there have been frequent global outbreaks of the influenza virus, which not only cause economic losses to all countries, but also severely threaten public health and security. Therefore, it is of great importance to realize fast diagnosis and timely surveillance on influenza viruses as far as the guarantee of human health is concerned. At present, molecular biology technology with high sensitivity, good specificity, rapid detection, and high-throughput detection, such as RT-PCR and real-time RT-PCR, have been widely applied to the rapid detection of influenza viruses, identification of viral subtypes, and analysis in their epidemic trend. With the further deepening of investigations, molecular biology technology can also achieve rapid detection of newly identified subtypes of influenza virus and fulfill early detection, early report, early treatment, and early prevention, which can help with providing ideas for disease diagnosis and control. It is of great significance to improve further the level for monitoring influenza virus in China.

1.5 Current Situation of Vaccine Researches

Recent years have witnessed the continuous development of the poultry breeding industry in China, from decentralized to centralized with the scale expanding continuously. Therefore, the outbreak of influenza will do great harm to the poultry breeding industry. The current prevention of avian influenza virus, which is common in human being, mainly rely on vaccination. Vaccines available in the Chinese market include inactivated vaccine, attenuated live vaccine, and split vaccine. Due to their limitations including the risk of relapse and poor cross immune-protection, these vaccines unable to cope with the influenza epidemic. With the uninterrupted development of biological technology, novel vaccines will replace the traditional ones. Main categories of vaccines in preventing avian influenza in China mainly include inactivated virus vaccine, attenuated live vaccine, DNA vaccine, subunit vaccine, and virus-like granular vaccine [11–13].

Inactivated vaccine: influenza inactivated vaccine is a kind of vaccine produced via viral proliferation through chicken embryo followed by inactivation with formaldehyde. It can be categorized into inactivated virus vaccine, subunit inactivated vaccine, and cleavage inactivated vaccine. The inactivated vaccine has complete antigen molecules and can provide immune-protection for birds. Owing to features of good immunization efficacy and prolonged duration of immunity, these vaccines have been approved for sale in many countries. After immunization with the vaccine, the body will not only produce neutralizing antibodies that specifically bind to HA and Na antigens, but also be induced to produce cytotoxic T lymphocyte (CTL) response. H5N1 influenza vaccine for human use is an important measure to prevent the influenza virus from infecting human beings, but a great limitation exists if only inactivated vaccine is used to prevent from influenza outbreak. Now inactivated vaccines for human use are already available in the market that has been approved for sale, such as H1N1/H3N2 trivalent influenza virus inactivated vaccine, etc. H5N1 influenza inactivated vaccine for human use can induce effective neutralizing antibodies in 54% of the subjects. The main inactivated vaccines for animal use in China are H5N1 avian influenza inactivated vaccine, H9N2 avian influenza inactivated vaccine, H5N1/H9N2 avian influenza bivalent inactivated vaccine, etc. Both H5N1 influenza cleavage inactivated vaccine and H5N1 virus inactivated vaccine can stimulate the systemic humoral immune response. With the continuous development of cellular technology, the cellular proliferation of the influenza virus has replaced the traditional way of proliferation, which has laid the foundation for formulating efficient and safe avian influenza vaccine. Therefore, it is an urgent to develop a safe, low-cost, and less time-consuming technology to manufacture vaccines. The inactivating agent contained in the inactivated vaccine may cause some adverse reactions, such as redness, swelling, pain, etc. Cross-protection should be considered, due to the high mutation rate of influenza virus and the presence of multiple branch strains of AIV. Though capable of providing effective immune-protection and reducing the incidence of avian influenza, the inactivated vaccine has no cross-protection, which makes it impossible for the inactivated vaccine to prevent from large-scale outbreak of avian influenza.

Live Attenuated Vaccine: Suguitan et al. inoculated mice with H5N1 live attenuated vaccine, performed challenge tests with homogenous and heterogenous viral strains, and found that these vaccines had cross-protection. Jin used H5N1 live attenuated vaccine to immunize mice, conducted safety evaluation and toxicology experiment and found its safety is good without toxicity or side effects. Compared with conventional live vaccines, live attenuated vaccine uses intranasal administration method, which is convenience, speediness, no necessity of operation by professionals, strong immunogenicity of the vaccines, and presence of cross-protection.

Virus-Like Granular Vaccine: Influenza VLP vaccines include subtypes of H5N1, H3N2, H1N1, H5N3, and H9N2, all of which have been confirmed by animal immunity experiment to induce systemic effective immune response. H3N2 VLP and H9N2 VLP, two vaccines developed by Lee et al., were evaluated in Beagles and SPF chickens respectively, finding that single dose of either H9N2 VLP or H3N2 VLP might induce the body to produce high titer of neutralizing antibodies and protect animals from being attacked by homogenous viral strains. Park et al. developed the unpurified avian influenza H5N1 VLP vaccine by using baculovirus expression system and conducted immune evaluation in SPF chickens. Although H5N1 influenza VLP is not purified, it has high immunogenicity and can protect SPF chickens from being infected by the homologous H5N1 virus. After immunizing pigs, the H1N1 VLP vaccine developed by Pyo et al. might induce humoral immune response and mucosal immune response. It was found in researches that VLP containing M1 protein could stimulate $CD8^{+}T$ cells and make them proliferate and activated to generate factors such as IFN-γ and TNF-α. For example, it was found in the research by Kang et al. that the H5N1 VLP vaccine could increase significantly titers of IgG2a and IgG2b antibodies of H5N1 in immunized animals in vivo. Good humoral and cellular immune response could be induced after the animals were immunized with H5N1 VLP and H9N2 VLP prepared with baculovirus expression system, using adjuvants including liposome, white oil, and chitosan microspheres, which could act as a reference for the development of VLP vaccines.

References

1. Chen X, Zhai C. A research on molecular epidemics of inter-species infection and variation of avian influenza virus. Int J Epidemic Infect Dis. 2006;33(2):90–2.
2. Gao D, Li J, Hu S, et al. Epidemiological investigation and analysis of the first case of highly pathogenic avian influenza in Chinese mainland. Pract Prev Med. 2006;13(2):238–40.
3. Chen H, Deng G, Li Z, et al. The evolution of H5N1 influenza viruses in ducks in southern China. Proc Natl Acad Sci USA. 2004;101(28):10452–7.
4. Kandasamy M, Furlong K, Perez JT, et al. Suppression of cytotoxic T cell functions and decreased levels of tissue resident memory T cell during H5N1 infection. J Virol. 2020.
5. Bi Y, Chen Q, Wang Q, Gao GF. Genesis, evolution and prevalence of H5N6 avian influenza viruses in China. Cell Host Microbe. 2016;20(6):810–21.
6. Yang L, Zhu W, Li X. Genesis and dissemination of highly pathogenic H5N6 avian influenza viruses. J Virol. 2017;91(5).
7. Chan PK. Outbreak of avian influenza A(H5N1) virus infection in Hong Kong in 1997. Clin Infect Dis. 2002;34(Suppl 2):S58–64.
8. Lin M, Lu B, Zhu Z. Progress in molecular biological technology on influenza virus. J Dis Surveill Control. 2017;11(1):36.
9. Li X, Xu J, Yang X. A research on the etiological diagnosis of influenza-like illnesses by rapid detection of influenza virus. Beijing Med. 2009;31(5):280–3.
10. Tan W, Li M, Xie Z. Surveillance and diagnosis of avian influenza virus. Chin J Zoonoses. 2014;30(11):1002–2694.
11. Liu Q, Chen F. Vaccine of H7N9 avian influenza virus and its control. Chin J Infect Control. 2015;14(12):865–8.
12. Deng W, Xu L, Bao L. Establishment of animal model of ferrets infected with H7N9 avian influenza virus. Chin J Comp Med. 2014;24(1):68–71.
13. Qin C. The current situation of investigation on H7N9 avian influenza research and the future thinking. Acta Lab Anim Sci Sinica. 2014;22(1):1–7.

2 Epidemiology

Gui-lin Yang, Kai Zhou, Yong-xiang Yi, and Chen Qiu

2.1 Outline of the Epidemics

Avian influenza, commonly known as fowl plague, was proved to be induced by the influenza A virus in 1955. Since the first isolation of subtype H5N1 of avian influenza from chicken in 1959, the virus has caused many outbreaks of avian influenza. Historically, avian influenza mainly infected vertebrates such as domestic fowls and wild animals. However, in recent years, human infection of avian influenza has been taking place continuously, attracting global attraction.

Subtypes of avian influenza viruses confirmed so far to be capable of infecting directly human beings including H5N1, H5N6, H7N1, H7N2, H7N3, H7N7, H7N4, H9N2, H7N9, and H10N8. Among them, the highly pathogenic subtype H5N1 and the subtype H7N9, the new avian virus identified firstly in human being in March 2013, were of particular interest, which not only caused high human casualties, but also hit the poultry industry hard. In recent 5 years, highly pathogenic subtype H5N6 has gradually replaced H5N1 to become the main pathogenic strain in poultry in Southern China. All human influenza viruses can cause influenza in birds, but not all avian influenza viruses can cause influenza in humans. Subtypes of avian influenza viruses of H5, H7, and H9 among avian influenza viruses may infect human beings, and H5 is highly pathogenic. Avian influenza viruses can be categorized into 198 subtypes (HxNx) based on their features, and the subtype H7N9 is the main strain causing human avian influenza.

A strain of influenza A virus was isolated from a 3-year-old child living in Hongkong China on May 9, 1997, which was confirmed etiologically to be virus subtype H5N1. In the same year, infection of H5N1 avian influenza was confirmed totally in 18 persons in Hongkong, including six deaths. This was the first report of direct human infection by avian influenza viruses, arousing global shock and concern [1–3]. Six hundred and twenty-two cases of highly pathogenic H5N1 avian influenza have been reported in the world, including 371 deaths, as of March 2013 since the first occurrence of human infection by H5N1 subtype of avian influenza viruses in Hongkong in 1997. These cases were distributed among 15 nations, including 45 in China with 30 deaths. Most sufferers of human infection of avian influenzas H5N1 are young people and children [4]. It is considered by WHO to be one of the diseases with the greatest potential threats to humans.

In addition, more than 100 cases of human avian influenza of subtypes of H9N2, H7N2, and H7N7 have been reported worldwide. Five cases of H9N2 infection were identified in the Chinese mainland in 1998. Moreover, in March 2003, H7N7 avian influenza viruses were identified in six farms in the eastern Netherlands adjacent to the German frontier, and an outbreak of human infection of H7N7 avian virus occurred in the Netherlands during February to April 2003 with 89 cases and one death [5]. A 57-year-old Dutch veterinarian was infected with the virus when he tested the sick chicken and died of pneumonia complications caused by

The original version of the chapter has been revised. A correction to this chapter can be found at https://doi.org/10.1007/978-981-16-1429-3_17

G.-l. Yang (✉)
Department of Infectious Diseases, Shenzhen People's Hospital, The Second Clinical Medical College of Jinan University, The First Affiliated Hospital of Southern University of Science and Technology, Shenzhen, Guangdong, China

K. Zhou
Shenzhen Institute of Respiratory Diseases, Shenzhen People's Hospital, The Second Clinical Medical College of Jinan University, The First Affiliated Hospital of Southern University of Science and Technology, Shenzhen, Guangdong, China

Y.-x. Yi
The Second Hospital of Nanjing, Nanjing University of Chinese Medicine, Nanjing, China

C. Qiu
Department of Respiratory Diseases, Shenzhen People's Hospital, The Second Clinical Medical College of Jinan University, The First Affiliated Hospital of Southern University of Science and Technology, Shenzhen, Guangdong, China

C. Qiu et al. (eds.), *Avian Influenza in Human*, https://doi.org/10.1007/978-981-16-1429-3_2

bird flu. Since then, H7N7 avian influenza has spread throughout Europe, with cases of avian influenza virus infection reported in Belgium and Germany, the two countries adjacent to the Netherlands.

In March 2013, cases of human infection of H7N9 avian influenza were found in both Shanghai and Anhui in China, which were identified firstly as the new subtype of influenzas infecting humans in the world [6]. In this Chinese epidemic occurring in Shanghai and Anhui, 33 infections were diagnosed, including nine deaths. Later this epidemic spread rapidly to Southern and Northern China, with outbreaks occurring in Guangdong and a number of cases of infection subsequently observed in Fujian, Hunan, etc. The epidemic spread so fast that more than 100 patients were diagnosed within only 2 months after the virus was isolated firstly, and most of the sufferers were the aged. Most patients had no history of direct exposure to birds and manifested a mild onset, but some of the patients progressed dramatically into severe pneumonia or respiratory failure within 1 week since the disease onset. The source of human infection of H7N9 avian influenza has not yet been fully clarified, and the exposure to sick birds and their living environment is considered to be the most likely route of transmission. One thousand five hundred and sixty-seven cases of laboratory-confirmed human infection of H7N9 avian influenza have been reported via the route of International Health Regulations since the years of 2013–2018, including 615 deaths with an accumulative mortality of 39.2%. In 2017 alone, 589 confirmed cases of human infection of H7N9 avian influenza were reported in the Chinese mainland with 259 deaths showing a mortality of 44%, and the proportion of severe cases rose significantly than before. Based on data published from March 2013 to April 2017 concerning human infection of H7N9 avian influenzas, there were totally 1416 cases of this disease in China with 559 deaths and a mortality of 39.5%. The year 2016 witnessed 127 confirmed cases of human infection of H7N9 avian influenza, with a mortality rate of 57.5%. The epidemiology of 127 cases of human infection of H7N9 avian influenza showed that the exposure to live birds prior to the onset of the disease was confirmed in 66% of the cases but 31% of transmission route remained unknown. About 70% of the cases had the exposure to poultry within 10 days prior to the onset, showing the exposures to live bird market and scattered poultry are still the two main routes of transmission. Compared data in the past 10 years about human infections of avian influenza such as H5N1, H7N7 or low pathogenic H9N2, H7N9 seems more likely to infect mankind, which may be explained by some of its molecular markers adaptive to mammals, such as the change of receptor binding site, the deletion of HA glycosylation site, and E627K mutation in PB2. Though non-lethal to birds, virus subtype H7N9 may induce rapid aggravation of pneumonia symptoms after infecting humans and cause dyspnea or severe respiratory distress syndrome. Based on related researches, H7N9 has a virulence weaker than H5N1 but stronger than H9N2, while it induces an inflammatory response weaker than H5N1 but stronger than H9N2. On the other hand, victims of H5N1 infection are mainly children and young persons, while those infected by H7N9 comprise mainly adults and the aged. Once acquiring the capability of inter-human transmission through evolution or mutation, it will inevitably cause a pandemic of avian influenza. The presence of multiple family-clustering cases, as observed in this epidemic in human populations, implies that H7N9 is of probability inter-human transmission.

Subtype H5N6 of influenza virus, a hypovirus coming from birds, does not cause severe disease in birds, but induces severe clinical manifestations after infecting a human. Risks are quite low for infection and transmission induced by subtype H5N6 in human beings, and evidence for human-to-human transmission has not been found.

Positiveness was identified for the nucleic acid of H5N6 avian influenza virus when detecting pharyngeal swab specimen from a patient with severe pneumonia in Nanchong City, Jiangsu Province in May 2014, which was confirmed further to be H5N6 avian influenza virus by the Chinese Center for Disease Control and Prevention. The patient was a 49-year-old male with a history of exposure to poultry that had died from sickness. He was diagnosed with acute severe pneumonia and died after the rescue failed despite every effort made by provincial and municipal joint expert group for diagnosis and treatment [7]. Positiveness was identified for the nucleic acid of H5N6 avian influenza virus in a patient with severe pneumonia in Guangdong Province on December 22, 2014, and the result of further re-examination by the Chinese Center for Disease Control and Prevention was also positive for the virus. The mutation of site 627 of H5N6 virus polymerase was identified, which made it easy for the virus to infect human beings. The patient was a 58-year-old male with a history of surgery of colon cancer and manifested a severe infection. He was cured successfully and then discharged.

Three cases of confirmed human infection of H10N8 avian influenza have been reported totally from January 2013 to February 2014 in Jiangxi Province, with two deaths [8]. All these three patients had definite exposure history to birds. The first patient died from the deterioration of disease after 7-day hospital stay. The second patient was admitted on January 15, 2014, and discharged after the condition was improved under treatment. The third patient, a 75-year-old retired worker confirmed globally suffering from H10N8 highly pathogenic human avian influenza, was admitted in February 2014. The patient bought chickens at the poultry market on January 29th, 2014, and slaughtered them by himself. The patient's tracheal aspirates and blood samples at the visit were sent respectively to the Disease Control Center of Jiangxi Province and Disease Control Center of China for detection. The results showed that detection of nucleic acids of H10N8 avian influenza virus by Reverse Transcription-Polymerase Chain Reaction (RT-PCR) assay was positive, and the diagnosis of H10N8 highly pathogenic human avian influenza was confirmed. Bedside chest X-ray showed large consolidation of the lung. The patient died on February 8, 2014, after the rescue failed due to the dangerous condition which progressed very rapidly.

A patient diagnosed with human infection of H7N4 avian influenza was admitted by the Third People's Hospital of Changzhou City, Jiangsu Province, on January 1, 2018 [9, 10]. Human infection of H7N4 avian influenza shares many similarities in clinical features with that of H7N9. This patient was found to have a history of exposure to live birds and admitted with a diagnosis of severe pneumonia. The nucleic acids of the H7N4 virus were examined positive by the CDC of Jiangsu Province, and confirmed by the Chinese CDC. The diagnosis of human infection of H7N4 avian influenza was made by the expert group organized by the National Health and Family Planning Commission considering comprehensively the clinical manifestations, epidemiological investigations, and laboratory findings of the patient. Before this, cases of human infection of H7N4 avian influenza have never been reported in the world. The patient was discharged after the disease was cured through cooperative medical treatment by the Intensive Care Unit and Infection Unit of the Third People's Hospital of Changzhou City, Jiangsu Province. The patient had a history of hypertension and manifested symptoms including fever, cough, and expectoration as well as viremias such as fatigue and muscle soreness. The disease progressed rapidly into severe pneumonia and respiratory failure within a very short period. Laboratory findings at the early stage showed the decrease of total leukocyte count, lymphocyte count, and platelet count; blood biochemical showed the rise of C-reactive protein, lactate dehydrogenase, CK, and AST. All these clinical characteristics and changes in the related laboratory were not significantly different from those of severe cases of human infection of H7N9 avian influenza. Findings of chest CT in this patient seemed similar roughly with those for H7N9 infection and manifested localized patchy opacity at the lower right lung at the early stage, which progressed into large patches of opacities distributed diffusively in both lungs. There was gradual absorption of the exudative lesions, though the absorption was slow and complicated with fibrosis of trace of pulmonary tissues.

Five cases of subtype H9N2 virus infection were identified in the Chinese Mainland in 1998, and two cases of this disease were identified in Hongkong China in 1999. All these patients survived, and the evidence showed that poultry was the source of infection. In 2000, subtype H9N2 virus was separated from a 22-month-old influenza-like child in Guangdong China. A child in Hongkong China was proved to be infected with subtype H9N2 virus in the same year, who recovered completely after treatment during a hospital stay. As of January 2017, 21 cases of human infection of H9N2 avian influenza had been reported in China's mainland, including one death. These 21 cases of human infection of H9N2 avian influenza were characterized clinically and epidemiologically in: (1) unobvious seasonal peak in onsets, with 1, 6, 8, and 6 cases, respectively, in spring, summer, autumn, and winter, (2) distribution of these 21 cases in 10 provinces including 11 males and 10 females with the range of age from 7 months to 84 years; (3) grouping and underlying diseases, with 17 mild cases (including 14 manifesting influenza-like symptoms and 3 manifesting pneumonia) and one death with severe underlying diseases; (4) the epidemiological history with 16 cases (76.19%) identified through routine monitoring for influenza-like patients, 11 cases having exposure to live poultry market or environment of live poultry prior to onset, 8 cases without exposure to live poultry and 2 cases with unknown epidemiological history.

2.2 Infection Source

The main infection source is the bird such as chicken, duck, and goose suffering from avian influenza or carrying avian influenza virus, especially the chicken. This disease spreads mainly through the respiratory tract, and also via close contact with secretion and excreta of infected poultry and water polluted by the virus. The infection may also occur due to direct contact with the virus in the laboratory. Populations at high risks are those who are engaged in poultry breeding, and those who have been to places such as poultry raising, selling, and slaughtering within 1 week before the onset of the disease, especially those exposed to sick or dead poultry. In a few cases, exposure to poultry feces is also considered as a source of infection when children play in areas frequented by free-range poultry.

I. *Domestic Poultry*

Poultries such as chickens, ducks, gooses, and doves suffering from avian influenza or carrying avian influenza virus are the important infection sources, especially chickens. Avian influenza virus exists widely in many poultries (such as turkey, chicken, guinea fowl, goose, duck, quail, pigeon, pheasant, ostrich, pheasant, parrot, etc.), and it can be carried by the secretions and excreta, feathers, tissues, organs and eggs of birds.

II. *Wild Birds*

H5N1 virus can infect several kinds of wild birds, and wild waterfowl (mostly covert infection) plays an important role in the natural transmission of avian influenza.

Wild birds (such as swans, terns, wild ducks, geese, puffins, turtledoves, and peacocks), waterfowls (such as swans, seagulls, and wild ducks), and migrating waterfowls (especially wild ducks) have the greatest opportunity to expelling avian influenza viruses.

There exist multiple species of birds in large quantities, and most of them are used to living in groups, which forms the conditions in favor of prolonged survival of the viruses.

Because all different subtypes of influenza A viruses identified so far can almost be found in birds, some researches consider that waterfowl is a huge natural reservoir of genes of influenza virus, and an important material basis for the origin of new subtypes of influenza A viruses.

However, the possibility of other birds or pigs becoming the source of infection cannot be excluded. It is generally believed that wild migrating waterfowl, especially wild ducks, are the natural hosts for avian influenzas, and the secretion, excreta, tissues, organs, and eggs of wild birds may contain virus and spread them to poultry for domestic cultivation and for sale.

III. *Birds*

Birds (such as swallows, grouse, spotted geese, crows, sparrows, and herons) can also act as the source of infection. Migration of migratory birds plays an important role in the spread of avian influenza.

IV. *Mammals*

Influenza A virus is also found in humans, horses, pigs, monkeys, domestic cats, mice, tigers, and leopards, and occasionally in minks, ferrets, seals, whales, and other mammals. In 1970, Kundin identified antibodies for subtype H3N2 in a pig herd and isolated similar virus. In 1976, an inter-human epidemic of classical swine influenza virus occurred in New Jersey, USA, while H1N1 and H1N2 strains coming from birds were found in pig herds in Europe; Some researchers isolated the H3N8 avian influenza virus from horses for the first time in 1989 and confirmed that H3 gene of equine influenza virus originated from avian influenza strains. These studies suggest that influenza A virus may happen in different hosts to some extent, i.e., induce direct or indirect transmission among humans, birds, horses, pigs, and other animals, which is also an important condition for the emergence of variation of influenza A virus and the origin of new subtypes. At the same time, virus A has been proved capable of spreading in poultries including chickens, ducks, and geese as well as livestocks including pigs, pigeons, horses, and domestic cats. Domestic cats used to be considered resistant to H5N1 virus. Kuiken et al. found, however, continuous excretion of H5N1 virus was identified in domestic cats fed with chicken infected with this virus, so that cats became the source of infection through expelling H5N1 viruses continuously, implying that domestic cats could also play an important role in the process of H5N1 virus epidemic, and should be paid attention to in the control of the epidemic. H5N1, the highly pathogenic avian influenza virus, infected tigers in Thailand in October 2004, causing 45 deaths. H5N1 virus can also infect mammals, such as monkeys, mice, pigs, ferrets, leopards, horses, minks, and cetaceans, which may act as the intermediate hosts to transmit the virus to humans or other mammals. Whether the H5N1 virus has acquired the ability necessary for breaking through species barrier and infecting a variety of mammals other than poultry remains to be further studied.

V. *Human Beings*

Whether human beings can be the source of infection needs to be confirmed further. It hasn't been determined whether human patients with avian influenza might be the source of infection. The possibility of human-to-human transmission of subtype H5N1 has been suggested by multiple family-clustering onsets, a confirmed case of children-mother transmission, and cases of diseases in multiple family members infected by one individual in Thailand and Indonesia. An 11-year-old girl was infected with avian influenza virus post to her exposure to a sick chicken, as reported in Thailand, and her mother and aunt got avian influenza successively after looking after her. It was considered by researchers that the virus infecting her mother and aunt spread probably through human-to-human transmission. So far, the risk of transmission in hospitals among medical staff remains low, even if appropriate isolation is not used. During the epidemic of H5N1 human avian influenza in 1997 in Hong Kong, it was found in a retrospective study that in 217 healthcare workers exposed to patients with H5N1 human avian influenza, anti-H5N1 antibodies were identified in serological test in two cases with mild or no symptoms, suggesting the epidemiological proof for human-to-human transmission and the probable presence of human with asymptomatic infection. Moreover, an occurrence of severe pneumonia was reported in a nurse prior to the exposure to an infected patient in Vietnam. However, epidemiological and virologic researches are needed for confirming further these results, despite the presence of individual cases.

VI. *Reservoir Hosts for Avian Influenza*

It has been confirmed that avian influenza viruses are widely distributed in many poultry (including turkey, chicken, guinea fowl, grouse, partridge, quail, pigeon, pheasant, ostrich, goose, and duck) and wild birds (including wild ducks, swans, and various sea birds) all over the world. More viruses have been isolated from migratory waterfowls, especially wild ducks, than from other birds. The disease in domestic chickens and turkeys induced by the avian influenza virus is the most serious. The covert infection of avian influenza exists in poultry, which may last for several months. Avian influenza virus can survive for at least 18 days on feathers, 1 week in feces, and 1 month in water. There is still no evidence for the invertebrate as a storage host.

2.3 Transmission Routes

The mechanism for rapid transmission either regional or international for avian influenza virus remains unclear. Some people think that migratory birds play an important role in this process, speculating that migratory birds carrying the virus may transmit the virus along their migration path, though there is no enough evidence. Virus can be contained in the corpse of sick birds and their secretions, excreta, tissues, organs, and eggs. The feces, containing the largest amount of virus, is the main vector for transmitting avian influenza. AIV (avian influenza virus) is transmitted mainly through routes including feces, contaminated drinks, drinking water, egg trays, bedding, chicken embryos, seed eggs, aerosols, dust, cages, eggs of birds, sprouts, clothing/hats/boots, and means of transportation. The virus is transmitted through the human respiratory tract, digestive tract, aerosol, skin damage, and conjunctiva, dominated by the respiratory tract and digestive tract. Direct contact with sick poultry or indirect contact with viral pollutants is also considered as the main route of infection; any object containing viruses such as secretions, feces, and dead poultry corpses may spread the epidemic mechanically; direct contact with virus strains (laboratories) can also induce the infection of this disease. The relative efficiencies of different transmission routes have not been determined yet. It is generally believed that human beings are not susceptible to the avian influenza virus. The phenomenon of multiple family-clustering cases of human avian influenza H5N1 and H7N9 suggests that the human-to-human transmission has already existed despite the necessary further confirmation, and the human-to-human transmission will be the focus of global experts [11].

Avian influenza virus can survive for several weeks in dried blood and tissues and remain infectious in frozen meat and bone after 287 days and 303 days respectively. Such a long survival period not only increases the opportunity of re-infection of poultry post to pandemic, but also raises risks of contact with wild birds and of remote viral transmission.

(I) *Respiratory Transmission*

The way of respiratory transmission includes inhalation of infectious droplets and droplet nucleus, and human infection of AIV is mainly caused by inhalation of virulent viral particles. AIV spreads with the air, and the viral particle inhaled may cause disease by attaching to the human upper respiratory tract, post to human direct contact with the sick birds or symptomatic infected birds and their secretions, excreta, and polluted environment. The spread via droplets is the focus under investigation at present. It was found in researches that mice infected with virus strains isolated from the human body manifested an obvious weight loss. Some virus strains can spread among ferrets via droplets, and the susceptibility of ferrets is similar to that of human beings. However, the possibility of transmission among ferrets was proved to be limited by experiments. Based on researches, infectivity exists in eyes, pharyngeal secretion, and feces in mice post to the infection, with the highest level in pharyngeal secretion, suggesting the possible presence of droplet transmission.

(II) *Contact Transmission*

Direct or indirect contract is also the transmission route for avian influenza virus. Human being can be infected through contacting closely feces of poultry or livestock infected with the H5N1 virus. The virus can be auto-inoculated on the mucous membrane of the upper respiratory tract and conjunctiva or skin wound through direct contact and possibly indirect contact with pollutants. Contact infection may occur when handling and processing sick poultry, catching and holding cockfights, or playing with poultry, such as asymptomatic but infected ducks. Nosocomial transmission through close contact is defined as an infection due to treatment, visit, care of patients and living together with patients, or directly contact with patients' secretions or body fluids of the infected patient.

(III) *Digestive Tract Transmission*

The spread of avian influenza via the digestive tract is mainly caused by the air polluted by a large number of viral particles contained in the feces. For example, the cases of human avian influenza in Vietnam that caused deaths were proved to be mainly transmitted through the feces of poultry. WHO warns that similar risk exists in human beings no matter what kind of sick chicken they are exposed to, because feces containing the virus will be discharged within at least 10 days by the survival poultries of viruses. Avian influenza virus can be transmitted via digestive tract due to contaminated hands, water, toys, etc. In addition, the infection can also be induced by intaking raw chicken, duck blood, or uncooked poultry food. Virus can also be discharged along with feces and spread through the fecal-oral pathway via water contaminated by feces.

(IV) *Transmission Through Skin Injury*

Contamination with the virus may also occur at injuries at skin or mucous membrane, which is similar to the inoculation of virus onto dermal injuries.

(V) *Ocular Conjunctival Transmission*

Virus particles contained in the infected or asymptomatic birds and their secretions, excreta, and polluted environment may cause infection by attaching to human conjunctiva. Auto-inoculation of virus onto conjunctiva occurs through direct contact or possibly indirect contact with pollutants.

(VI) *Aerosol Transmission*

AIV proliferates greatly in the respiratory tract, and exfoliated cells containing infectious virus are discharged via respiration, cough, and sneeze by the patient and suspended in the air to form the aerosol of avian influenza virus. Cough and sneeze are the good force to generate the aerosol of avian influenza virus, though whether the virus can be transmitted via aerosol need further confirmation based on epidemiological studies.

(VII) *Blood Transmission*

H5N1 influenza virus can be detected in the blood of patients infected with highly pathogenic avian influenza, and the virus content in the dead is higher than in the survivals, so there exists the possibility of blood transmission. However, it is of little epidemiological significance, because of the short duration of viremia in avian influenza and the low probability of avian influenza infection through blood route in human beings.

(VIII) *Vertical Transmission*

Avian influenza virus H5N1 could pass through the placental barrier, as reported by a research on a mice model, and viral RNA could be detected continuously in the nervous system of mice. Two cases of pregnant women infected with avian influenza virus H5N1 were reported in Anhui Province, China. One of them died, and the other woman was rescued successfully, though artificial abortion was performed. Therefore, further pathological and immunohistochemical studies are needed to determine whether the fetus is infected with H5N1. The number of pregnant women infected with H5N1 of avian influenza virus is still rare so far, so it is difficult to conclude whether the virus can spread vertically.

(IX) *Laboratory Transmission*

Laboratory safety standards in some countries and regions are not very strict, so there is the possibility of laboratory transmission. In 1981, keratitis occurred in a refresher in an American laboratory due to infection with the H7N1 strain. In 2003, a 57-year old Dutch veterinarian was infected with the virus when examining the sick chicken and finally died of the complication of pneumonia caused by H7N7 avian influenza. Laboratory infection may occur in the case of exposure to respiratory secretions, blood, throat swabs, and tracheal aspirates of patients with avian influenza. The key to control effectively cases of laboratory infection is to improve laboratory safety standards and achieve early detection and timely quarantine.

(X) *Vehicle Transmission*

In the epidemic of SARS, remote transmission through civil aircraft and land vehicles plays an important role, especially the enhancement of the global rapid epidemic by civil aircrafts, which is of great significance for reference when considering the spread of avian influenza. On the one hand, aircrafts can transport birds with avian influenza to any part of the world within 24–48 h, accelerating the spread of epidemics, and on the other hand, land vehicles can also bring the virus to other areas over long distances. The H5N1 avian influenza epidemic in Hong Kong in 1997 was spread by means of road transportation importing sick chickens from Guangdong Province. Most of the imported cases were transmitted by means of transportation vehicles. For example, in the outbreak of avian influenza in Hong Kong in February 2003, two members of a Hong Kong family who traveled to Fujian got sick after coming back to Hong Kong and one of them died.

(XI) *Nosocomial Infection*

Despite the low risk of nosocomial infection of H5N1 up to now, an infection suspicious of H5N1 did occur in a nurse in Vietnam in 2005. The positive rate of H5N1 antibody was 3.7% in medical practitioners working in medical wards admitting patients with avian influenza in Hong Kong, compared with 0.7% in those working in wards not serving these patients in a same hospital and 12% in relatives of avian influenza patients, showing the significant difference. This suggests that human avian influenza has an occupational correlation with nosocomial infection.

(XII) *Other Routes*

Transmission routes remain still unclear in some of the patients, such as those in Indonesia and Thailand, as well as Guangdong and Shenzhen in China with their transmission routes unidentifiable. Unknown communicators should be enquired if they live in the environment polluted by birds, which may cause transmission. For example, some of the cases in Vietnam and Indonesia had no definite history of exposure to sick birds, and it was speculated that the patients might be infected through contacting lake water and/or chemical fertilizer polluted by feces of birds.

Human-to-human transmission for human avian influenza still lacks direct and powerful evidence so far. Most evidences involved in the researches imply that there exists surely avian-to-human transmission, possibly environment (polluted by avian feces)-to-human transmission, and in small number the discontinuous H5N1/H7N9 inter-human transmission. Despite the occurrence of multiple family-clustering cases, the virus has not been identified to have the ability of sustainable inter-human transmission.

2.4 Susceptible Populations

(I) Susceptible populations

It is generally believed that human beings are not susceptible to the avian influenza virus. Although there have been outbreaks of human avian influenza in different scales successively all over the world, reports of human infection have been rare. According to the small number of human avian influenzas that have occurred, the infection may happen at any age. The proportion of children under the age of 12 seems higher with the severer condition, and there is no gender difference. The high-risk populations are those who are engaged in poultry breeding or have been to places of cultivation, sales, and slaughtering of poultry within 1 week prior to the onset, and the laboratory workers who are exposed to the materials of avian influenza virus infection. Human being generally lacks the immunity to avian influenza. Most patients were children, as shown by analysis on the age of avian influenza patients in history. This might be explained by much more opportunities for children in exposure to chickens and birds and their excreta, or children's low resistance to the virus because of their under-developed immune system. The positive rate of antibodies against H5N1 is about 10% in employees in the poultry industry, about 3% in those participating in the slaughter of sick poultry, 3.7% in medical practitioners working in wards admitting avian influenza patients, 0.7% in those working in wards not treating these patients in the same hospital, and 12% in the relatives of avian influenza patients. This suggests the high occupational correlation of these diseases and the presence of latent infections.

(II) *Immunity Post to Healing*

The current data shows that this disease is an acute self-limited infectious disease. The neutralizing antibodies against avian influenza can be detected in 2–3 weeks after the healing, but the changes and duration of the neutralizing antibody need further investigation. Genetic variation or antigenic shift may occur in avian influenza virus, and whether the patient will be re-infected or get sick will need prolonged observation and study.

(III) *Vaccination*

The most effective way to prevent avian influenza is to vaccinate humans and birds with the influenza vaccine. Susceptible populations and high-risk populations should be vaccinated with influenza vaccine 1 month before the occurrence of influenza. The influenza vaccines for humans produced every year are routinely used to protect human beings during the epidemic season. Although these vaccines cannot prevent infection by the H5N1 avian influenza virus, they can prevent the spread of human virus strains after inoculating high-risk populations, thereby reducing the risk of their simultaneous infection with human influenza virus and avian influenza virus, and lowering the chance of genetic exchange between human and avian influenza viruses. The key populations requiring influenza vaccination include: infants and children aged between 6 and 35 months; the aged older than 60 years; patients with chronic diseases; personnel engaged in poultry breeding, sales and slaughter, and those who may be exposed to risky materials with avian influenza virus, including laboratory workers, medical practitioners, and healthcare workers, especially those in front-line positions; as well as primary school students and children in kindergartens. In an unpredictable influenza epidemic in the future, the vaccine of human avian influenza is likely to be the only effective way to curb the influenza epidemic. At present, the vaccine of human avian influenza mainly includes inactivated vaccine, attenuated live vaccine, DNA vaccine, subunit vaccine, and virus-like particle vaccine.

2.5 Epidemiological Features

I. *Epidemiological Seasons*

Epidemic of human avian influenza may happen all the year round, but mainly in the transition between winter and spring or between autumn and winter. It often takes place when cold current attacks and temperature changes abruptly, and its incidence drops obviously after the climate becomes warm. As of the end of 2003, H5N1 human avian influenza in the world has occurred in November, December, January, February, and March. Generally speaking, it seldom occurs in summer, though there are sporadic cases in summer, such as the first case of H5N1 avian influenza which happened in June 2006 in Shenzhen, China. The analysis on the onset time of 23 highly pathogenic cases of H5N1 human avian influenza that have happened in the Chinese Mainland shows 3, 4, 4, 4, 2, 2, 2, and 2 cases occurring respectively in November, December, January, February, March, April, June, and October, with the incidence peaks observed in January, February, November, and December. All cases of H5N1 human avian influenza in 1997 in Hongkong took place in November and December, except for the first case that occurred in May. Ten cases of human avian influenza of H5N1 reported in Vietnam in 2004 occurred mainly in December and January. In 2004, 12 cases of human avian influenza occurred in Thailand from January to March. Eight cases of human avian influenza in Azerbaijan happened from February to March, while 8 family-clustering cases in Indonesia took place from July to October. As of May 1, 2013, 30 cases of human infection of H7N9 avian influenza had been reported in Hangzhou, China, and the onsets of diseases had been concentrated mainly in April [12]. Five cycles of the epidemic of H7N9 human avian influenza had occurred from March 2013 to September 2017, as far as the temporal distribution is concerned. Five peaks appeared in April 2013, January to February 2014, January 2015, January 2016, and January 2017. The second peak is higher than the first, the third dropped somewhat, the fourth seemed the lowest among all these five peaks and the fifth exceeded any previous peak. However, all these peaks indicate that winter and spring are the seasons with the climax of the epidemic. Cases of human infection of H5N6 avian influenza during 2013–2018 in Guangdong in China happened mainly in winter and spring, but they manifested mainly sporadic onsets because of the small number of the cases.

II. *Features in Spatial and Temporal Distribution*

Human avian influenza happens mainly in vast rural regions in various countries, such as Vietnam, Thailand, China, and Indonesia, which is related to the extensive breeding of birds, the pandemic of avian influenza, and lots of opportunities of the population in exposure to dead birds due to sickness. The occurrence of the avian influenza epidemic in human being is closely related to that in birds. Generally, avian influenza precedes (about 1 month, with an interval of 15–45 days) human influenza. Most epidemics of highly pathogenic human avian influenza in China happens in rural areas and regions around provincial capital cities. Main environmental factors include low temperature, higher relative humidity, and higher atmosphere pressure, with the obvious geographical aggregation of epidemic zones. Factors such as highly intensive environment for poultry cultivation and relatively humid market environment accumulated excessively with multiple kinds of birds provide conditions for the high frequency of genetic mutation and recombination of avian influenza virus. Factors precipitating the spread of epidemic include a warm and humid environment rich in the water source, dense population with great mobility, weak immunity defense, poor condition in breeding poultry, and absence of scientific defensive measure as for sanitary conditions, complicated with mixed breeding of all kinds of poultry. Human's close contact with dead birds due to diseases and their excretion and excreta provides the main route for transmission of human avian influenza.

III. *Features of Population Distribution*

(I) *Distribution of Gender and Age*

Children and young adults occupy a high proportion of patients with H5N1 human avian influenza, with the youngest aged 3 months and the oldest aged 75 years. Eighteen cases of H5N1 in Hongkong in 1997 had a male/female ratio of 8:10 and 11 children patients. Children accounted for a considerable proportion of H5N1 cases in Vietnam and Thailand. In ten cases of H5N1 in Vietnam, 60% were male, 40% were female, and 60% were aged below 14 years old, with the range of age of 5–13 years old; young patients occupied 40% with the range of age of 16–24 years. In 12 cases of H5N1 avian influenza in Thailand, there were 7 children aged below 14 years old and 5 adults, with a male/female ratio of 4:8. The majority of 21 cases of H5N1 avian influenza in China were young adults (n = 17), in addition to 5 children and one old person, with a male/female ratio of 7:14 with females significantly higher than males. The incidence rate of human infection with H7N9 avian influenza was higher in adults and elderly patients [13]. The mean latent duration was 5.0 ± 1.3 days (4 ~ 7 days) from exposure to onset, and 6.6 ± 3.2 days (1 ~ 10 days) from exposure to admission, with a latent duration of 4–7 days. The interval from onset to admission was more than 1 week in five patients and 1–5 days in the other three patients. The higher incidence observed in the females and children might be correlated to their vulnerability to infection because of their relatively weak immunity.

(II) *Occupational Distribution*

Data from Hong Kong of China, Vietnam, Thailand, Indonesia, and Turkey showed primary school students occupied a higher percentage among all patients. From the perspective of the occupational composition of 23 cases of H5N1 human avian influenza in China, the proportion of farmers (9/23, 39%) and rural students or children (6/23, 26%) seemed higher, which might be correlated to the raised opportunity of infection due to their higher risks in exposure to dead bird because of disease.

IV. *The Influence of Natural Factors upon Epidemic Process of Human Avian Influenza*

Webster et al. proposed that whether the avian influenza virus can cause a large-scale epidemic depends on both the virus itself and host. At present, influenza viruses with high prevalence including H5N1, H7N9, H7N3, H7N7, and H9N2 all have the possibility of infecting humans, among which H5N1 and H7N9 seem the most serious. Natural factors include climate, geography, migration of migratory birds, and the interacting course between host and virus.

(I) *Influence on Epidemic by Migration of Migratory Birds*

In the western hemisphere, many subtypes of AIV can be easily isolated from Alaska Lake in North America by ITO et al. Therefore, the Alaskan lake can be considered as the place where AIV proliferates in migrating waterfowl in North America. From the perspective of the eastern hemisphere, however, South China has a vast area of water, and it is the place where the migratory birds must pass by. Therefore, it is also the main area for recombination, proliferation, and diffusion of AIV. Wild waterfowl are natural repositories of all influenza A viruses, carrying low pathogenic viruses but not manifesting symptoms. From May to June 2005, thousands of migratory birds were found to be infected with HPIV H5N1 in Qinghai Lake, China. The migration of these birds covers Siberia, Southeast Asia, and India. The migration of birds can bring the virus to all areas of the world, so that it is impossible to perform effective control and prevention.

(II) *Influence on Epidemic by Geography and Environment*

Most of the outbreaks of highly pathogenic avian influenza in China occur in the provincial capitals and their adjacent areas, and are distributed mainly in the first-class rivers, lakes, and coastal areas; the main environmental factors in favor of the occurrence of the epidemic are low temperature, high relative humidity, and high air pressure, and the epidemic area is characterized in obvious regional aggregation.

(III) *Host Factors*

1. Hosts of different ages differ in severity of infection of avian influenza. At present, there is a consensus that children are more susceptible than young adults, but the disease in children is milder. The old and pregnant women seem also susceptible, with severe disease and higher mortality rate. The study shows that the clinical process of children is milder, while the mortality of the elderly is higher than others.
2. Whether different ethnic groups differ in susceptibility. There is no identified evidence supporting the different susceptibility in different ethnic groups.
3. Pregnancy. Pregnancy has long been considered as an important risk factor for the onset and death of influenza virus infection. During the two human influenza pandemics in 1918 and 1957, the mortality of pregnant women with influenza was as high as 45%.
4. Immunity. The immunity of hosts differing in immune status determines the different outcomes of the interaction between the body immune system and avian influenza virus. The disease is severer with raised mortality in patients with poor immunity (such as children, pregnant women, and the elderly), taking immunosuppressive drugs, or having other complications. The compromised immune function leads to a great replication of the virus in the body, raised viral excretion from the body, and high mortality. It has been confirmed that viral excretion from the body was higher significantly in the dead than in the survival. Compared with the survival, the level of cytokines in the plasma of the patients that have died from H5N1 infection was higher and the level of IP-10, MCP-1, MIG, and IL-8 significantly increased. These cytokines play an important role in the pathophysiological mechanism of ARDS.

(IV) *Factor of Virus*

1. Viral load. Higher viral content in throat secretion, sputum, or nasopharynx secretion there is, the stronger infectivity the virus has. The viral load of avian influenza in the throat is the highest during the symptomatic period (about day 8 of the disease course), so infectivity is the strongest during this period and drops gradually thereafter. It has also been found in the researches that the viral load in pharynx, larynx, or blood is higher in lethal avian influenzas than in non-lethal ones, especially for the blood where the viral load increases significantly ($P < 0.01$). These findings suggest that viral load correlates closely to the severity of disease and mortality.
2. Among different subtypes of strains, strong pathogenicity is observed in H5 and H7, but weak pathogenicity in H9, N2, and N3. Historically, all highly pathogenic avian influenzas were caused by H5 and H7, but not all H5 and H7 are strong-virulent strains.

3. Strains with different virulence. The pathogenicity and disease severity depend on the number of splicing sites for viral hemagglutinin by the host. For example, the virus is capable of replicating at every part of the body with strong infectivity and pathogenicity if there are multiple splicing sites for viral hemagglutinin. On the contrary, the virus will have the low replicating capability and weak pathogenicity if there is only one splicing site.

(V) *Influence on the Epidemic by Social Factors*

Influences on the epidemic by social factors are usually complicated and changeable, including social status, medical insurance, sanitation and anti-epidemic system, living conditions, medical conditions, economic and cultural level, health and customs, religion, and social stability.

Government and sanitation/anti-epidemic systems play the important role for avian influenza, and the emergency-response ability of anti-epidemic department directly determines the epidemic situation of the disease. Early detection, early report, early isolation, and early treatment shall be carried out for epidemic prevention and control, and effective disinfection shall be performed for epicenters. The 3-km area around the epicenter of the highly pathogenic avian influenza shall be designated as the epidemic area, and all poultry in this area shall be killed. Meanwhile, urgent vaccination must be performed for all susceptible birds within 5 km around the epidemic area, and an immune isolation belt shall be established within 30 km around the epidemic area. It is the most effective measure to control the spread of avian influenza, which can control the epidemic within a small range.

Educational level of patients and the importance attached to the disease will also affect the prevalence of the disease. Generally speaking, people with higher education will see a doctor earlier when they have symptoms, otherwise, isolation and treatment would be delayed, causing the spread of the disease. Therefore, it is necessary to strengthen health education and popularize knowledge related to avian influenza. In order to prevent the widespread of avian influenza, it is of great importance to strengthen macro-control and focus by the government, implement traffic control, prohibit trading in live poultry market, implement necessary martial law when necessary in the worst-hit areas, slaughter birds infected by the influenza virus, and carry out national mobilization. It is also vital for WHO to communicate and cooperate with governments and health administrative departments of all countries and share information with them to control the epidemic of avian influenzas.

References

1. Luo R, Zhu Y, Xu Z, et al. The report of the first case of H5N1 human avian pneumonia in Chinese Mainland. Chin J Pediatr. 2006;44(5):342–5.
2. Yang G, Huang C. Epidemic and countermeasures of avian influenza. Forum Prevent Med. 2005;11(3):312–4.
3. Yu H, Chen Y, Shu Y, et al. Investigation and confirmation of the first case of human avian influenza (H5N1) in Chinese Mainland. Chin J Epidemiol. 2006;27(4):181–287.
4. Ahmet FO, Ali B, Sukru A, et al. Avian influenza A(H5N1) infection in eastern Turkey. N Engl J Med. 2006,21:2179–85.
5. Zhang Y, Lu H. Recent researches on avian influenza. Foreign Med; Epidemiol Infect Dis. 2005;32(6):332–4.
6. Han D, Han C, Li L, et al. Epidemiological features of human infection of H7N9 avian influenza 2013-2017 China. Chin J Epidemiol. 2018;39(1):44–6.
7. Wang X, Hou M, Mei Y. Analysis on laboratory findings for the first human infection of H5N6 avian influenza in Hubei Province. Chin J Zoonoses. 2017;33(1):89–91.
8. Shen M, Liu Z. Nursing of a patient with H10N8 highly pathogenic human avian influenza. Chin J Pract Nurs. 2014;30(23):47–8.
9. Tong X, Wu X, Xue F. Analysis of clinical treatment of the first case of human infection of H7N4 avian influenza in the world. Chin J Epidemiol. 2018;36(3):129–32.
10. Jin Q, Zhang L, Yang L. CT manifestations of the first case of human infection of H7N4 avian influenza pneumonia in the world. Electron J Emerg Infect Dis. 2018;3(1):45–8.
11. Sun H, Tong H, Cui D. Progression in researches on human infection of H7N9 avian influenza. Chin J Clin Infect Dis. 2017;10(1):68–75.
12. Xie L, Ding H, Sun Z, et al. Analysis of distributional characteristics and exposure source of human infection of H7N9 avian influenza in Hangzhou City. 2013;34(9):944–5.15.
13. Gao Z, Liu W, Muti M. Epidemiological analysis on cases of human infection of H7N9 avian influenza in Xinjiang. Chin J Zoonoses. 2008;34(11):1056–8.

3 Etiology

Zhi-gang Song, Yu-xin Shi, Hua-bin Yin, Jun Chen, and Hong-zhou Lu

3.1 Discovery of the Pathogen and Confirmation of Pathogeny

Avian influenza in human is an acute respiratory infectious disease caused by human exposure to avian influenza viruses contained in feces or secretions discharged by birds infected with these viruses or their tissues.

I. *Discovery of the Pathogen*

The first strain of avian influenza virus (H5N1) was isolated in Hongkong China in May 1997, when 18 patients infected with H5N1 avian influenza were diagnosed, including six deaths. Since 1997, epidemics of human avian influenza have outbroken in many parts of the world, including those of multiple subtypes of viruses such as H7N1 and H9N2 [1]. Eight hundred and sixty-one confirmed cases in total of highly pathogenic H5N1 avian influenza in humans have been reported globally from January 2003 to May 2019, including 455 deaths. These patients have been distributed among 16 countries/regions, and 53 cases have been reported in China, including 31 deaths. (https://www.who.int/influenza/human_animal_interface/2019_05_10_tableH5N1.pdf?ua=1).

In March 2013, human infection with novel H7N9 avian influenza virus was identified firstly in Shanghai, China [2, 3]. 1567 human infections of H7N9 have been diagnosed accumulatively in the world including 615 deaths, as of February 6, 2019. The sufferers of H7N9 avian influenza were mostly the aged, with more male patients than female ones.

II. *Etiological Diagnosis*

The first strain of H5N1 (A/HongKong/156/97) was isolated through MDCK from influenza-like patients in Hongkong China in May 1997, and identified through hemagglutination inhibition test, using serums of different subtypes of avian influenza virus. It was found by researchers that this virus had hemagglutination inhibition only with serums of subtype H5 and subtype H1, in the neutralizing tests involving 23 different anti-HA antigen serums and 9 NA-antigen serums. Further identification was performed, using subsequent tests including RT-PCR, nucleotide sequencing, and immunofluorescence, concluding that this virus was H5N1 avian influenza virus. The same identification and confirmation were performed for 18 strains of H5N1 viruses isolated from this epidemic [1].

Multiple epidemics of novel avian influenzas in humans have outbroken globally since 1997. Nine human patients infected with H9N2 influenza were diagnosed in total in Guangdong Province in 1998, which were the first cases reported globally of human infections with this virus [4]. The year 2003 witnessed the discovery of H5N1 and H9N2 avian influenzas in Hongkong China and that of H7N3 in the Netherlands. H7N3 was discovered in 2004 in Canada. In 2005 and 2006, H5N1 avian influenza outbroke in multiple regions. Human infections of the H7N9 avian influenza virus occurred in Shanghai City and Anhui Province in March 2013, and human infections of H10N8 were discovered in Nanchang City of Jiangxi Province in December 2013. Human infec-

The original version of the chapter has been revised. A correction to this chapter can be found at https://doi.org/10.1007/978-981-16-1429-3_17

Z.-g. Song
Department of Biosafety, Shanghai Public Health Clinical Center, Shanghai, China

Y.-x. Shi
Department of Radiology, Shanghai Public Health Clinical Center, Shanghai, China

H.-b. Yin
Department of Radiology, Shanghai Fifth People's Hospital, Fudan University, Shanghai, China

J. Chen · H.-z. Lu (✉)
Department of Infectious Disease and Immunology, Shanghai Public Health Clinical Center, Shanghai, China
e-mail: luhongzhou@shphc.org.cn

C. Qiu et al. (eds.), *Avian Influenza in Human*, https://doi.org/10.1007/978-981-16-1429-3_3

tions of the H5N6 avian influenza virus occurred in multiple regions in Guangdong and Yunnan from 2014 to 2017, and human infections of H7N4 avian influenza virus was observed in Jiangsu Province, China in 2018 [5, 6]. Other avian influenza viruses that have infected humans as of March 2019 include also H10N8, H9N2, H7N9, H7N7, H7N4, H7N3, H7N1, H7N2, H5N6, and H5N1 [7–10].

3.2 Morphological Structure and Physical/Chemical Profiles of the Viruses

I. *Morphological Structure and Profiles*

Avian influenza virus belongs to Orthomyxoviridae, which has many subtypes and spherical virus particles. Some strains of influenza viruses usually have the filamentous appearance at their initial isolation, with different lengths and even up to several microns. However, both filaments and spheres are similar in diameter (80–120 nm). However, the polymorphous viral particles at the first isolation may turn into spheres gradually after successive passages in chicken embryos or cells. RNA accounts for 0.8–1.1% of influenza virus, with protein for 70–75%, lipids for 20–24%, and sugars for 5–8%. Most of the lipids are phospholipids, which are located on the viral membrane and contain a small amount of cholesterol and glycolipids. The sugars inside viral particles include ribose, galactose, mannose, fucose, and glucosamine, existing mainly in the form of glycoprotein and glycolipid. Lipid chains and sugar chains of viral proteins are determined by host cells. The viral envelope has a spiral nucleocapsid inside and its surface is covered with fibroids, generally about 10–12 nm long. Both HA, the rod-shaped trimer capable of agglutinating red blood cells, and NA with an appearance of a mushroom-shaped tetramer correlate to viral infection and its pathogenicity, despite they differ in functions. The nucleocapsid of the influenza virus seems helically symmetric, and the total length of the RNA fragment is 13.6 Kb. The nucleic acids are covered exteriorly with nucleocapsids, which are arranged spirally and comprise mainly nucleoprotein, with a diameter of 9–15 nm. HA, NA, and matrix protein M2 are all embedded inside the lipid capsule, which is the cell membrane deriving from the host. M1 tubercle protein is directly under the capsule and forms a spherical nucleocapsid composed of one or several molecules, enclosing viral RNA molecules, and responsible for RNA replication and transcription together with NP nucleoprotein and three polymerases including PB1, PB2, and PA [6].

II. *Stability in External Environment*

Highly pathogenic avian influenza viruses, such as H5N1 and H7N9, have poor resistance to the external environment. They are sensitive to UV, high temperature, and chemical disinfectants such as various alcohols, and easy to inactivate.

1. *Stability in Natural Environment*

Influenza viruses show a strong resistance to low temperatures in the natural environment. They can be stored for more than 2 months under minus 10 °C to minus 40 °C, but this temperature often causes them to lose their hemagglutination activity. The viruses can be preserved for several years under minus 70 °C, and for prolonged period under 4 °C post to lyophilization. The viruses in feces can survive for 30–35 days under 4 °C, and maintain their infectivity within 7 days under 20 °C. Influenza viruses may also survive in lakes and ponds for a prolonged duration, though how long they may survive remains unknown.

The viruses can survive for a prolonged duration in the natural environment, especially under cool and humid conditions. Influenza viruses can often be isolated from lakes or ponds where waterfowls live. In summer, influenza viruses do not survive for a long time in the water of pond without waterfowls.

2. *Sensitivity to Temperature*

Generally, the viruses can be inactivated within 30 min if heated up to 56 °C and 70 °C 2 min. As for the sequence of inactivation, the infectivity of viral particles is first inactivated, followed by neuraminidase activity, and then the Hemagglutination activity. The viral activity is unstable under 4 to 40 °C.

3. *Sensitivity to Sunlight and Ultraviolet*

Avian influenza virus is so sensitive to ultraviolet rays that direct exposure to sunlight within 40–48 h is enough to inactivate the naked virus, and it can be destroyed rapidly if irradiated directly by ultraviolet.

4. *Sensitivity to Chemical Factors*

Avian influenza virus as an envelope virus is sensitive to oxidants, halogens, heavy metals, detergents, ethanol, and formaldehyde, as well as organic solvents such as chloroform, ether, and acetone. Moreover, it can also be inactivated by acetic acid and lactic acid. The virus will lose its infectivity if treated overnight with 20% ether at 4 °C. The viral particle can be split after being treated with ether in equivalent amount for 2 h under 4 °C. In addition, the virus is also sensitive to 0.1% peracetic acid, 1% sodium hypochlorite, and 0.1% Bromogeramine.

Inactivators and inactivating methods that are commonly used include 3-min inactivation with 1‰ mercuric chloride and 1‰ potassium permanganate; 30-min inactivation with 1‰ formaldehyde; 5-min inactivation with 75% ethanol; and 3-min inactivation with 1% hydrochloric acid and 1‰ iodine.

3.3 Molecular Biological Characteristics of the Virus

The genome of the avian influenza virus contains eight single-segmented negative-strand RNAs. The total length of nucleic acid is 13.6 kb. It can encode ten kinds of proteins, including haemagglutinin (HA), neuraminidase (NA), nuclear protein (NP), RNA polymerase (PB1, PB2, PA), matrix protein (M1, M2), and nonstructural protein (NS1, NS2) [11]. All genetic segments have the same nucleotide sequence at the 5′ end and the 3′ end. The 13 conservative sequences at the 5′ end is 5′-AGUAGAAA-CAAGG, and the 12 conservative sequences at the 3′ end is 3′UCG(U/C)UUUCGUCC. Reverse complementarity exists in these common sequences and may form the handle-like circular structure, which is the nucleotide recognition site necessary for the combination of RNA polymerase of influenza viruses [11].

I. *Polymerase Protein*

The RNA polymerase of the avian influenza virus is composed of three subunits including two basic proteins (PB2 and PB1) and an acid protein PA. These three proteins existing in the viral particle with a ratio of 1:1:1 are connected together through noncovalent bonds, without covalent connection among them. Three polymerases, an NP protein and a vRNA (viral RNA; vRNA) segment of the virus form together with the ribonucleoprotein (RNP). In addition, matrix protein M1 as one of the components of RNP also participates in the formation of RNPs by combining with 3′ end of the genomic segment. RNP is contained in every genomic segment, so every particle of the influenza virus has eight RNP complexes.

PB1, PB2, and PA share a common characteristic in their amino acid sequence, i.e., the specific nucleophilic amino acid sequence region, which makes it easy for the proteins synthesized in the cytoplasm to enter the cell nucleus of the host. After being infected by the viruses, the nucleus of human somatic cells will have these three polymerase proteins. Despite their small quantity during viral replication after the cells are infected, these three polymerase proteins are essential for the replication and expression of viral genes. At the initial stage of RNA transcription, PB2 recognizes and combines with 5′-end cap, and also has restriction endonuclease activity, participates in the slicing of mRNA cap of the host, and acts as the primer in synthesizing viral mRNA [12, 13].

Genes PB1, PB2, PA, M2, and NP of avian influenza virus are important determinants of host specificity. The change of nucleotide in the PB2 gene adapts the virus to different hosts, thereby determining the range of hosts suitable for viral colonization. For example, locus 627 of gene PB2 encodes glutamic acid in the avian influenza virus, but it is changed to encode lysine in the human influenza virus. That is to say, the substitution of lysine for glutamic acid encoded by locus 627 of PB2 gene will adapt reproduction of avian influenza virus to intracellular environment of mammals. It was inferred from genetic analysis on avian influenza virus in Hongkong 1997 (A/Hong Kong/156/97) performed by Kat ZJM et al. that changes occurred in amino acids encoded by loci 199, 627, 661, and 667, and lysine encoded by locus 355 was changed to glutamic acid. These mutations of PB2 were considered as the cause of the high pathogenicity on both mice and human being. In 2001, Yao et al. investigated genetics principles for the range of hosts for subtype H7 of avian influenza virus using the H7 influenza model and found that Dobson 4H showed a difference of six amino acids encoded by PB2 genetic sequence including loci 132, 461, 482, 611, 647, and 701 when compared with Dobson adaptive strain, and a difference of 23 amino acids encoded when compared with Rostock adaptive strain. All these strains had the glutamic acid encoded by locus 627, which was the attribute of genes of avian viruses. Loci 362–581 of gene PB2 encoding amino acids were shown to be the key sequences essential for viral replication in mice cells, while amino acids encoded by loci 647 and 701 were found correlated to the proliferation capacity of viruses in mouse cells [12].

The structure and functions of subunit PB1 of polymerase protein. Subunit PB1 is not only the center of RNA polymerase, but also the catalytic center of the polymerase. PB1 is mainly responsible for the initiation of synthesis of mRNA and its prolongation, as well as synthesis and prolongation of vRNA and complementary RNA (cRNA). In all viruses with RNA-dependent RNA polymerases and RNA-dependent DNA polymerase, PB1 proteins all have four conservative regions and each region has a conservative amino acid. During replication and transcription of the viral genome, the phenomenon of conformational transformation may exist in the RNA polymerase. PB1 may synthesize cRNA or messenger RNA (mRNA) when it maintains the vRNA-binding conformation and may synthesize vRNA when it maintains the cRNA-binding conformation [12].

PB1 protein is essential for the replication of the influenza virus, and the amount of its expression varies greatly in different types of cells. It is mainly distributed in the endoplasmic reticulum of cells. The C-terminal of PB1 protein, consisting of three-dimensional helix bundles, can combine with PB2 protein to form a stable helix, which plays an important role in nucleotide polymerization.

PB2 protein, one of the components of trimer polymerase, has many functions. When the virus is infecting cells, PB2 determines the host specificity by shuttling between the nucleus and cytoplasm, and the amino acid at the site of 702 is the key site of this characteristic. The amino acid residue at site 627 of the PB2 subunit is closely related to the pathogenicity of the virus. D701N mutation can affect the interspecies transmission of the virus, which may be due to the destruction of the salt bridge connecting NSL of PB2 to arg753 and the change of the aggregation of three polymerase subunits. PB2 subunit can recognize the 5′ terminal of the RNA promoter of the virus and initiate specific binding, acting as an endonuclease. Then it cuts the mRNA of the host cell into the transcription primer to initiate the transcription process of the virus genome, though this conclusion needs further study [12].

PA protein regulates the stability of the protein and has the activity of the endonuclease. Meanwhile, it can also combine the cap and promoter structure, playing an important role in maintaining the structure of polymerase. In the process of transcription and replication of viral RNA, PA protein participates in viral RNA replication together with PB1 and Pb2, the two polymerase proteins. It acts as a protein kinase during the process of synthesis of viral RNA and has also the function of helicase. PA has polymerase activity and participates in the process of transcription and replication. At the initial stage of transcription, the endonuclease cuts the capped RNA primer and participates as a factor in the replication process in RNA synthesis. PA can specifically bind to the promoter of vRNA and of cRNA. PA has the function to enhance the activity of PB1 protein in binding to 5′-terminal viral RNA and strengthen PB1-RNA interaction.

The process of transcription and replication of the genome of the avian influenza virus is catalyzed by RNA polymerase of the virus itself. In cells, the assembly of the RNA polymerase complex proceeds step by step. Firstly, PB1 and PA are assembled into a dimer. Secondly, PB1-PA dimer and PB2 are respectively transported into the nucleus and assembled into the complete polymerase complexes. The trimer formed performs the function and the effects during the process of transcription and replication [12].

II. *Hemagglutinin (HA)*

HA, encoded by genetic segment 4, is in a length of 1.7 kb. It is not only the main glycoprotein over the viral surface, but also the main component of the viral envelope, playing an important role in viral adsorption and membrane penetration. Every viral particle contains about 500 HA proteins. Hemagglutinin has the immunogenicity capable of stimulating the body to produce neutralizing antibodies to neutralize the infectivity of the virus and resist viral infection and its pathogenicity. It is one of the main determinants of the virulence of the influenza virus [11]. Influenza viruses can be categorized into 18 subtypes (H1–H18), based on the difference in the antigenicity of HA.

Hemagglutinin is a type-I glycoprotein, which is one of the main components of viral capsular protrusion [14]. HA protein consists of signal peptide, cytoplasmic region, transmembrane region, and extracellular region. A mature HA molecule cannot be formed unless the translated HA is cleaved by lyase followed by glycosylation and the processing with acetylation of fatty acids. HA firstly binds to the membrane receptor, and the signal peptide breaks off to become HA0. Then HA0 is broken down by the pancreatin in the host cell into subunits HA1 and HA2, followed by linkage of them by a disulfide bond before being delivered onto Golgi Complex to complete glycosylation. Finally, after acetylation is completed in the cytoplasm, the two subunits are transported to the cellular membrane and embedded there and brought onto the viral capsule when viruses are released [13, 15].

HA, a trimer formed by three subunits, has a head-stem structure. The head is composed of subunit HA1, and the stem is composed of HA2 and partial HA1 fragments. HA may agglutinate with red blood cells of multiple animals including human being, bird, pig, and guinea pig, so it is called agglutinin and the main determinant of pathogenicity and host specificity of avian influenza virus, playing an important role in viral adsorption and membrane penetration. Cleavage by lyase, glycosylation, and acylation of fatty acids are the three main processes of post-translational processing of HA. The splitting process of HA0 is the cleavage into two subunits of HA1 and HA2 by a lysozyme in the host that functions similarly to a pancreatin. The cleavage of HA0 into HA1 and HA2 is the prerequisite of infection and very important for the infectivity and virulence of viruses. As the epitope and receptor-binding site, HA1 mediates mainly the combination between virus and receptors of host cells. As the main target of the immune system of the host, it may induce the host to produce neutralizing antibodies. The free amino terminal of HA2 can mediate the fusion of cell membrane and viral capsule, promote the entry of ribonucleoprotein complex of the virus into cells, and cause cellular viral infection [15].

III. *Neuraminidase (NA)*

Neuraminidase NA is encoded by gene fragment 6, about 1.4 kb long. Each virus particle contains about 100 Na molecules [14]. Avian influenza viruses can be categorized into 11 subtypes (N1–11) according to the different antigenicity of NA. NA is a mushroom-like tetrameric sialidase with discontinuous distribution on the surface of virus particles and capable of catalyzing the hydrolysis of sialic acid. NA is an n-glycoprotein and another important antigen on the surface of virus particles. NA can destroy the sialic acid residue at the receptor end of the influenza virus on the cell surface when the virus is infecting cells, thereby making the virus enter the cells. NA destroys cellular receptors, opens up channels for viral budding, and promotes the maturation and release of virus particles, thereby facilitating the free spread of the virus in the host. Anti-NA antibody (NI) has a protective effect on the host and the neuraminidase activity can be blocked by antibodies or specific inhibitors, so that viral replication is inhibited.

IV. *Nucleoprotein (NP)*

NP is encoded by segment 5 with the genetic sequence about 1.5 kb long. This sequence is the most conservative one with type specificity, encoding 498 amino acids [14]. Influenza virus can be divided into four serotypes (A, B, C, and D) according to the difference of nucleoprotein NP and matrix protein M, which are also important determinants of host specificity of avian influenza virus [13]. NP, a phosphorylated polypeptide in large amount, is the second most abundant in virus particles. NP is capable of forming RNP together with viral RNA and RNA polymerases PB1, PB2, and PA, and exists in two forms: one is phosphorylated form capable of entering the nucleus, and the other is non-phosphorylated one remaining in the cytoplasm. Nucleoprotein NP and matrix protein M not only form the nucleocapsid of the virus, but also stabilize viral RNA by forming viral RNP, so as to prevent it from being digested by RNA enzyme. Moreover, NP also acts as a switch controlling the transcription and replication of viral RNA. NP is an internal structural protein, which can act as the target antigen in cellular immunity. The host can induce specific cytotoxic T lymphocyte (CTL) reaction against to NP protein, and generate cross-reactions among different viral subtypes.

V. *Matrix Protein 1 (M1) and Matrix Protein 2 (M2)*

M1 and M2 are encoded by genetic segment 7 in a length of about 1 kb. Each viral particle contains about 3000 matrix proteins [14]. Segment 7 has two Open Reading Frames (ORF), encoding respectively M1 and M2, the two matrix proteins. M1 is the protein with the highest content in viral particles, accounting for 42% of the whole particles. M1 consisting of 252 amino acid residues is the main structural protein of the virus and the main component of the nucleocapsid. It has type specificity and plays a key role in the process of viral budding and assembly. M1 has type specificity and its antigenicity is the main basis for categorizing avian influenza viruses. The monoclonal antibody of M1 has no neutralizing capacity and cannot provide passive protection for animals. M2, a transmembrane ion channel protein comprising 97 amino acids, is a tetramer and one of the main protein components on the envelope of the virus. It is abundant on the surface of infected cells, but scarce in mature viral particles and on the surface of capsule, where there are only 40–63 molecules for each viral particle [15].

VI. *Non-Structural Protein 1 (NS1) and Non-Structural Protein 2 (NS2)*

NS1 and NS2 are encoded by segment 8 with a genetic sequence of about 838 bp. This segment has two reading frames, which translate respectively NS1 and NS2, the two nonstructural proteins. Both are situated mainly in the nucleus and cytoplasm, but not in viral particles [14]. NS1 is synthesized in great amount in the early stage of cell infection, and NS2 is not synthesized until the late stage. NS1 protein has the effect to block the host's antiviral activity mediated by interferon. The main function of NS2 protein is to mediate the transference of assembled RNP from the nucleus into the cytoplasm. NS2 protein not only has the function of error adjustment, but also possibly regulates the synthesis of nonstructural protein when NS2 remains in the cytoplasm. Now the functions of NS1 and NS2 have not been fully elucidated, and further researchers are needed in the future.

3.4 Virus Cultivation and Animal Models

I. *Isolation and Cultivation of Virus* [16]

Avian influenza viruses are usually isolated by two methods: cell cultivation and chicken embryo inoculation. Caution: ① Specimen can be collected from anal swab, nasal swab, pharyngeal swab and tissues/organs (such as trachea, lung, liver, heart, spleen, kidney, intestine, and brain); ② Swabs collected should be put instantly into a centrifuge tube containing PBS (pH 7.0–7.4, spiked with antibiotics) or normal saline. Feces and anal swab should firstly undergo filtration and sterilization, and the supernatant is reserved under −70 °C until usage; ③ specimen collected or treated should be stored under 2–8 °C for no more than 24 h; or be kept in a −70 °C refrigerator for a prolonged storage. Repeated freezing and thawing should be avoided (no more than 3 cycles).

Avian influenza virus can grow in primary culture cells of animals, such as human embryonic kidney, bovine kidney, chicken embryonic kidney, monkey kidney, and hamster kidney. However, the method that the most commonly used to isolate influenza virus is subculture cell lines, such as MDCK and bovine kidney cells

(Madin–Darby bovine kidney Madin–Darby bovine kidney (MDBK). Both have oncogenes, and the influenza virus isolated using either method cannot be used to manufacture human vaccines. Obvious cytopathic effect (CPE) can be observed when the influenza virus is proliferating in cells, i.e., the cells manifesting patchy networks, with the increase of intracellular granules, and rounding and detachment of cells.

Procedures for isolating virus: the MDCK cells are inoculated into a cell culture bottle or onto a plate for cultivation during 24–48 h under 35 °C in 5% CO_2, to form a single-layer of cells. When inoculating the sample, first wash it with PBS or serum-free basic cell medium (DMEM) for three times, and inoculate the sample according to 10% of the culture volume. The specimen inoculated is put in a 35 °C constant-temperature shaker under 150 rpm for 60-min incubation. The inoculum is aspirate and the cell side is rinsed twice with serum-free EMDM, added with virus culture medium, and incubated under 35 °C in 5% CO_2, with a continuous observation for 5–7 days. When CPE appears in the cells, hemagglutination test is performed to determine HA titer of influenza virus, using usually 1% blood cells of animals such as guinea pigs, chickens or horses, or human type-O blood cells. Two blind passages can be carried out if CPE does not appear after 7 days; those without the appearance of CPE and hemagglutination at the second passage is determined to be negative.

The avian influenza virus is an animal virus to which chicken embryo is susceptible, so chicken embryo culture is often used in isolation and incubation for it.

Chicken embryo culture is characterized by rich sources, simple inoculation, and easy accessibility in large quantities. However, it can be polluted easily by pathogens such as chicken leukemia virus, and antigenic variation easily takes place in the influenza virus in the case of isolation or passage. The sites the most commonly used for inoculation onto chicken embryo include the allantoic cavity, amniotic cavity, and yolk sac.

Procedures: ① Selection of chicken embryo for inoculation. Chicken embryos aged 9–11 days are chosen for amniotic inoculation through the approach of the upper part of the air chamber. Embryos aged 6–8 days are chosen for inoculation inside the yolk sac through the approach of the upper part of the air chamber. Embryos aged 10–12 days are chosen for membrane cavity inoculation through the approach of penetrating the allantoic cavity into the amniotic cavity. ② The growth of the chicken embryos is observed with an egg lighter, and a marker is used to mark important parts such as the air chamber, embryo, and large blood vessels as well as the position for inoculation. ③ Disinfect the inoculation position with 3% iodine and wipe it with 75% alcohol swab once. ④ Use a punch to drill a hole at the position of inoculation, through which 0.1 mL of liquid is inoculated using a syringe, followed by incubation for 3–7 days under 35–37 °C, with the daily observation of the growth of the chicken embryo. ⑤ Before the harvest, the embryo is kept under 4 °C overnight or under −20 °C for 2 h. The dead chicken embryos with their allantoic fluid are collected and centrifuged under 3000 rpm for 5 min to eliminate the blood cells, and then perform hemagglutination test. Different samples are collected for different inoculation sites, with allantoic fluid for allantoic fluid inoculation, amniotic fluid for amniotic cavity inoculation, and the yolk fluid and yolk membrane for the yolk sac inoculation.

II. *Animal Models*

1. *Mice* [17, 18]

Mice are the mammalian models commonly used for avian influenza virus infection, with BALB/C, ICR, and NIH mice as the common ones. BALB/C mice are sensitive to all subtypes of avian influenza virus, and the species the most frequently used. Now, seasonal influenza models such as H3N2 and H1N1 have been successfully established with BALB/C mice, as well as mice models for avian influenza viruses such as H5N1 and H7N9.

Mice are not the natural host for the avian influenza virus, but they are more susceptible to almost all influenza viruses. A variety of influenza strains in the experiment can infect mice or even cause death. Subtypes of human influenzas including H1N1 and H3N2 as well as subtypes of avian influenza virus including H5N1, H7N9, H7N9, and H9N2 may infect mice through intranasal inoculation under experimental condition. Their clinical manifestations are similar to those of the patients, such as weight loss, pneumonia, and bow back. Pathological changes observed in mice include metamorphic pneumonia, alveolar septal rupture, necrosis and exfoliation of epithelial cell, and inflammatory cell infiltration in the alveolar septum, as well as some pathological changes observed in a small number of animals including septal thickening, pulmonary edema, and proliferation of epithelial cells. In addition, some strains including subtype H5N1 avian influenza virus with high pathogenicity and 1918 Spanish influenza virus may cause high infection rate and mortality after infecting mice. Avian influenza viruses with high pathogenicity may even invade multiple organs/tissues of mice, such as lung, brain, liver, and kidney, as well as their nervous system. However, almost all influenza viruses cannot be spread horizontally among mice, so the mice are not the ideal model for investigating the transmission of influenza viruses.

The pathogenicity of the avian influenza virus in mice can be categorized into two types: high pathogenicity and low pathogenicity. The former induces a high mortality after infecting mice, with viral replication and discharge occurring in many organs throughout the body besides lungs, while the latter manifests a low mortality rate, with the replication observed only in the upper and lower respiratory tract and minor damage of extrapulmonary organs.

Mice can be used as models for animals infected with various avian influenza viruses, with the advantages of low price, clear genetic pedigree background, availability of lots of pure strains, and complete matching reagents for testing and identification. The disadvantages include its identity not being the natural host for influenza, the inability of mice model to simulate sufficiently clinical symptoms caused by influenza viruses, its manifestations of hypothermia instead of fever when infected with most of the strains, the failure of viral transmission among mice and the dependence of infectivity upon species of mice.

2. *Ferrets* [17, 18]

Ferrets, sensitive to various influenza viruses both human and avian, manifest clinical symptoms similar to those observed in human being, such as similar traits in fever, pulmonary function, morphology of respiratory tract, and categories of epithelial cells. Therefore, they are considered as the most ideal animal models for investigating the infection with influenza viruses. Among models of small animals, the ferret is the only one manifesting fever after infection. Similar to human beings, the ferret respiratory tract is distributed with α—2,6 sialic acid receptors of influenza virus, which extends from the upper respiratory tract to the lower ones, with α—2,3 sialic acid receptors mainly distributed in the bronchioles of the lower respiratory tract. These characteristics of distribution are similar to those of influenza receptors in the human respiratory tract.

Ferret, susceptible to most influenza viruses, is an ideal model for investigating infection and transmission of avian influenza virus. The clinical manifestations may occur in ferrets infected with human influenza H3N2 and H1N1 and avian influenza virus H5N1, H7N9, and H9N2 through intranasal inoculation, including symptoms of the common cold such as fever, weight loss, sneezing, and cough as well as changes in pulse and respiratory rate. Severe disease sometimes occurs in ferrets infected with highly pathogenic avian influenza viruses, even causing them death. Also, the ferret is a good model for transmission of influenza viruses, which may realize horizontal or vertical transmission for not only highly pathogenic avian influenza viruses such as H5N1 and H7N9, but also lowly pathogenic ones such as avian influenza virus H9N2, and human influenza virus subtypes of H1N1 and H3N2.

The advantages of the ferret model include its similarities in the distribution of sialic acid receptor, the clinical symptoms, and the pathological changes of the respiratory tract when compared with humans. The disadvantages are the high cost of purchasing and breeding, high requirement on the breeding environment, the lack of matching reagents and antibodies, the lack of SPF-grade individuals, and insufficient standardization for experimental ferrets.

3. *Non-Human Primates* [17, 18]

From the perspective of genetic evolution, non-human primates are the most similar creatures to human beings in physiology, pathology, and genetic sequences, and they are ideal animal models for investigating pathogens such as influenza viruses. At present, non-human primates including both Old World Monkeys (rhesus monkeys and macaques) and New World Monkeys (capuchin monkeys) have been used to study the avian influenza virus. Non-human primates are susceptible to many influenza viruses. The clinical symptoms include loss of appetite or weight loss, fever and pneumonia after the primates are infected with subtypes H1N1 or H3N2 of human influenza virus or subtypes H5N1, H7N9, or H9N2 of avian influenza virus subtypes via intranasal inoculation. Lethal infection may occur post to the infection with the subtype H5N1, the highly pathogenic avian influenza virus. Almost no influenza viruses, however, can spread horizontally among non-human primates, so they are not the ideal models for investigating the transmission of influenza viruses.

The advantages of non-human primates used as infection models include their approximation in genetic evolution, their similarity in anatomical structure, living habits, physiology, and biochemistry, their analogy in clinical symptoms, and their likeliness in pathogenesis, histopathology, and viral replication, as compared with human beings. Their disadvantages include high price, difficulties in experimental operation, the great limitations by animal ethics, clinical symptoms in correlation to viral categories, host populations and ways of attacks, and similar distribution of sialic acid receptors compared with humans.

Unlike ferrets and guinea pigs, non-human primates showed a viral adsorption pattern in vivo significantly different compared with the human respiratory tract. Viruses are not adsorbed at the trachea, bronchi, or bronchiole in non-human primates infected with influenza viruses such as H3N2 and

H5N1, which is the reason for the unobvious clinical symptoms after infection with human H3N2 viruses. The reason for the lowered susceptibility in non-human primates to seasonal viruses might be the different distribution of receptors in them compared to that in humans.

4. *Tree Shrew* [19, 20]

   Tree shrew, the close relative of primates, is the novel animal model established and developed during recent years. As for animal models for influenza viruses, ferrets and guinea pigs are sensitive but hard to obtain with high price, while the mouse model needs mouse-adaptive strains. Tree shrew shares the similar distribution of receptors of avian influenza virus, similar clinical symptoms, and similar pathological mechanism with human being. Using intranasal inoculation, Chinese and foreign researchers have established three models (A, B, and C) of tree shrews infected with influenza during recent years, which are capable of simulating effectively production of antibodies and viral discharge. Most of the infected tree shrews are complicated with symptoms of respiratory infection in mild or moderate degrees, and irregular temperature curves.

   Tree shrews as the model for influenza infection have the advantages of small body size as a small mammal with a bodyweight lower than 300 g, low cost, easy operation, easy taming and breeding, and wide distribution in South Asia, Southeast Asia, and Southern China. Compared with experimental rodents commonly used such as rats and mice, tree shrews have higher similarity with human in respect of physiological and biochemical characteristics and in biology, taxonomy, genomics, and immunology. Tree shrews have the advantage of susceptibility to multiple viruses. Due to its close relationship with human beings in taxonomic status and evolutionary degree, tree shrews are highly similar to human beings in respect of many virus-related immune factors (such as MHC, lymphocyte, cytokine, etc.), and they are potentially excellent new experimental animal models for viral infection.

5. *Guinea Pigs* [17, 18]

   Guinea pig is an ideal model for investigating transmission, and susceptible to influenza viruses, especially distant strain Hartley of guinea pig which has been applied widely to investigation on the transmission of influenza viruses. Models of guinea pigs that have been established now include subtype H1N1 of seasonal influenza, epidemic strain H1N1 of influenza virus 2009, epidemic strain H1N1 of influenza virus 1918, subtype H3N2 of seasonal influenza virus, subtype H5N1 of highly pathogenic avian influenza virus, highly pathogenic H7N9 avian influenza virus 2013, etc. The upper respiratory tract is the main place for replication of the influenza virus in guinea pigs in vivo, but the virus becomes undetectable in the lungs and nasal cavity respectively since days 5 and 8 after the infection. Although the viral titer is higher in their respiratory tract, the clinical symptoms are no so severe in guinea pigs post to infection with influenza viruses. Guinea pigs infected with seasonal influenza viruses or H1N1 influenza virus 2009 will not cause the symptoms such as fever, weight loss, cough, or sneeze. Even if the dosage inducing the infection is raised, only a few symptoms may happen after 4 days post to the infection. Horizontal transmission among guinea pigs can be achieved for the virus, including contact and aerosol transmission. Guinea pigs can be adopted as the animal model for influenza transmission, though they may vary due to differences in viral subtypes and strains. Advantages/disadvantages: no symptoms occur in guinea pigs post to infection, so they cannot be applied to the evaluation of efficacy of drugs and vaccines. Viral replication post to the infection happens in the respiratory tract of guinea pigs. None but detection on changes of antibodies and nasal lavage are needed, while sacrifice and anatomy of animals are not required in order to analyze viral content and discharge. Therefore, the model of guinea pig can be applied to not only the investigation of environmental factors influencing viral replication, but also the evaluation of resistance to drugs and transmission of epidemic strains.

6. *Birds* [17, 21]

   Birds such as chickens, ducks, and gooses are often used to investigate the pathogenesis and transmission of avian influenza viruses. For example, pneumonia and symptoms such as red strips on leg joints and reddening of the beak may occur in goose infected with avian influenza virus. Severe hemorrhage may be observed in dead goose, and low and high titer of viruses is detectable respectively in the blood and the brain. Specific Pathogen Free (SPF) chicken aged 4–10 weeks are often chosen when pathogenesis of avian influenza viruses is evaluated or vaccines are developed.

7. *Other Animal Models* [17, 18]

   Dogs and cats can also be used as animal models of influenza virus infection, though they are rarely used. Certain susceptibility can be observed in dogs and cats to multiple subtypes of influenza viruses. It has been observed in preliminary researches that seasonal H1N1 and H3N2 influenza, avian influenza virus subtypes H5N1, H6N1, and H9N2 may infect dogs, while seasonal H1N1 and avian influenza virus subtype

H9N2 may infect cats. Dogs and cats manifest similar clinical symptoms post to infection, including fever, runny nose, and occurrence of pneumonia. The influenza viruses may spread horizontally among dogs.

3.5 Pathogenicity of Viruses

The avian influenza virus is adsorbed onto respiratory epithelial cells through HA. HA is hydrolyzed under the action of protease, and the virus infects cells through merging with them. Multiple basic amino acids exist at endonuclease sites of highly pathogenic avian influenza virus and are easily hydrolyzed by proteases existing widely throughout the body, thereby having many types of cells infected. The human influenza virus and avian influenza virus differ in the receptors, with the former binding the receptor containing 2–6-sialic acid galactose, and the latter binding the receptor containing 2–3-sialic acid galactose. The upper respiratory tract is mainly distributed with glycol receptors with 2–6 connection, while the distribution of glycol receptors with 2–3 connection is observed in the lower respiratory tract and pulmonary ugh tissue. It is implied by researches in vitro that H5N1 can also infect the epithelial cells in the nasopharynx and in the upper respiratory tract, suggesting the possible presence of other binding receptors [6].

Different from infection caused by other influenza viruses, infection with subtype H1N1 of human avian influenza virus is characterized by systemic infection dominated by that in the lower respiratory tract, with pulmonary interstitial infiltration by the great amount of monocytes/macrophages and lymphocytes. The virus may disseminate further and infect monocytes/macrophages, and the macrophages and lymphocytes under the stimulation of viruses and cytokines are over activated, featuring not only enhanced phagocytic functions and the production of a large amount of pro-inflammatory factors, such as IL-1, IL-6, TNF-α, and chemokines, but also activation and proliferation of T lymphocytes releasing a great amount of IFN-γ. Meanwhile, there is selective hypofunction or scarcity of immune cells (such as NK cells and cytotoxic T cells). These "cytokine storms" do harm to tissues and organs by inducing hypoxia, lymphocytopenia, and multiple organ failure, thereby causing the death of patients.

It has been found in experimental animal models that multiple animals such as mice, monkeys, cats, and ferrets can be infected with subtype H5N1, the highly pathogenic avian influenza virus. Studies have shown that inter-human transmission of H5N1 is weak. Most of the cases identified by the World Health Organization have a history of contact with sick birds. Silent infection induced by avian influenza virus exists in the population, but its ratio remains very low. It has been proved by experiments in vitro that the high pathogenicity of H5N1 is closely related to polymerase gene PB1 and genetic sequence NS encoding the nonstructural proteins.

The latent period of avian influenza patients generally does not exceed 7 days, and the body temperature of most patients is persistently above 39 °C. It has the acute onset, with its early symptoms similar to those of common influenza, manifesting mainly fever, runny nose, nasal obstruction, cough, sore throat, headache, and general discomforts. Some patients might have conjunctivitis. A few patients might have alimentary symptoms, such as complications of nausea, stomachache, diarrhea, and watery stool. Half of the patients have the sign of pulmonary consolidation. Decreased lymphocytes and normal platelet can be observed in most patients and raised ALT in some patients. X-ray shows unilateral or bilateral pneumonia in half of patients, and pleural effusion in a few patients. Most patients with avian influenza virus have short disease course and rapid recovery, without sequela post to healing. However, the rapid deterioration may occur in a few patients especially the aged with delay in their treatment, and the disease may be fatal due to rapid progression into multiple complications including pneumonitis, acute respiratory distress, pulmonary hemorrhage, pancytopenia, renal failure, septic shock and Reye Syndrome [22]. This disease has no gender difference and may occur in populations at any age, but children are more susceptible to it.

The highly pathogenic avian influenza virus (HPAIV) can be discharged along with secretions of eyes, nose and mouth and feces, so the virus can be transmitted mechanically via any secretions and feces containing the virus, or via any object polluted by the dead poultry bodies, such as forage, drinking water, air in henhouse, furniture, equipment for feeding and management and transportation vehicles, insects and various birds carrying the virus [23]. It is generally considered that the whole human population is susceptible to the avian influenza virus, regardless of gender or age. Nevertheless, the higher incidence is observed usually in children younger than 12 years with severer diseases. High-risk populations are those in close contact with the dead poultry of unknown cause or poultry suspected to be infected with avian influenza virus [24]. Detection performed by Beare and Webster on volunteers in 1991 showed that it was hard for the avian influenza virus to replicate in the human body. Viral replication can only be seen under great amount of doses of viral infection, but it does not cause inter-human transmission. Now it has been confirmed that avian influenza virus can be transmitted through close communication with respiratory droplets. Similarly, high viral load and high inflammatory response in the host have been identified as the main lethal factors of the patients, as concluded by analysis on fatal cases [23].

3.6 Sources of Avian Influenza Virus

Under natural circumstances, influenza viruses have host specificity, and different influenza viruses can only infect hosts in a certain range. Influenza viruses can be distinguished according to the difference of their hosts, such as human, avian, swine, horse, and dog influenza viruses. The hosts of viruses, however, are not limited absolutely within a certain range, and cross-species transmission has been found for various types of influenza viruses. Up to now, the original sources of avian influenza virus infecting humans have been animals, and they are zoonoses.

From 1997 to 2018, there were a number of outbreaks of avian influenza in humans in the world, which were confirmed to be of animal origin, especially poultry and waterfowl [4, 25]. The nucleotide sequence of all eight RNA fragments of subtype H5N1 of avian influenza virus prevalent in Hong Kong China in 1997 had a homology above 99% with avian influenza virus, while its homology with any other known human influenza virus was up to 95%. H5N1 of avian influenza viruses isolated from patients, chickens, and other animals are related closely with each other, so it is probable that they have come from a common ancestor. Subtype H7N9 of avian influenza virus prevalent in Shanghai and Anhui China in 2013 had a genetic sequence originating from multiple reassortments among different subtypes of avian influenza viruses, wherein fragment HA might come from duck H7N9 influenza in Zhejiang China in 2011, NA gene might come from duck H4N9 and H11N9 influenza, while other six fragments of viral genes such as PB1, PB2, PA, NP, M, and NS came from two different subtypes of H9N2 avian influenza virus. Except for the NS gene that originated from the chicken H9N2 subtype in Jiangsu Province China, all other five genes originated from the H9N2 avian influenza virus in Shanghai [3, 26].

Multiple kinds of avian influenza viruses are preserved globally in many birds, including turkeys, chickens, ducks, wild birds, etc., and these birds are the reservoir hosts of the avian influenza virus. Based on their pathogenicity in chickens and turkeys, avian influenza viruses can be categorized into high, middle, low/nonpathogenic avian influenza viruses [6, 7]. Generally, the avian influenza virus cannot break through interspecies barrier, infect people or cause disease in human. Avian influenza virus in humans, however, cannot happen unless the virus acquires the capability to infect humans due to structural changes or gene rearrangement of genetic fragments in the process of virus replication. Now avian influenza viruses infecting humans include mainly the subtypes H5N1, H9N2, H5N6, H7N1, H7N2, H7N3, H7N4, H7N8, H7N9, and H10N8 [10, 27–29]. Birds carrying viruses are the main sources of the original infection of poultries. These birds have a virus-carrying period up to 30 days post to infection and discharge viruses via feces without any symptoms of diseases [4, 30].

According to the antigenic differences of HA and NA which encoded two surface protein genes, influenza viruses can be categorized into different subtypes. Up to now [5, 6], it has been found that HA has 18 subtypes, NA has 11 subtypes, and HA and NA may form different genetic subtypes, such as viruses H5N1 and H2N2 (https://www.cdc.gov/flu/avianflu/influenza-a-virus-subtypes.htm). Except for H17N10 and H18N11 that exist only in bats, all other subtypes of avian influenza viruses can be isolated from birds [31]. Influenza viruses prevalent in populations are mainly subtypes H1, H2, and H3, wherein H1 and H3 are mainly observed in pigs, and H3 and H7 mainly in horses [6]. Birds are the reservoir hosts of influenza viruses. Most of the influenza viruses in humans and other animals originate from birds. In most cases, genetic recombination and reassortment happen in domestic poultries and water birds in vivo. Therefore, birds have great importance in the transmission and variation of influenza viruses.

References

1. Qian H, Liu J, Huang Y. A newly found influenza – H5N1. Chem Life. 2001;21(2):134–6.
2. Gao HN, Lu HZ, Cao B, et al. Clinical findings in 111 cases of influenza A(H7N9) virus infection. N Engl J Med. 2013;368(24):2277–85.
3. Gao R, Bin Cao B, Hu Y, et al. Human infection with a novel avian-origin influenza A(H7N9) virus. N Engl J Med. 2013;368(20):1888–97.
4. Munir I, Tahir Y, Kolli R, et al. Novel genotypes of H9N2 influenza A viruses isolated from poultry in Pakistan containing NS genes similar to highly pathogenic H7N3 and H5N1 viruses. PLoS One. 2009;4(6):e5788.
5. Sarker RD, Sarker RD, Giasuddin M, et al. Serological and virological surveillance of avian influenza virus in domestic ducks of the north-east region of Bangladesh. BMC Vet Res. 2017;13(1):180.
6. Ma X'e, Yang C. Molecular biological characteristics of highly pathogenic avian influenza and its viruses. Anim Husb Feed Sci. 2006;27(1):25–7.
7. Venkatesh D, PoenAM J, Bestebroer BTM, et al. Avian influenza viruses in wild birds: virus evolution in a multihost ecosystem. J Virol. 2018;92(15):e00433–18.
8. Song K, Feng L. Overview of avian influenza in human. World J Crit Med. 2004;2:145–50.
9. Wang G, Xu S. Research progress on avian influenza in human. Clin Focus. 2004;19(13):777–9.
10. Tweed SA, Skowronski DM, David ST, et al. Human illness from avian influenza H7N3. Br Columb Emerg Infect Dis. 2004;10(12):2196–9.
11. Jin Y, Li J, Zhang L, et al. Research progress on molecular biology of avian influenza virus. Adv Anim Med. 2003;24(1):12–5.
12. Ge Y, Deng G. Research progress on polymerase of influenza virus A. Chin J Prev Vet Med. 2009;31(2):161–4.
13. Gao L. Molecular biological features of avian influenza virus and its research progress. Yunnan Anim Husb Vet. 2003;2:10–2.

14. Li L, Wei P, Wei T, et al. Molecular biological characteristics of avian influenza viruses and research progress of its detection technology. Genom Appl Biol. 2005;24(4):347–51.
15. Pasick J, Handel K, Robinson J, et al. Intersegmental recombination between the haemagglutinin and matrix genes was responsible for the emergence of a highly pathogenic H7N3 avian influenza virus in British Columbia. J Gen Virol. 2005;86(Pt 3):727–31.
16. Deng G. Complete gene cloning of isolation strain of avian influenza virus A/Chicken/Xinjiang/1/96(H14N5) and its sequence analysis. Northeast Agriculture University; 2000.
17. Yu Z, Sun W, Zhang X, et al. Animal models for influenza virus infection and their application. Inf Infect Dis. 2016;29(3):133–8.
18. Zhang C, Zhu D, Liu H. Research progress on establishment of experimental animal models for with influenza virus infection. J Guangxi Med Univ. 2011;28(5):808–11.
19. Zhou F, Li R, Yuan B, et al. Research progress of tree shrew applied to animal models for viral infectious diseases. Chin J Comp Med. 2018;6:115–20.
20. Zhou F. A research on influence by multiple cytokines on immune response to influenza virus infection in tree shrews. Kunming University of Science and Technology; 2018.
21. Wang M. A research on lentiviral-vector-mediated siRNA/shRNA in inhibiting avian influenza virus in transgenic chickens. Nangjing Agriculture University, 2008.
22. Hu Y, Lu S, Song Z, et al. Association between adverse clinical outcome in human disease caused by novel influenza A H7N9 virus and sustained viral shedding and emergence of antiviral resistance. Lancet. 2013;381(9885):2273–9.
23. Jiang K, Zhong L, Wang X, et al. Research progress on airborne transmission of influenza virus. China Poultry. 2015;37(13): 43–9.
24. Varga C, Pearl DL, Mcewen SA, et al. Incidence, distribution, seasonality, and demographic risk factors of Salmonella Enteritidis human infections in Ontario, Canada, 2007-2009. BMC Infect Dis. 2013;13:212.
25. Li C, Wan J. Source and research of influenza. Bull Biol. 2005;6:9–11.
26. Zhao J, Wang T, Yao W, et al. Research progress on novel recombinant H7N9 avian influenza. Chin J Vet Drug. 2018;52(9):64–9.
27. Koopmans M, Wilbrink B, Conyn M, et al. Transmission of H7N7 avian influenza A virus to human beings during a large outbreak in commercial poultry farms in the Netherlands. Lancet. 2004;363(9409):587–93.
28. Sun Y, Lou X, Zhang L, et al. Research progress on etiology of novel H7N9 avian influenza virus infecting human. Zhejiang J Prevent Med. 2014;26(5):481–5.
29. Baas C, Barr I, Fouchier R, et al. A comparison of rapid point-of-care tests for the detection of avian influenza A(H7N9) virus, 2013. Euro Surveill. 2013;18(21):20487.
30. Fang M. A research on subtype identification of avian influenza virus in winter ducks in Jiangsu Province and the main genetic information. Nanjing Agricultural University, 2009.
31. Campos ACA, Góes LGB, Moreira-Soto A, et al. Bat influenza A(HL18NL11) Virus in Fruit Bats, Brazil. Emerg Infect Dis. 2019;25(2):333–7.

4 Pathogenesis and Pathological Changes of Avian Influenza in Human

Yan-ling Feng, Xiao-hua Le, and Shi-pin Wu

4.1 Pathogenesis

Both human influenza virus and avian influenza virus are classified as influenza A virus of Orthomyxoviridae. Influenza A Virus is a category of the virus with envelope, a staged RNA genome, and the high affinity to mucoproteins on the cellular surface of human or some animals. Influenza viruses can be classified into four types including A, B, C, and D, based on the difference in M1 antigenicity of their nucleoprotein (NP) [1]. Mutation often occurs in Influenza Virus A due to its multiple hosts and structural features. An important antigenic variant appears every 2–3 years under population immunity pressure, inducing general susceptibility in populations to this disease and causing seasonal epidemics. Human being is the natural host of Influenza Virus B with few mutations, which may cause seasonal epidemics. Influenza Virus C infects human, dogs, and pigs, and its structure is more stable compared with Virus B and C. Antibody against Influenza Virus C becomes detectable in 80% of the population as young as 7–10 years. Influenza Virus D infects mainly pigs, oxen, etc., and human infection with it has not been reported yet. Influenza virus A has two kinds of viral proteins embedded in its lipid bilayer: hemagglutinin (HA) and neuraminidase (NA), based on which Virus A can be categorized further into various subtypes, including 18 HA subtypes (H1–H18) and 11 NA ones (N1–N11). All subtypes exist in birds, so avian influenza viruses can be understood as the repository of human influenza viruses. The main subtypes of human influenza viruses include subtypes H1, H2, and H3, while most of highly pathogenic avian influenza viruses with serious harms are subtypes H5, H7, and H9. The gene of influenza virus A has a very high mutation rate, because its RNA polymerase lacks the ability of self proof-reading. In addition to local variation within the gene, the vulnerability to genetic rearrangement due to nucleotide segmentation is also a cause for the formation of new viral subtypes when the replacement of genetic segments of influenza virus results in antigenicity conversion and antigenicity drift of main antigen genes of HA and NA, thereby leading to the lack of immunity in the population against the newly emerging strains and inducing subsequently outbreak of influenza virus [1, 2]. Studies have shown that the simultaneous infection with both the human influenza virus and avian influenza virus in pigs may cause staged gene rearrangement of the influenza virus. Subtypes of avian influenza occurring during recent years mainly include H5N1, H5N6, H9N2, H7N2, H7N3, H10N8, and H7N9, wherein H5N1 and H7N9 capable of inducing the severe diseases with high mortality are called highly pathogenic influenza in human [3]. They have been challenging human being greatly, despite their pathogenesis has not been elucidated completely.

I. *Pathogenesis of Direct Harm Caused by Avian Influenza in Human*

Coupled receptor with HA active in fusing with the target cell membrane makes viruses enter the cell. The neuraminidase of the virus destroys the neuraminic acid at the end of glycoprotein on the surface of cells infected with viruses, thereby causing hydrolysis of mucin, promoting the budding and the release of mature viral bodies, and exposing glycoprotein receptors. At this time, the influenza virus initiates the infection by utilizing its

The original version of the chapter has been revised. A correction to this chapter can be found at https://doi.org/10.1007/978-981-16-1429-3_17

Y.-l. Feng (✉)
Department of Pathology, Shanghai Public Health Clinical Center, Shanghai, China

X.-h. Le
Department of Pathology, The Third People's Hospital of Shenzhen, Shenzhen, Guangdong, China

S.-p. Wu
Department of Infectious Diseases, Shenzhen People's Hospital, The Second Clinical Medical College of Jinan University, The First Affiliated Hospital of Southern University of Science and Technology, Shenzhen, Guangdong, China

C. Qiu et al. (eds.), *Avian Influenza in Human*, https://doi.org/10.1007/978-981-16-1429-3_4

hemagglutinin (HA) to bind the surface of epithelial cells containing sialic acid receptors [4].

Despite avian influenza virus and human influenza virus share the similarity in affinity to human respiratory epithelial cells, they differ in their identifiable categories of sialic acid of receptor glycoproteins. The human influenza virus identifies α-2-6 cross-linked sialic acid, while the avian influenza virus identifies α-2-3 cross-linked sialic acid, with the former manifesting dominance in the expression in human respiratory epithelium.

Compared with the human influenza virus, the avian influenza virus (AIV) shows a significantly lower capability to replicate and transmit in human respiratory epithelium. However, receptor specificity of AIV is not the sole determinant that limits cross-species communication of AIV. It has been found by researchers that the specific receptors of all H5N1 viruses including human isolates are α-2-3 cross-linked sialic acid, but not α-2-6 cross-linked sialic acid that is identifiable by the human influenza virus. Accumulating evidences imply that AIV is breaking through species barrier and acquiring gradually the capability to infect human being. Under the joint action of antigen drift and antigen transformation, surface glycoproteins HA and NA of influenza virus will keep evolving to obtain higher activities to identify sialic acid and membrane fusion and to achieve a new balance of HA- and NA-activities, thereby having stronger infectivity and replication. The receptors of anthropophilic influenza virus exist in upper and lower respiratory tracts, mainly in bronchial epithelial tissue and type I alveolar cells, while the receptors of avian influenza virus are distributed in distal bronchiole, type II alveolar cells, and alveolar macrophages [5]. It has been found by researchers that H7N9 avian influenza virus may combine bothα-2-3 receptor and α-2-6 receptor of sialic acid, and invade into type II alveolar epithelial cells and epithelial cells in the lower respiratory tract. Virus membrane protein post to complete processing and decoration is embedded into cellular membrane, and the nucleocapsid binds tightly to the cellular membrane embedded with viral specific membrane protein, thereby releasing progeny viral particles in budding mode. Neuraminidase (NA) eliminates sialic acid between the virus and cellular membrane and sialic acid in the mucus of the respiratory tract, to facilitate the arrival of viral particles at other epithelial cells. Finally, the protease of the host hydrolyzes HA into HA1 and HA2, thus imparting infectivity to viral particles. A fusion peptide is situated at the N-terminal of the HA2 subunit and mediates the fusion between the viral envelope and lysosomal membrane. Having infected successfully a few cells, the influenza virus replicates a great deal of new progeny viral particles, which spread through the respiratory tract mucosa and infect other cells. Having proliferated in the upper respiratory tract, influenza viruses induce vacuolar degeneration and cilia loss and spread toward adjacent cells, thereby causing finally necrosis and exfoliation of the mucous epithelium of the respiratory tract, as well as failure and loss of respiratory barrier function [6, 7].

Viremia or extrapulmonary infection is observed in rare cases of seasonal influenza. Cases of avian influenza in human, with the viral load higher in the lower respiratory tract than in the upper and higher in the throat than in the nasal cavity, manifest sometimes viremia, gastrointestinal infection, extrapulmonary transmission, and occasionally, infection in the central nervous system. The virus can be detected in heart, liver, spleen, kidney, adrenal gland, muscle, and meninges, and sometimes in cerebrospinal fluid of patients with symptoms of the central nervous system. Inflammatory reactions and abnormality in pulmonary function post to infection caused by influenza viruses may last for weeks or months. Restrictive and obstructive ventilatory dysfunction can be found in researches on pulmonary function, complicated with abnormal alveolar gas exchange, decrease in diffusion capacity of carbon monoxide, and airway hyperresponsiveness [8].

II. *Mechanism of Immunopathological Injury Mediated by Avian Influenza Virus*

The invasion of the influenza virus can stimulate systemic production of interferon and the release of lymphokines by immunocompetent cells. Both H5N1 and H7N9 may induce cytokine storm effect, causing immunopathological injury in a way characterized in overproduction of inflammatory cytokines and their dysfunctions.

Firstly, the avian influenza virus enters epithelial cells in the respiratory tract and initiates systemic immune response. Secondly, macrophages under the effect of viral peptides and immune receptors activate T cells to produce proinflammatory cytokines. Meanwhile, the macrophages activated produce further chemokines and proinflammatory cytokines, and the uncontrolled strong immune response causes finally acute respiratory distress syndrome. Following cytokines have been described in researches. ① Interleukins: there is mainly the overexpression of IL-6 and IL-8, activating respectively macrophages and neutrophils to release a great deal of metabolites of proteolytic enzyme, oxygen free radical, and arachidonic acid (such as prostaglandin, leukotriene, and thromboxane A2), which induce diffusive damages of alveolar capillary wall and increased permeability, followed by pulmonary edema, cellulose exudations, and formation of the hyaline membrane. The type II alveolar epithelial cells are damaged, and alveolar surfactant decreases or disappears, causing lung collapse. These foresaid changes can cause oxygen dispersion disorder in alveoli, imbalance of ventilation/blood flow ratio, hypoxemia, and respiratory distress. IL-6 and IL-8 are called lethal cytokines [9]. ② IFN-γ. It participates in antiviral immune response if it is in normal level, while inducing the production of mononuclear factors if in high level, and harming lungs indirectly, with correlation to the severity of the damages [10]. ③ IP-10: IFN-γ-inducible protein 10 (IP-10) derives mainly from more than 30 categories of cells, such as activated fibroblasts, epithelial cells, monocytes/macrophages, endothelial cells, and T cells. Genetic expression of human IP-10 in vitro needs the stimulus by IFN, with its expression level dependent on IFN dosage and time. On the other hand, IP-10 in vitro may induce peripheral blood mononuclear cells to express IFN, while recruiting cells excreting IFN to the site of the inflammatory response in vivo, thereby making the excretion of IP-1O to be a process with continuous enhancement. Significant increase of serum IP-10 was observed in our researches in H7N9 patients in the early stage, and IP-10 was expressed in the whole lungs, which initiated the immunopathological process. However, the obvious increase of IP-10 in lungs and serum without the rise of IFN-γ suggests the rise of IP-10 in humans infected with H7N9 is not dependent upon IFN and its mechanism needs further exploration [11], ④ Chemokines MIP-1α,MIP-2, and MCP-1. These chemokines are detectable in blood and nasal lavage of patients infected with avian influenza as well as in tissues of the dead and induce chemotaxis of inflammatory factors to the inflammatory sites to cause pathological injuries of corresponding organs. ⑤ $CD8^{+}$T cells: Avian influenza virus can induce apoptosis of lymphocytes in the body, so that the RATIO of $CD4^{+}/CD8^{+}$T cells is significantly reduced, and then promote the spread of the virus, which is one of the reasons for the high pathogenicity of avian influenza virus. However, only some lymphocytes in the tissues are infiltrated. Some researches showed that the dosage of viral infection influenced obviously the effect of $CD8^{+}$T cells. $CD8^{+}$T cells had a protective effect in the case of low dosage of viral infection and correlated to severe pathological injuries and fatality in the case of high dosage. In fact, the most obvious immunopathological injuries occurred when viral load could not be effectively controlled by $CD8^{+}$T cells. This dose effect in $CD8^{+}$T cells response could also be confirmed in the experiment on adult mice. It was interesting that adult mice might control viral load effectively in the case of an infection of low-dose viruses, while the infection with a stronger strain might induce more obvious fatality and pathological injury, which was limited within pulmonary tissues but without harm to extrapulmonary tissues. ⑥ $CD4^{+}$T cells. They play an important role in eliminating avian influenza viruses, through amplifying responses of $CD8^{+}$T cells and B cells. However, the disease can be deteriorated due to the small number of $CD4^{+}$T cells and their insufficiency in antagonizing viruses post to infection of influenza viruses, and its mechanism is still in discussion [12].

III. *Mechanism of Complement-Mediated Immunopathological Injury*

Complement plays an important systemic role in vivo for immunity and physiology in humans and induces diseases or injuries in the case of its abnormal expression caused by some factors. The Institute of Microbiology and Epidemiology under the Academy of Military Medical Sciences, in cooperation with the Experimental Animal Center and Team of Basic Medical Research under this Academy, Shanghai Fudan University and German InflaRx GmbH company, carried out scientific research and discovered a new pathogenic mechanism of human infection with H7N9 avian influenza virus, that virus might cause over activation of human type I immune protein molecule-complement system, thereby inducing acute pulmonary injury. Based on this discovery, they confirmed the efficacy of a novel therapeutic strategy, the modification of molecular expression level of complements using an antibody-drug targeting at anaphylatoxin C5a, in lowering dramatically "inflammatory factor storm" and relieving significantly pathological injuries in lung tissue, thereby treating effectively severe pneumonitis induced by viral infection and providing a new approach to ameliorate the diseases of patients and saving their lives [13, 14].

4.2 Pathophysiology

Viral infection may cause damages to cellular structure and functions and induce apoptosis of cells. Meanwhile, a great amount of specific proteins from pathogenic avian influenza viruses act as the superantigen polyclone to activate the systemic immune system and keep it in a highly activated state, thereby stimulating the release of a great deal of inflammatory cytokines and causing massive destruction in normal cells and tissues of human. Statistics show that about 60–70% of human avian influenza are severe cases, which may progress clinically into Acute Lung Injury (ALI) or Acute Respiratory Distress Syndrome (ARDS), with simultaneous degenerations and necrosis observed in liver, kidneys, heart, gastrointestinal tract, and adrenal parenchymal cells, suggesting the complication of multiple organ dysfunction syndrome (MODS). Some of the patients may progress further into multiple organ failure (MOF), with an extremely high mortality.

I. *Pathophysiology of Acute Lung Injury Caused by Avian Influenza in Human*

The pathological change due to acute lung injury in patients with avian influenza is characterized by increased pulmonary capillary permeability, alveolar atrophy (micro atelectasis), interstitial and alveolar edema, and formation of hyaline membrane, which will inevitably lead to pathophysiological changes including the increase of pulmonary vascular resistance and airway resistance, imbalance of ventilation/blood flow ratio, progressive hypoxemia, and decreased lung compliance.

(I) *Change of Permeability of Lung* Capillary

Possible reasons for the change of lung capillary permeability include: ① the infection in capillary endothelium by the avian influenza virus, which may induce directly destructive injury; ② a functional increase of vascular permeability, which is mediated by inflammatory mediators such as arachidonic acid metabolites including prostaglandin, leukotriene, and thromboxane, or cytokines; ③ the increased permeability caused by the destruction of the vascular wall due to damage of capillary endothelial cells and basement membrane, which is mediated by inflammatory cells, Gram-negative bacilli endotoxin (co-infection), fibrin and its degradation products, complement, polymorphonuclear granulocyte, platelet, free fatty acid, bradykinin, proteolytic enzyme, lysosomal enzyme, high-concentration oxygen inhalation, and micro-thrombosis.

(II) *Pulmonary Interstitial Injury and Retention of Edema Fluid*

Inflammatory cells may aggravate pulmonary injuries through infiltrating pulmonary interstitium and releasing inflammatory mediators, which manifests the increase of permeability caused by capillary endothelial injury in pulmonary interstitium complicated with the increase of liquid escape but without the corresponding rise of lymphatic drainage, thereby causing liquid retention that induces interstitial and alveolar edema. In addition, after the capillary endothelial permeability increases, the interstitial edema is made severer by the lowered intravascular plasma osmotic pressure due to the increase of protein content in interstitial fluid and its approximation to the level in plasma, while the formation of edema is aggravated because of alveolar collapse and the rise of interstitial negative pressure.

(III) *Injury of Alveolar Epithelial Cells*

In case of acute pulmonary injury, inflammatory cells and mediators may result in directly structural and functional damages of type I and II alveolar epithelial cells, with the destruction of the basement membrane. Tissue fluid, protein, and inflammatory cells all can leak into alveoli, causing pulmonary edema. The functions to repair type I alveolar epithelial cells and to synthesize anti-injury factor abates or disappear, which aggravates further pulmonary edema and ventilatory dysfunction [15].

II. *Pathophysiological Changes of Respiratory Function*

(I) *Increased Ventilatory Capacity in the Early Phase*

Besides emotional stress, trauma, and pain, hypoxia is its main reason. In addition, when shock occurs, the low blood flow and insufficient perfusion of chemoreceptors in the carotid sinus and aortic arch may also induce reflex stimulation upon the respiratory center and cause hyperventilation.

(II) *The Decrease of Diffusive Function of Alveolar Capillary*

In the case of ALI or ARDS, hyperplasia of alveolar epithelium and formation of the alveolar hyaline membrane due to interstitial and alveolar edema in lungs cause disturbance of air exchange between alveoli and capillaries with the imbalance of ventilation/blood flow ratio, thereby causing severe hypoxemia.

(III) *Reduced Functional Residual Capacity*

Reasons include: ① paravascular interstitial edema reduces the normal negative pressure of the interstitium and increases the tendency of small airway collapse, thereby inducing atelectasis; ② pulmonary edema decreases the pulmonary surfactant and reduces its activity, so as to make the alveoli shrink or collapse; ③ pulmonary blood vessels are congested with increased pulmonary blood volume.

(IV) *Decrease of Lung Compliance*

Lung compliance is the change of lung volume induced by the change of unit pressure. When acute lung injury caused by avian influenza occurs in human, the decrease of functional residual capacity, congestion, and edema of pulmonary interstitium and alveolar wall and decrease of surfactant result in the decrease of pulmonary compliance, dramatic increase of oxygen demand for respiratory movement, shallow and speedy breathing with reduction of tidal volume, lowered effective alveolar ventilation, and the aggravation of hypoxia. In the late stage of pulmonary fibrosis, pulmonary fibrosis is further reduced.

III. *Pathophysiological Changes of Pulmonary Circulation*

(I) *Pulmonary Hemodynamic Changes*

The accelerated blood flow shortens the duration of the perialveolar blood flow when hypoxia occurs, compared with the normal level.

Meanwhile, the timepoint when the equilibrium of gas exchange arrives is postponed compared with the normal, because of the hyperplasia of alveolar capillary membrane.

Therefore, the venous blood flowing through the alveoli cannot be oxygenated sufficiently, and a certain amount of mixed venous blood returns to the left heart.

(II) In case of the increased intrapulmonary shunt or ARDS, sufficient oxygenation cannot be achieved for venous blood circulating in capillaries, resulting in the significant rise of venous blood (even up to 30%) mixed in arterial blood flowing back to the left heart, due to imbalance of ventilation/blood flow ratio and insufficient alveolar ventilation.

(III) *Acid-Base Imbalance*

In the early stage of severe patients, mixed alkalosis often occurs due to hyperventilation. In addition, there are factors causing alkalosis, including reduced alkali discharge capacity, insufficient blood volume, decreased glomerular filtration rate, sodium reabsorption in renal tubules impelled by the increase of aldosterone post to injury, and continuous acid discharged by kidneys. However, in the advanced stage, a great amount of metabolites produced by anaerobic metabolism in tissue enter the circulation, thereby inducing severe metabolic acidosis. Respiratory acidosis occurs in the respiratory failure in the end stage. Therefore, the rule for the acute pulmonary injury or acid-base imbalance in ARDS is characterized in conversion from the transient alkalosis either metabolic or mixed in the early stage to the mixed acidosis in the advanced stage [15].

IV. Multiple Organ Dysfunction Syndrome (MODS) Related to Avian Influenza in Human.

Generally, avian influenza in human goes through systemic inflammatory response syndrome (SIRS) and thereafter develops into MODS, and finally, multiple organ failure (MOF) occurs in severe cases.

(I) *Inducing Mechanism of MODS*

Abundant inflammatory cells and bioactive mediators exist in the lung and various organs in the body, most of which are concentrated in the microcirculation system of each organ. These inflammatory mediators are activated, in case of ALI or ARDS, causing a comprehensive microcirculation damages in lungs, and then in extrapulmonary organs, and starting to trigger the outbreak of SIRS, which damages seriously the structure and function of organs. The most important inflammatory mediators include tumor necrosis factor (TNF), interleukin (IL-1, IL-6, and IL-8), prostaglandins (PGs), platelet activating factor (PAF), and thromboxane A_2 (TXA_2). SIRS is characterized by excessive inflammatory response, i.e., the systemic inflammatory response, high dynamic circulation, and persistent metabolism caused by excessive release of multiple inflammatory mediators and their interaction. Its occurrence is a waterfall-like chain reaction that is not easily controlled, and other organs vulnerable to this damage include kidneys, liver, heart, gastrointestinal system, hematological system, and cerebral-nervous system.

(II) *Renal Failure*

Several changes may occur as follows, due to ischemia and insufficient oxygen provision caused by shock and hypovolemia.

① Sympathetic excitation: the contraction of renal afferent and efferent arterioles increases the resistance of the renal vessels, reduces the renal blood flow, and lowers glomerular filtration rate, thereby stimulating the pituitary baroreceptor to release antidiuretic hormone and to promote water reabsorption at the distal renal tubules and collecting ducts. ② Activation of renin-angiotensin-aldosterone system: The main inducement is the activation of sensilla compacta in the distal convoluted tubule, which leads to the increase of renin release and improves water reabsorption. The above compensatory changes, together with the increased endothelin release and the decreased synthesis of vasodilator substance in case of hypovolemia also lead to renal vasoconstriction. Along with the further decrease of renal blood flow, therefore, redistribution of intrarenal blood flow occurs, involving firstly renal cortex manifesting cortical ischemia, and if it is not corrected in time, the damage of renal function will aggravate gradually, and acute renal failure will occur. ③ Harms induced by toxins and inflammatory mediators: toxins and mediators act directly upon renal tubular cells, endothelial cells, and mesangial cells in case of bacterial infection and sepsis occurring secondarily in patients with avian influenza, so as to decrease the production of reduced glutathione and induce the overload of free calcium, resulting in increased production of oxygen free radical and disturbance of its elimination, which harm directly renal tubular cells and cause renal failure. Upon this secondary impact, renal function will deteriorate dramatically, and manifest change in urine volume, metabolic disorder, and other complications.

(III) *Disorders in Gastrointestinal Function*

Common gastrointestinal symptoms of avian influenza in human include nausea, vomiting, stomachache, and diarrhea. Upon overwhelming attacks such as shock or infection, patients with severe diseases may have unstable circulatory function, and selective contraction of visceral vessels occurs sometimes to guarantee blood perfusion for vital organs, which induces ischemic injury of gastrointestinal mucosa. Moreover, the xanthine oxidase system contained abundantly in gastrointestinal mucosa may induce reperfusion injury caused by the superoxide.

The central links of gastrointestinal dysfunction are disturbed intestinal mucosal barrier and bacterial translocation, which manifest: ① Impaired mechanical barrier: ischemia and shedding of intestinal mucosal epithelium occurs, which increase permeability of intestinal wall, and prolonged fasting causes atrophy of intestinal mucosa; ② Impaired chemical barrier: bacterial propagation in gastrointestinal tract is caused by reflux of intestinal juice and bile, slow peristalsis of intestines, and neutralization of gastric acid by excessive anti-acid drugs; ③ Impaired immune barrier: the potency to kill foreign pathogenic bacteria is weakened due to the decreased quantity of secretory IgA antibodies, and the biological barrier is impaired; ④ The irrational use of clinical antibiotics causes the imbalance of intestinal ecological environment, inhibition of intestinal probiotics, the proliferation of drug-resistant exogenous pathogens in large quantities, and their translocation into abdominal cavity through the intestinal mucosa, followed by their entry into the systemic circulation through mesenteric lymph nodes and portal vein. Now it is considered that impaired barrier of the gastrointestinal mucosa and bacterial translocation are important causes inducing sepsis. These actions lead to complications including toxic enteroparalysis, stress ulcer, and gastrointestinal bleeding in patients with severe avian influenza.

(IV) *Liver Dysfunction*

Damage of liver cells and disorders in energy metabolism are caused by viral infection and overactive immune response in humans infected with avian influenza. Liver dysfunction is complicated in 60–70% of patients with avian influenza, as shown by statistics, manifesting minor elevation of ALT and AST. This injury occurs most often in week 2 to 3, suggesting a low probability of direct harm by viruses.

(V) *Heart Dysfunction*

Clinical manifestations of cardiomyopathy may occur in some of the patients, including chest tightness, insidious precordial pain, palpitation, and shortness of breath. About 20–40% of the patients have bradycardia, mild and moderate elevation of myocardial enzymes CPK and LDH, and abnormal ECG, and cardiac arrest may occur in those with severe diseases. The main reason might be respiratory failure, myocardial ischemia and hypoxia and excessive release of inflammatory mediators, or the viruses harm directly myocardium in a few patients.

(VI) *Hematological Changes*

Main hematological changes in avian influenza in humans include decrease of lymphocytes and platelets, lowering of hemoglobin, and prolongation of prothrombin time, and in a few patients, the disseminated intravascular coagulation (DIC). Mechanism of hematological changes may involve many aspects including the phenomena of reactive hemophagocytic syndrome caused by extensive phagocytosis of red blood cells, white blood cells, and platelets by macrophages in various organs of the body, excessive systemic immune response, redistribution of blood components in vivo, secondary bacterial infection, sepsis, apoptosis, and medication with corticosteroids and/or antiviral drugs.

(VII) *Changes in Nervous System*

Severe hypoxia may cause cerebral edema in various degrees. In addition, some of the children or adolescent patients may manifest nausea and vomiting complicated with severe headache, followed by symptoms of the central nervous system, such as drowsiness, coma, or delirium, complicated with hepatomegaly and elevation of transaminase but without jaundice, which is called (Reye's syndrome RS). With a mortality above 50%, RS has a pathogenic mechanism involving mitochondrial damage in hepatocytes, carnitine deficiency, abnormal cytokines and chemokines, and elevated blood ammonia.

(VIII) *Disorders in Immune System*

Immune system is the important organ targeted by immune attack medicated by highly pathogenic avian influenza virus in humans. Pathological examinations reveal severe damages in immune organs including spleen and lymph nodes and in hematopoietic tissue in bone marrow, with significant decrease of immune cells including $CD4^+$ T lymphocytes, NK cells, and DC cells in peripheral blood, showing a greater drop in case of greater severity and faster progression. Meanwhile, the capability of immune cells to secrete antibodies is reduced and systemic immune is in a state of inhibition or inability, so the secondary double infection often occurs in patients with severe diseases.

(IX) *Changes in Energy Metabolism*

The main manifestation is high catabolism, showing the autophagy, which cannot be curbed generally by supplying exogenous nutrients. General consumption of both oxygen and energy at rest is higher obviously than the normal level. The utilization of sugar, lipids, and amino acids is increased, with enhanced muscular proteolysis, lifted urea nitrogen, and elevated protein metabolism. There was a negative nitrogen balance of protein metabolism in the body. Due to increased oxygen consumption, tissue oxygen uptake decreases, resulting in lactic acid accumulation, which further leads to a vicious cycle, aggravating the functional damage of major organs throughout the body [16, 17].

4.3 Pathological Changes

Highly pathogenic avian influenza in human caused by avian influenza virus is a disease manifesting mainly acute respiratory lesions. Its main pathological changes can be summarized as severe pulmonary lesions, toxic changes of immune organs and other organs, and secondary infection, as shown by literature retrieval both domestic and abroad.

I. *Lungs*

(I) *Gross Inspection*

The lung tissue is swollen with increased weight. Both lungs seem in dark red with obvious consolidation, especially in the lower lobes (Fig. 4.1). There may be slight adhesion between the lungs and the parietal pleura. Obvious congestion and edema are observed at lung sections, with spillage of light red foam-like liquid. Hyperemia is observed at mucosa the trachea and bronchi, with light red foam-like exudates inside the lumens. A small amount of light-yellow effusion can be seen in the pleural cavity.

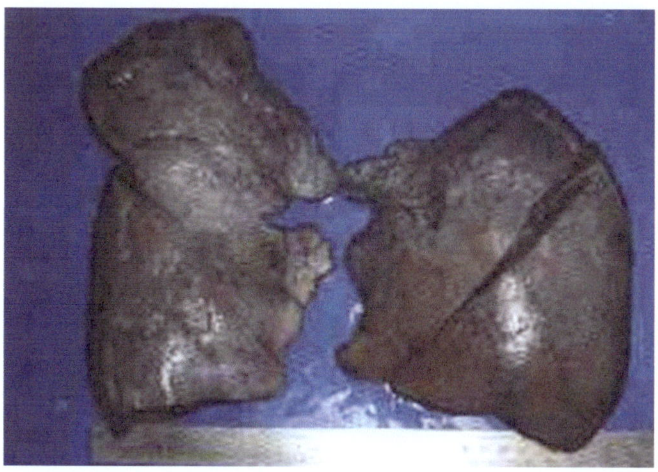

Fig. 4.1 Gross anatomy of both fixed lungs at autopsy in the patient with H5N1 avian influenza

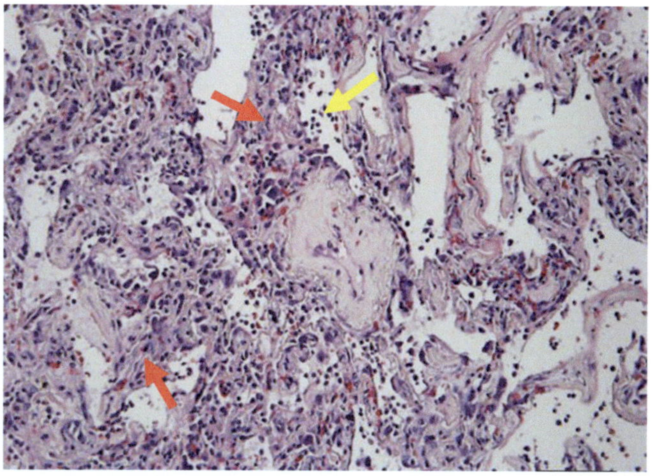

Fig. 4.2 Inflammatory cell exudation (yellow arrow) within the alveolar cavity and alveolar septal broadening (red arrows) of a patient with H7N9 avian influenza. HE×200

(II) *Microscopic Observation*

The manifestations of the lesions in the early stage are diffuse alveolar injuries in both lungs, dominated by acute diffuse exudative lesions. The alveolar cavities are filled with exudate in light red or pink and the different amount of inflammatory cells, dominantly lymphocytes, plasma cells, and macrophages, with the widened alveolar septum (Fig. 4.2). Hyperplasia of type II alveolar epithelium is observed, and the alveolar cavity shrinks (Fig. 4.3). In the alveolar cavity, there are exfoliated, degenerated and necrotic alveolar epithelial cells, together with fibrin exudates. The necrotic alveolar epithelium and fibrin concentrate to form the alveolar hyaline membrane (Fig. 4.4). Bleeding foci can be seen in some alveolar cavities or pulmonary interstitium (Fig. 4.5). Neutrophil infiltration can be observed, if it is complicated with infection (Fig. 4.6). The disease in the middle stage manifests proliferative changes; besides the lesions in the early stage, there are focal pulmonary fibrosis and consolidation. In the advanced stage, there are reactive fibroblast proliferation, fibrosis, consolidation, and organization of the exudate, and hyperplasia of type II alveolar epithelium and hyaline membrane are still observable (Figs. 4.7 and 4.8). Alveolar collapse or compensatory emphysema are observed in some cases. Transparent thrombus is found in pulmonary interstitial capillaries, with the formation of DIC. Inflammatory changes are found in the walls of bronchi and bronchioles, with mucoid inflammatory secretions observable in bronchiole cavities [14, 18].

II. *Immune Organs*

(I) *Lymph Nodes*

Decrease is observed in number of lymphocytes, which manifest sporadic distribution with

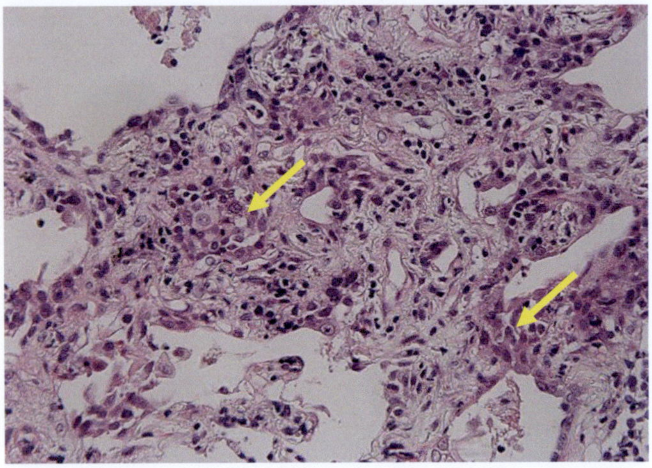

Fig. 4.3 Interstitial inflammatory cell infiltration in pulmonary tissue, alveolar type II epithelial cell hyperplasia (yellow arrow), and alveolar lumen narrowing of the patient with H7N9 avian influenza. HE×400

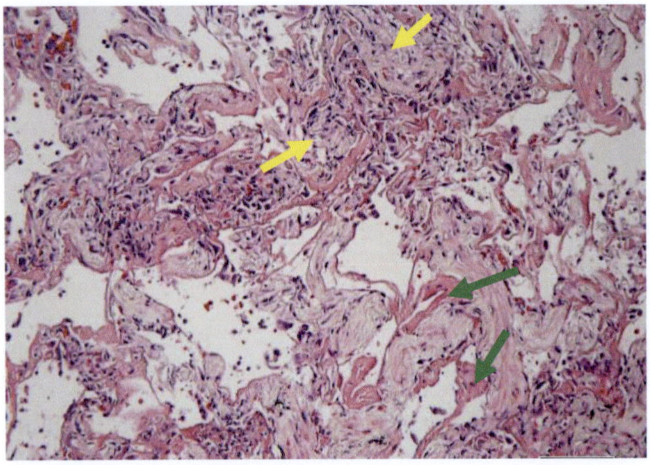

Fig. 4.4 The exudate organization (yellow arrow) in some alveolar cavities, transparent membranes formation in many fields (green arrow) of the patient with H7N9 avian influenza HE×200

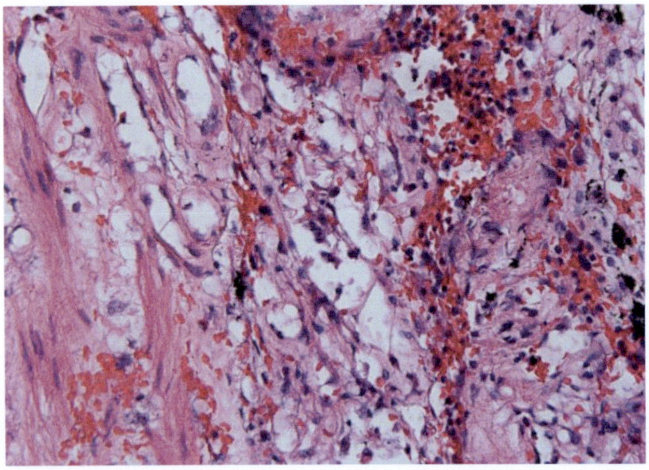

Fig. 4.5 The hemorrhage in the alveolar cavity and pulmonary interstitial tissue of the patient with H7N9 avian influenza. HE×400

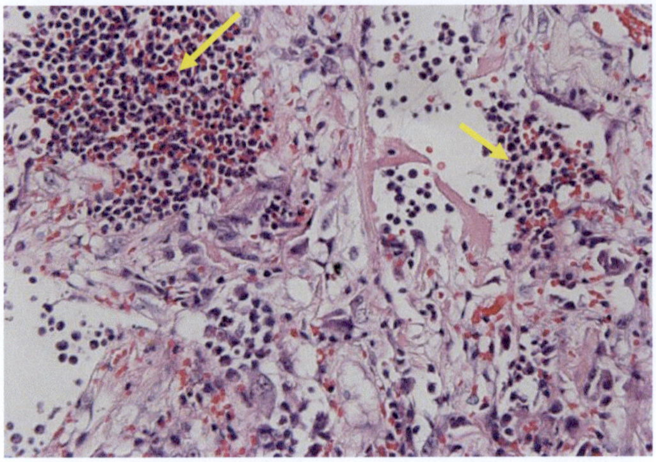

Fig. 4.6 The neutrophil infiltration in alveolar spaces and pulmonary tissues in patients with H7N9 avian influenza (yellow means neutrophils indicated) HE×200

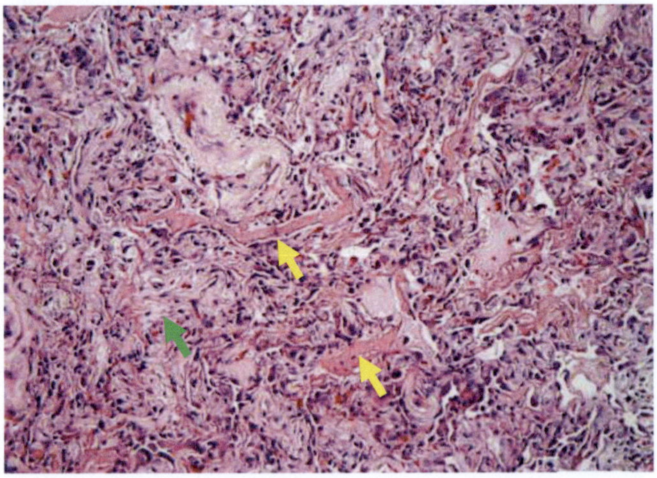

Fig. 4.7 The fibrosis of the pulmonary tissue and formation of consolidation (green arrow), the transparent membrane is visible (yellow arrow) HE×200

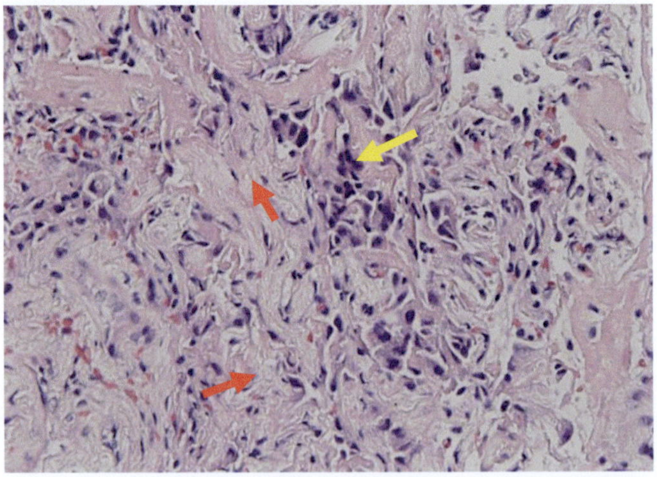

Fig. 4.8 The fibrosis of pulmonary tissue and formation of consolidation (red arrows), the transparent membrane has organized, alveolar type II epithelial hyperplasia is visible (yellow arrow) HE×400

enlarged lymphatic sinus and possibly focal necrosis. Histiocytosis can also be observed, with erythrophagocytosis and lymphocyte.

(II) Atypical lymphocytes are found at the peripheral of the white pulp of the spleen. Infiltration of small amount of inflammatory cells and histiocytosis can be found in some of the splenic sinuses, with hemophagocytosis.

(III) *Bone Marrow*

Reactive histiocytosis and hemophagocytosis can be observed in the bone marrow.

III. *Other Important Organs*

(I) *Cerebrum, Cerebellum, and Spinal Cord*

Congestion of blood vessels is observed on the surface of the brain, and the gyrus is widened slightly. The enlargement of gaps is observed between cerebrum/cerebellum and nerve cells in the spinal cord/small blood vessels, and there is congestion of blood vessels.

(II) *Heart*

Dark brown blood clots can be found in intracardiac cavities. Microscopically, vacuolar degeneration of cardiomyocytes is observed, while cardiomyocytes manifest swelling and disappearance of striations. Pyknosis appears in some of the cardiomyocytes. There is mild edema in the interstitium with congestion within blood vessels.

(III) *Liver*

The surface of the liver seems smooth in grayish red with homogeneous sections. Structure of the hepatic lobule is normal, while mild hydropic degeneration, fatty degeneration, and focal necrosis of the hepatic lobule are observable (Fig. 4.9). There is mild congestion in the interstitium, with infiltration of a little amount of lymphocytes in the partial portal area.

(IV) *Kidneys*

Kidneys are swelling, with easily peelable capsules. The boundary between cortex and medulla seems still clear, with slight congestion in the medulla. Microscopically, dilation and congestion can be observed in most of the glomerular capillaries, with renal tubular necrosis. There is renal interstitial blood stasis and thrombosis [19, 20].

IV. *Molecular Pathology*

(I) *Immunohistochemistry*

Positiveness in $CD3^{+}$T cells and $CD8^{+}$T cells is expressed in a little amount of lymphocytes in the alveolar septum and alveolar cavity in human patients with avian influenza, without expression of $CD4^{+}$T cells and $CD20^{+}$T cells (Figs. 4.10, 4.11 and 4.12). $CD68^{+}$T cells positiveness is observed for monocytes (Fig. 4.13), and neutrophils show the positiveness of $CD15^{+}$T cells and MPO. Positive expression of SPA is found in type II alveolar epithelial cells (Fig. 4.14). In addition, the expression of C4d of the complement is positive (Figs. 4.15 and 4.16).

(II) *In Situ Hybridization*

It is found by in situ hybridization that the expression of H7N9 RNA is positive in pulmonary epithelial cells and macrophages (Figs. 4.17 and 4.18). IL-6 and IP10 are expressed positively (Fig. 4.19) [14].

(III) *RT-PCR*

Influenza virus-specific RNA: it is not detectable in other tissues.

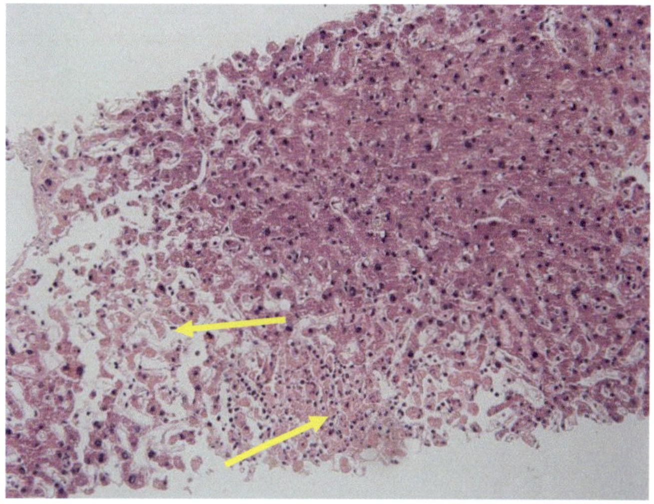

Fig. 4.9 The focal necrosis of hepatocytes with inflammatory cells infiltration (yellow arrow), with a small number of hepatocyte vesicular steatosis HE×200

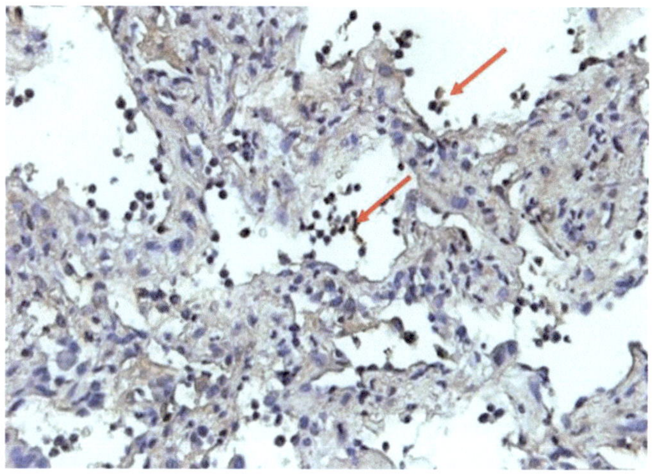

Fig. 4.10 The CD3 expression in the pulmonary tissue of patient with human infected with H7N9 avian influenza (red arrow) IHC × 200

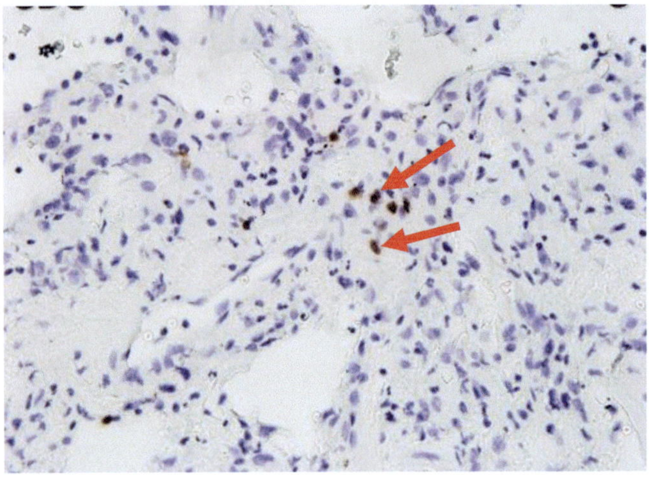

Fig. 4.11 The CD8⁺T cells expression of T lymphocytes in the pulmonary tissue of patients with human infected H7N9 avian influenza (red arrow) IHC × 400

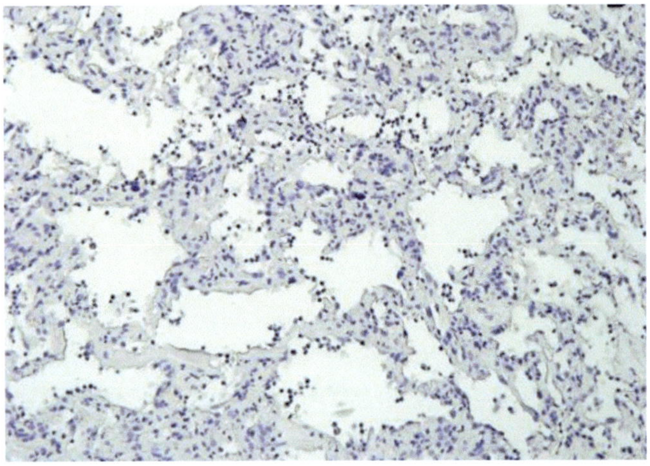

Fig. 4.12 The negative expression of CD4 T lymphocytes in the pulmonary tissue of patient with H7N9 avian influenza IHC × 100

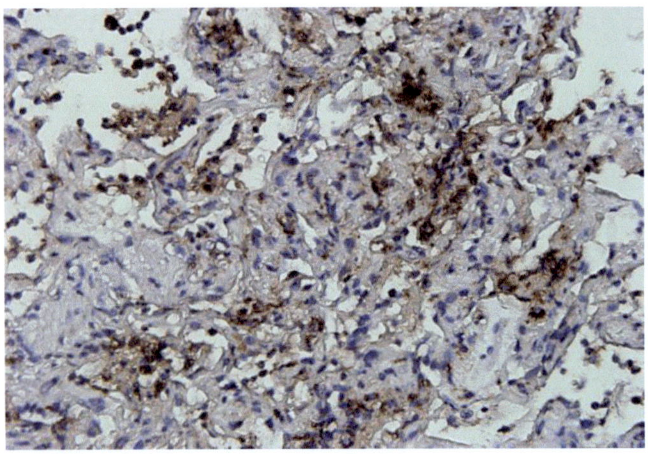

Fig. 4.13 The KP1 is expressed in macrophages in the pulmonary tissue of patients with H7N9 avian influenza, and the positive cells are brownish yellow IHC × 200

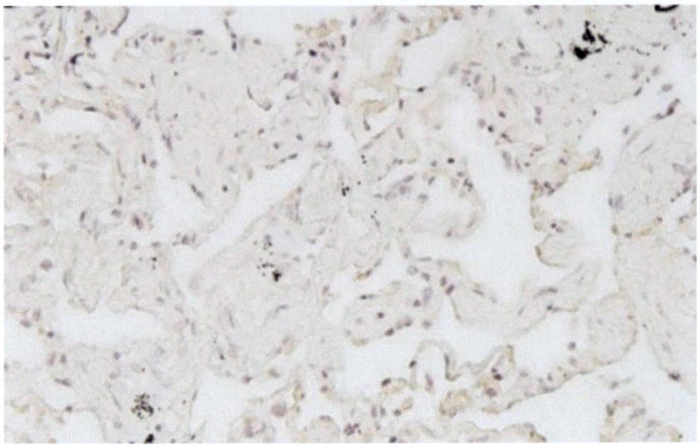

Fig. 4.14 The SPA expression in hyperplastic II type alveolar epithelium and partially transparent membrane in the pulmonary tissue of patients with avian influenza IHC × 400

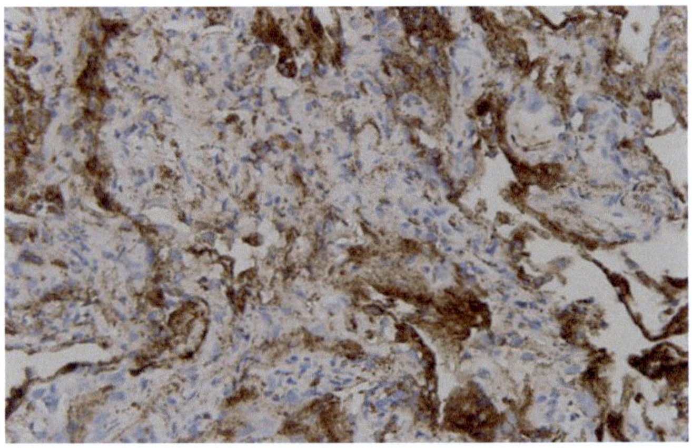

Fig. 4.15 The slightly positive expression of C4d in the pulmonary of patients infected with H7N9 avian influenza IHC × 200

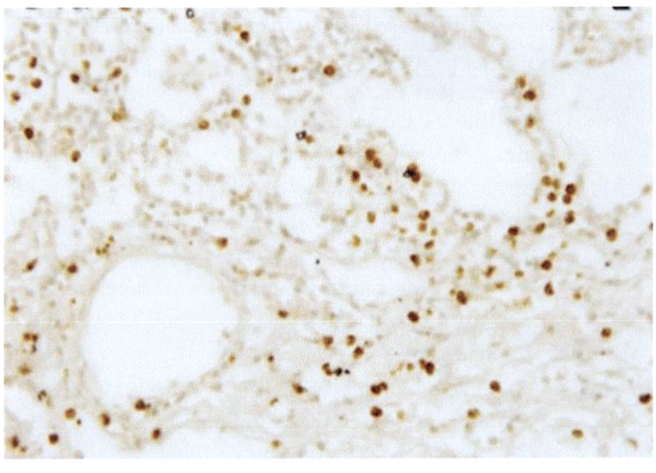

Fig. 4.16 C4d strongly positive expression in the pulmonary tissue of patients with H7N9 avian influenza IHC × 200

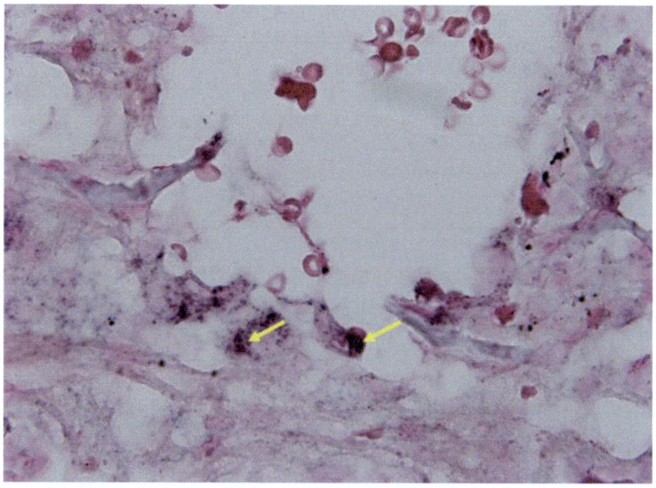

Fig. 4.17 Expression in situ of the H7N9 virus in the lungs tissue of patients with avian influenza, positive signal was blue, and the expression in the nucleus was stronger than that within the cytoplasm, in situ hybridization×400

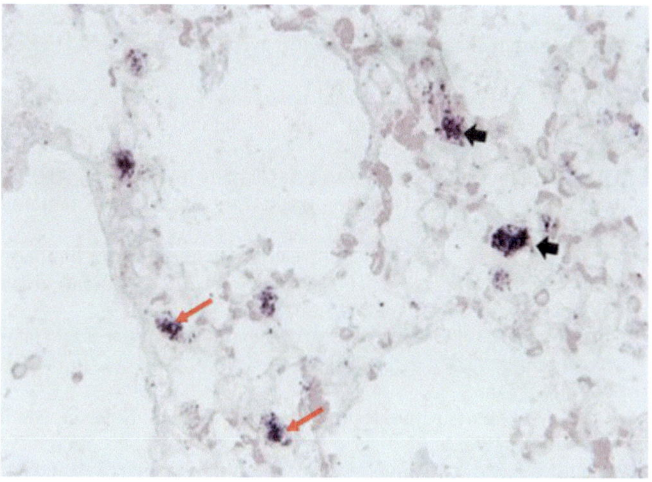

Fig. 4.18 The expression in situ of the H7N9 virus in lung tissue of patient with avian influenza, positive signal was blue, the expression of nuclear was stronger than that within the cytoplasm (as shown by red and black arrows), in situ hybridization×400

V. Differential pathological diagnosis of pulmonary lesions for avian influenza.

(I) *Contagious Severe Acute Respiratory Syndrome (SARS)*

Its pulmonary pathological change is similar to that of pneumonitis of avian influenza in humans. The difference lies in the appearance of viral inclusion bodies in cells and macrophages, which may be observed in contagious SARS but not in pneumonitis in avian influenza in humans. However, the latter disease may manifest hemophagocytosis of blood cells by histiocytes.

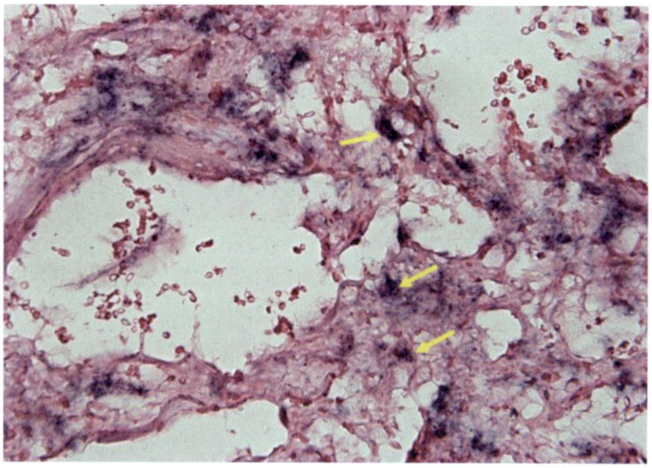

Fig. 4.19 In situ expression in pulmonary tissues in human infected with H7N9 avian influenza; positive signals are in blue, with stronger staining in nucleus than in the plasma, in situ hybridization ×400

(II) *Typical Viral Pneumonia*

It includes mainly interstitial pneumonitis, which shows mostly focal lesions. There is pulmonary interstitial congestion and edema, infiltrated with lymphocytes and monocytes. Significant widening is observed for the alveolar septum. There is exudate in bronchioles, but less exudates within alveolar cavities, which has hyaline membrane inside. Hyperplasia or formation of multinucleated giant cells can be found in bronchial and alveolar epithelium, with viral inclusion bodies observable in the epithelium and macrophages.

(III) *Rickettsial Pneumonia*

It shows diffuse lobar distribution and consolidations in various degrees in red hepatoid region, with the alveoli and bronchi containing neutrophils, monocytes, lymphocytes, and plasma cells. There is pulmonary interstitial edema. Pulmonary septum thickens because of cellular infiltration and has necrotic lesions. There is no formation of the hyaline membrane.

(IV) *Chlamydia Pneumonia*

The disease often begins at the hilum of the lung, manifesting a perivascular inflammation that expand around and causes not only lobular and interstitial pneumonitis, especially significant in the drooping parts of the lobes or segments of the lungs, but also desquamation and necrosis of bronchiole and bronchial epithelium, with exudate of inflammatory cells and edema fluid observed in alveoli, complicated with a little amount of hemorrhage. There is no formation of the hyaline membrane.

(V) *Pneumocystis Pneumonia*

There is foam-like or honeycomb exudates in the alveoli, with pulmonary interstitial infiltration by lymphocytes and plasma cells. Some of the patients manifest pulmonary epithelioid cell granuloma, focal multinucleated giant cell infiltration, obvious interstitial fibrosis, vasculitis, and severe alveolar infiltration by giant cells, together with the formation of hyaline membrane. Pneumocystis or trophozoites are detectable, using immunohistochemistry, in situ hybridization, PCR, silver hexamine staining, and PAS staining.

(VI) *Cytomegalovirus Pneumonia*

It is commonly seen in patients with immunosuppression. Microscopically, it shows inflammatory infiltration dominantly by monocytes with edema and alveolar epithelial hyperplasia. Diffuse lesions may be accompanied by spherical regions of hemorrhage and necrosis, with neutrophil infiltration. In most cases, large viral inclusion bodies are found in the infected nuclei. IHC CMV antibody can be used to detect the corresponding antigens.

(VII) *Herpes Simplex Virus Pneumonia*

The main manifestation is the change of interstitial pneumonia with mononuclear cell infiltration, alveolar epithelial hyperplasia, or necrotic branch gas Tube pneumonia. Intranuclear viral inclusion bodies are found in the cells at the edge of the necrotic zone, and multiple viral inclusions can be observed in one nucleus. Antigens against specific virus inclusion body could be detected by immunohistochemistry.

Inclusion, despite specific features for avian influenza in humans and for various pneumonias that need to differentiate, all of them do not have pathological changes based on which specific diagnosis can be established. The final diagnosis must depend upon a comprehensive analysis incorporating molecular pathology, secretion or serum etiology, RT-PCR laboratory detection, imaging, and clinical data.

References

1. Li M, Zhikai X. Medical microbiology. Beijing: People's Medical Publishing House.
2. Feng L, Yang P, Zhang T, et al. Technical guidelines for application of seasonal influenza vaccines in China (2014-2015). Chin J Epidemiol. 2014;35(12):1295–319.
3. Baigent SJ, McCauley JW. Influenza type A in humans, mammals and birds: determinants of virus virulence, host-range and interspecies transmission. BioEssays. 2003;25(7):657–71.
4. Qin C, Qin E. Pathogenesis, clinical characteristics and controlling strategy for g avian influenza in human. Chin PLA Med J. 2006;31(1):81–2.
5. Matrosovich MN, Matrosovich TY, Gray T, et al. Human and avian influenza viruses target different cell types in cultures of human airway epithelium. Pro Natl Acad Sci USA. 2004;101(13):4620–4.
6. Xu T, Dong W, Li J, et al. Researches progress in pathogenic mechanism of avian influenza in human. J Hebei North Univ. 2006;23(6):75–8.
7. Harvey R, Martin AC, Zambon M, et al. Restrictions to the adaptation of influenza A virus H5. 2004;78(1):502–7.
8. Ren G, Liu J, Jing X, et al. Epidemiological features of avian influenza in human and the controlling measures. Biotechnol Commun. 2013;24(4):568–72.
9. Lv J, Wang X. Researches progress in immunopathological injury mediated by infection with influenza virus. Progress in Biochemistry and Biophysics. 2009;36(8):961–7.
10. Zeng H, Belser JA, Goldsmith CS, et al. A(H7N9) virus results in early induction of proinflammatory cytokine responses in both human lung epithelial and endothelial cells and shows increased human adaptation compared with avian H5N1 virus. J Virol. 2015;89(8):4655–67.
11. Hui DS, Hayden FG. Editorial commentary: host and viral factors in emergent influenza virus infections. Clin Infect Dis. 2014;58(8):1104–6.
12. Wang Z, Zhu L, Nguyen THO, et al. Clonally diverse CD38^{+} HLA-DR^{+}CD8^{+} T cells persist during fatal H7N9 disease. Nat Commun. 2018,26;9(1):824.
13. Sun S, Zhao G, Liu C, et al. Treatment with anti-C5a antibody improves the outcome of H7N9 virus infection in African green monkeys. Clin Infect Dis. 2015;60(4):586–95.
14. Feng Y, Hu L, Lu S, et al. Molecular pathology analyses of two fatal human infections of avian influenza A(H7N9) virus. J Clin Pathol. 2015;68:57–63.
15. Chen W. Acute respiratory distress syndrome. Sichuan Med. 1997;18(3):180–2.
16. Chen M, Guan X. Pathophysiology of multiple organ dysfunction syndrome. Chin J Pract Gynecol Obstet. 2002;18(6):334–6.
17. Liu Z, Duan X. Clinical analysis of extrapulmonary injuries in patients with severe acute respiratory syndrome. Chin J Infect Dis. 2003;21(3):186–7.
18. Bai Y, Xu G, Gong Z, et al. Pathological analysis of autopsy of human infected with highly pathogenic avian influenza H5N1. Chin J Pathol. 2006;32:545–8.
19. Zhu L, Liu L, Zhang Y, et al. High level of neutrophil extracellular traps correlates with poor prognosis of severe influenza A infection. J Infect Dis. 2018;217(3):428–37.
20. Zhang W, Wen L, Lu M, et al. Analysis of clinical features of the first case of human infected with highly pathogenic H5N1 avian influenza in Jiangxi Province. Chin J Tuberculosis Respirat. 2006;29:300–6.

5 Laboratory Examination

Zhao-qin Zhu, Hong-zhou Lu, Yu-xin Shi, and Wan-shui Shan

What are the abnormalities in laboratory examinations for avian influenza in human? Here are the main results of laboratory examinations: ① peripheral he mo gram shows decrease or no elevation of total leukocyte count. In patients with severe diseases, a decrease of leukocytes and lymphocytes may occur, complicated with a decrease of platelets. ② Viral antigens and their genetic detection: samples from the respiratory tract are collected to detect nucleoprotein antigen of influenza A virus, M1 protein antigen, and subtype H antigen of avian influenza virus through immunofluorescence. RT-PCR can also be used to detect the gene of subtype-specific H antigen of avian influenza virus. ③ Virus isolation: avian influenza virus can be isolated from a specimen of respiratory tract of patients. ④ Serological examination: an elevation for four times or more has been found for titration of anti-AIV antibody in paired sera in recovery period than in initial period.

5.1 Determination of T Lymphocyte Subsets in Peripheral Blood

T lymphocytes, abbreviated as T cells, are lymphoid stem cells deriving mainly from bone marrow. After differentiating and developing into maturity in the thymus gland, they are distributed into systemic immune organs and tissues through lymph and blood circulation to play a role in immunity. T cells have multiple biological functions, and the immune response that they generate is cellular immunity, such as killing target cells directly, helping or inhibiting B cells' production of antibodies, responding to specific antigens and mitogens, and producing cytokines. The detection of lymphocyte subsets may help to understand whether the systemic immunity of the patient is in equilibrium. The abnormal percentage of a cellular subset suggests the possible presence of immunity disorder. Determination of peripheral T lymphocyte subsets is used mainly to know the immunity of patients with malignancy, genetic defects, severe viral infection, and autoimmune diseases.

The main changes of blood routine of human patients infected with avian influenza virus include the decrease of peripheral white blood cells and lymphocytes, and in some of the patients with severe diseases, the drop of platelets [1]. Avian influenza in humans is characterized by a decrease of peripheral leukocyte count, especially the drop of lymphocytes, as observed in laboratory examination differentiating with respect to influenza-like diseases. Moreover, the decrease of peripheral leukocytes and lymphocytes correlates to the occurrence of acute respiratory distress syndrome (ARDS) and its mortality [1–3].

Lymphocytes can be categorized into various subsets, based on the difference in surface-specific antigens, and some diseases may harm selectively certain subsets and cause an imbalance of the inter-subset ratio. The variation of absolute values and ratios of T lymphocyte subsets in patients with avian influenza has great influence upon and predictive value for the prognosis of this disease, and the dynamic change of lymphocyte count and of $CD4^+$/$CD8^+$T cells might be the prognostic index. The dynamic monitoring for peripheral T lymphocyte subsets in patients with avian influenza is helpful to study the pathogenic mechanism of highly pathogenic avian influenza virus, with great value in guiding the treatment, especially therapeutic schedule and dosage for glucocorticoids, and in prognosing the disease.

The original version of the chapter has been revised. A correction to this chapter can be found at https://doi.org/10.1007/978-981-16-1429-3_17

Z.-q. Zhu (✉)
Department of Clinical Laboratory, Shanghai Public Health Clinical Center, Shanghai, China

H.-z. Lu
Department of Infectious Disease and Immunology, Shanghai Public Health Clinical Center, Shanghai, China

Y.-x. Shi
Department of Radiology, Shanghai Public Health Clinical Center, Shanghai, China

W.-s. Shan
Department of Clinical Laboratory, The Third People's Hospital of Shenzhen, Shenzhen, Guangdong, China

C. Qiu et al. (eds.), *Avian Influenza in Human*, https://doi.org/10.1007/978-981-16-1429-3_5

5.2 Determination of Viral Antigen

I. *Immunofluorescence*

The known monoclonal specific antibody (primary antibody) is used to react with the specimen antigen, and then the anti-antibody labeled with FITC, i.e., the anti-globulin antibody (secondary antibody) is used to react with the specimen antigen to form an antigen–antibody–antiantibody complex, which shows apple green fluorescence in tissue or cells under fluorescence microscope, thereby helping determine the property and locality of the antigen, and quantify its content using quantitative technology.

1. The negative control must be the dark red cytoplasm in the whole vision, without any apple green fluorescence in the cytoplasm.
2. The positive signal is the apple green fluorescence in the cytoplasm, and the negative cells are shown as the part of the cytoplasm in dark red. The positiveness can be determined, in the case of more than three positive fluorescent signals.

Influenza virus infects mainly respiratory epithelial cells or the cells inoculated with the specimen, so the virus is contained in exfoliated cells from human respiratory tract specimens or in cells under detection that have been inoculated with specimens and have manifested cytopathic effect (CPE). The positive result illustrates that the influenza virus is contained in the patient or the culture, and can be determined directly to be the infection with influenza virus or its subtype that the experiment corresponds to. The advantage of this detection is that its specificity and sensitivity are superior to that of direct immunofluorescence assay.

II. *Colloid gold method*

The leaching liquor for the specimen in the kit is mixed with any clinical specimen to extract the viral antigen from the specimen, and the extract is dripped onto the detection membrane adsorbed with substrate solution and monoclonal antibodies against influenza virus A nucleoprotein labeled with alkaline phosphatase. The chromogenic reaction is induced under the catalysis of enzymes post to the sufficient reaction between antibodies and antigens.

This method, suitable for the rapid detection of influenza viruses A and B through the colloidal gold method, achieves qualitative determination of influenza viruses A and B in specimens including nasal aspirate, nasal swab, and throat swab. The reaction is induced according to procedures in the manual and determined in considering the purplish-red bands shown at positions C and T. Please perform the determination at the time points specified by the instruction. The detection is considered invalid if there is no purplish-red band at position C.

III. *Enzyme-linked immunosorbent assay (ELISA)*

Type H5 antibody is determined for serum specimen, using competitive inhibition. The monoclonal antibody is coated on the microplate of the kit, added with serum specimen and antigen reaction solution to form the complex of "coated monoclonal antibody–antigen–specimen antibody," and finally added with enzyme-labeled antibody. The obvious inhibition exerted by the serum specimen upon the combination between the enzyme-labeled monoclonal antibody and the antigen may suggest the presence of H5 antibody against avian influenza virus in the specimen.

1. Cutoff value: cutoff value = OD mean of negative control * 0.5;
2. Positiveness determined: it is determined to be positive if specimen OD < cutoff. Otherwise, it is negative.
   Clinical significance and precautions.
   (1) The elevation for four times or more of H5 antibody of serum in both the initial period after the onset and the recovery period may serve as diagnostic evidence.
   (2) The OD value should be ≤ 0.1 for the positive control post to balancing at room temperature for 30 min after the kit is taken out of the refrigerator.
   (3) Avian influenza virus mutates easily. Follow-up of serum test in convalescence is required for patients negative in serum test in acute stage, and a comprehensive determination is performed according to integrated clinical data.
   (4) All specimens and wastes should be treated as the source of infection.

IV. *Technology of molecular biology detection for avian influenza virus*

This technology includes mainly Quantitative Real-time PCR (RT-PCR), Reverse Transcription-Polymerase Chain Reaction (RT-PCR), Nucleic Acid Sequence-Based Amplification (NASBA), Gene Chip and LAMP Technology. Polymerase Chain Reaction (PCR), one of the methods of molecular biological detection, may detect nucleic acids of avian influenza virus in various specimens, such as blood, feces, respiratory secretions, and tissue sections. PCR can be used to amplify specific genes or DNA fragments for hundreds of thousands to millions of times within a period of only 2–3 h.

1. Real-Time PCR (RT-PCR) technology

   Real-Time PCR (RT-PCR) technology is a molecular biological detection technology frequently used in recent years. It is mainly based on a specific probe stained or labeled with the fluorescence for tracking the labeled PCR products, followed by the real-time online monitoring of reaction course, analysis on results using corresponding software, and calculation of the initial quantity of templates of the specimen under detection. This is a sensitive and rapid method capable of categorizing subtypes of avian influenza viruses, and it has been used in institutions diagnosing zoonotic diseases at corresponding levels.

2. RT-PCR technology

   RT-PCR, a molecular biological technology widely used, has a main rationale based on the direct detection of viral genes, using genetic amplification. It is a method for detecting the avian influenza virus at the genetic level, characterized by high sensitivity and high specificity. At present, there are many reports on the application of RT-PCR to the diagnosis of influenza virus, which separates out a variety of RT-PCR techniques according to details, and the common ones include RT-PCR, nested RT-PCR, and multiplex PCR.

3. Nucleic acid sequence-based amplification (NASBA)

   NASBA is a molecular biological technology specifically suitable for detecting RNA molecules. It is a rapid isothermal amplification using RNA as a template and has no cross-reactivity with phylogenetic systematics or clinically related viruses during the detection. This detection has high sensitivity, strong specificity, and easy manipulation, gaining valuable time for confirming the epidemics and taking preventive measures.

4. Gene chip

   Gene chip for avian influenza, a relatively systematic and perfect detection technology, provides a reliable technical reserve for dealing with new outbreaks of epidemic. Because influenza viruses have multiple types and subtypes, none of the diagnostic methods available now may achieve simultaneous accurate typing for all influenza viruses. Gene chip can detect thousands of genes, which provides a possible way for detecting and typing the influenza virus simultaneously. The establishment of this method not only contributes to the effective monitoring of various subtypes of avian influenza viruses but also detects accurately new mutations or new subtypes of avian influenza virus with gene rearrangement as soon as possible.

5. Loop-mediated isothermal amplification (LAMP)

   LAMP, another breakthrough of molecular detection technology, is very suitable for the detection at basic laboratory and large-scale farms. This detection is based on a nucleic acid amplification under constant temperature powered by strand replacement activity of Bst DNA, using two pairs of primers. This technology can be completed within dozens of minutes under constant temperature and does not require expensive instruments and equipment. With its results observable by naked eyes, this technology is characterized in convenience, rapidness, high sensitivity, and good specificity. During recent years, there have been literature about the successful detection of pathogens, using this technology [4–6].

5.3 Detection of Serum Antigens Against Viral Infection

The present detection methods used as diagnostic approaches include mainly detection of virus antigen/antibody, virus culture, and nucleic acid detection. Among them, the detection of virus antibody is commonly used, because of its high specificity and sensitivity, its relatively simple and mature manipulation, and more importantly, its long-term presence in vivo post to infection of multiple viruses. Virus isolation and determination, nucleic acid detection, and antigen detection are often used as auxiliary means when antibody detection cannot satisfy the requirement for the diagnosis of viral infection.

The definite diagnosis cannot be based on only the presence of an antibody or its titer in the serum of patients, due to the universality of influenza virus infection and the presence of cross-antigenicity in various degrees between variant strains in different eras of the same subtype. Serum must be collected for patients in the acute stage (3 days prior to onset) and convalescence (week 2–3 weeks post to onset) for determination under the same conditions. Only when the antibody titer in the serum of the convalescent stage is more than four times higher than that in the acute stage, can they be confirmed as influenza patients. In addition, the local epidemic strain at that moment plus the representative strain around the country is preferred when detecting the antibodies, because of the complexity of antigenic variation of the influenza virus.

The candidates for detection are the populations infected with the influenza virus. Serum antigen detection is not applicable to the early phase of the infection when antibodies have not been produced or their titer is lower than the detectable threshold. Serum methods for detecting antigens include hemagglutination inhibition test, neutralization test, complement binding test, and ELISA.

I. *Hemagglutination and hemagglutination inhibition test*

   (I) *Categories and rationale.*

   1. *Hemagglutination test.* Hemagglutinin of influenza virus may agglutinate selectively red blood cells of the certain animal(s). The phenomenon of coagulating red blood cells is called hemagglutination (HA), or direct hemagglutination reaction, and the test based on this profile is called hemagglutination test (HA). The hemagglutination by influenza virus occurs via the mutual adsorption between hemagglutinin on virus envelope and receptor glycoprotein on the surface of erythrocytes.

2. *Hemagglutination inhibition (HI)*. It is based on the addition of a specific antibody at first in a quantity sufficient to inhibit viral granules or its hemagglutinin, so as to make it impossible for surface receptors of erythrocytes to contact directly viral granules or its hemagglutinin and inhibit the hemagglutination of erythrocytes. This is called erythrocyte hemagglutination inhibition, or hemagglutination inhibition, and the test based on this profile is called the hemagglutination inhibition test.

   Procedures for hemagglutination–hemagglutination inhibition for avian influenza: these tests are applicable to the detection of antigen level in serum, and to the determination of infection status in populations not vaccinated. This is the popularized test for present global monitoring of influenzas performed by the World Health Organization and International Organization for Animal Health, featuring advantages including high cost-effectiveness, rapidness, reliability, easy manipulation, the capability to treat samples in large quantities, and to report the level of influenza virus antigens within a short period. It has become the method most commonly used among all procedures for immune antibody detection and monitoring of influenza epidemics carried out by basic veterinary laboratory at present. The test, vulnerable greatly to human operation, often yields a great deviation with poor repeatability due to nonstandard and/or unprecise operation.

(II) *Samples, reagents, consumable materials, and equipment*

1. Samples for detecting serum antibody against virus infection
   (1) Standard positive serum and strains of influenza virus
   (2) Isolated cultures (specimen)
   (3) Standard serum
   (4) Strains of all subtypes of avian influenza available for identification
2. Reagent consumables for routine identification
   (1) At least three antibodies of representative strains for influenza type A1, A3, and B.
   (2) Receptor destroying enzyme (RDE)
   (3) Suspension of erythrocytes (Preparation procedures: (a) Blood is sampled from the vein or heart of a normal healthy chicken, or from the heart of a guinea pig, kept in the Alsever's liquid and preserved under 4 °C. (b) Before usage, the sample is rinsed three times with normal saline, and the last rinsing is followed by a centrifuge of 2000 rpm for 10 min. (c) The erythrocytes are prepared into a suspension of concentration of 1% (chicken) or 1.5% (guinea pig).
   (4) PBS or normal saline
   (5) 96-well micro hemagglutination plate (V-shape plate for chicken blood cells, and U-shape plate for guinea pig).
3. Adjustable multi-channel or single-channel pipettes and their tips (Table 5.1).

Table 5.1 List of representative strains of various subtypes of avian influenza viruses

Type of influenza viruses	Representative strains
H1a	A/PR/8/34(H1N1)
H1b	A/FM/1/47(H1N2)
H1c	A/swine/IA/30(H1N1)
H2a	A/Japan/305/57(H2N2)
H3a	A/Hong Kong/1/68(H3N2)
H3b	A/equine/Miami/63(H3N8)
H3c	A/duck/Ukraine/63(H3N8)
H4	A/duck/Czech/56(H4N6)
H5	A/tern/So.Af/61(H5N3)
H6a	A/turkey/MA/65(H6N2)
H7a	A/equine/Prague/56(H7N7)
H7b	A/FPV/Rostock/34(H7N1)
H8	A/turkey/Ont./6118/68(H8N4)
H9	A/turkey/WI/66(H9N2)
H10	A/chicken/N/Germany/49(H10N8)
H11a	A/duck/England/56(H11N6)
H11b	A/duck/Memphis/546/74(H11N9)
H12	A/duck/Alberta/60/76(H12N5)
H13	A/gull/MD/707/77(H13N6)
H14	A/mallard/Ast./263/82(H14N5)
H15	A/sheatwater/W.Aus/79(H15N9)

(III) *Operational procedures*

1. Preparation

   Turn on the biosafety cabinet in advance, and confirm the presence of negative pressure in the cabinet and the normal operation of the directional airflow. Preparation of waste containers and disinfectants. Preparation of disposable disinfection paper pad containing 75% ethanol, which is spread onto the top of the cabinet. Experimental materials and samples to be used inside the cabinet are disinfected with 75% ethanol before being put into the cabinet.
2. Hemagglutination test (HA)

   A 96-well micro hemagglutination plate is added with normal saline with 0.9 mL in well 1, and 0.5 mL in each of the rest wells. 0.1 mL of separated culture or sample suspension is added into the well 1 (i.e., a 1:10 dilution), from which 0.5 mL of suspension mixed even is pipetted to well 2, from which 0.5 mL of suspension mixed

Table 5.2 Criteria for interpretation of hemagglutination test results

Phenomenon	Results
Thin layers of red blood cells in the form of fine sand or thin film are evenly tiled on the well bottom of the hemagglutination plate, which is considered to be 100% agglutination of erythrocytes	4+
Though erythrocytes are tiled on the well bottom in the form of fine sand, the edge seems irregular with a sinking trend, which is considered to be 75% agglutination of erythrocytes	3+
The erythrocytes form a ring on the well bottom with small agglutination blocks at the periphery, which is considered to be 50% agglutination of erythrocytes	2+
The punctiform sediment of erythrocytes is observed on the well bottom, with an unsmooth edge and small agglutination blocks at the periphery, which is considered to be 25% agglutination of erythrocytes	1+
The punctiform of erythrocytes is observed on the well bottom, with a smooth and tidy edge, without agglutination of erythrocytes	—

Note: the appearance of 2+ is adopted as the endpoint for agglutination titer, i.e., the 2+ agglutination among the viral solutions with the highest dilution times is considered to have one unit of viral agglutination unit

even is pipetted to well 3, followed by the same operation of double dilutions until well 8, from which 0.5 mL of suspension mixed even is discarded. In this way, the liquid volume in each well is 0.5 mL, with the dilution of 1:2, 1:4, 1:8… 1:256, respectively, from well 1 to 8, and well 9 is the control of normal saline. After dilution, 0.5 mL of erythrocyte suspension is added into each well in the sequence from well 9 to 1, vibrated gently and kept at ambient temperature for 30 min (for chicken blood) or 60 min (for blood of guinea pig). The samples should be handled gently to avoid vibration when the results are observed, and hemagglutination in each well is expressed with 4+, 3+, 2+, and 1+, with the dilution of viral suspension showing 2+ taken as the hemagglutination titer (Table 5.2).

3. Hemagglutination inhibition (HI)

Qualitative test: four wells are chosen from the agglutination plate, labeled, and added with corresponding reagents in turn, wherein 0.25 mL of viral solution contains four agglutination units. Contents in each well are mixed evenly and kept standing at ambient temperature for 45 min. The result is observed after the completion of sedimentation of erythrocytes. The hemagglutination inhibition test is determined to be negative for any obvious agglutination, while any test well without hemagglutination is expressed as positiveness, illustrating the type and subtype of virus are identical with those of the diagnostic serum in the well.

Quantitative test: serum from the patient is pre-treated firstly with cholera filtrate to eliminate nonspecific inhibitor in human serum. The procedures are as follows: one part of serum is added with four parts (or in an equal amount of) vibrio cholerae filtrate, kept in a water bath under 37 °C overnight, taken out on the next day, and heated under 56 °C for 30 min, and then the experiment is carried out. Now the serum is 1:5 diluted. Ten wells are chosen from a 96-well agglutination well and spiked, with well 1 to well spiked with 0.25 mL of normal saline for each and well 10 with 0.5 ml. 0.25 mL of pretreated serum of patient post to 1:5 dilution is added into well 1 for a 1:10 dilution, blown for three times and mixed even, and 0.25 mL is pipetted to well 2, followed by the same operation of double dilutions until well 7, from which 0.25 mL of suspension mixed even is discarded. Well 8 is the serum control, which is added with 0.25 mL of 1:5 diluted serum; well 9 is the virus control and well 10 is erythrocyte control, neither of which is added with serum. For wells 1 to 7 and well 9, each is spiked with 0.25 mL of viral suspension containing 4 agglutination units, while there is no spiking of viral suspension to well 8 (serum control) or well 10 (erythrocyte control). 0.5 mL of erythrocytes is added to each well, mixed even, kept under ambient temperature, and observed respectively at minute 30 and 45, and the result at the latter timepoint prevails (the result at minute 30 is referenced, if sliding of erythrocytes is observed).

II. *Complement fixation test (CFT)*

As early as 1906, the complement fixation test (CFT) was applied by Wassermann to procedures for diagnosing syphilis, i.e., the famous Wassermann reaction. With continuous improvement, this traditional test has been applied to detection and analysis for autoantibodies, tumor-associated antigens, and HLA, besides diagnosis of contagious diseases and investigation on epidemics.

1. Types and rationale

Autoimmune hemolysis. If complement participates, it will go through a series of activation to form finally the membrane attack complex (MAC). MAC may attack the membrane of erythrocytes and make the rupture of them, which is called intravascular hemolysis. In the immune hemolysis without complement, however, the antibody combining the antigen over the membrane of erythrocytes does not destroy erythrocytes but sensitize them. The sensitized RBC will be swallowed by phagocytes when passing through a reticuloendothelial system such as the spleen, which is called extravascular hemolysis.

Five components that participate in the reaction can be categorized into three systems: ① reaction system, i.e., known antigen (or antibody) and antibody (or antigen) under test; ② complement system; ③ indicator system, i.e., SRBC and corresponding hemolysin, which are often combined together in advance to sensitize red blood cells. The reaction system competes with the indicator system for the complement system, and the reaction system is prioritized by being added firstly to get a chance of combining complement. If the antibody (or antigen) under test exists in the reaction system, the antigen and antibody post to reaction may combine complement. When the indicator system is added, it is considered positive in the complement binding test due to the absence of hemolysis because there is no free complement anymore in the reaction system. If the antibody (or antigen) under test does not exist in the reaction system, there is still a free complement in the liquid. A negative complement binding test can be concluded if hemolysis occurs when the indicator system is added. Therefore, the complement binding test can be used to detect the corresponding antibody based on the known antigen or detect the corresponding antigen based on the known antibody.

2. Test method

Test methods frequently used include the total quantity method (3 mL), semi-quantity method (1.5 mL), small-quantity method (0.6 mL), and micro-quantity method (plastic plate method). Now antigens can be economized with the small-quantity method and micro-quantity method, with relative low consumption of serum samples, good specificity, and wide application. We will make a description based on the small-quantity method as follows (i.e., antigen, antibody, hemolysin, and sheep erythrocytes are spiked with 0.1 mL for each, and 0.2 mL of complement is spiked to yield a total volume of 0.6 mL).

Antigen applied to antibody determination should be purified properly, with higher purity and stronger specificity. If crude antigen is used, a normal tissue post to the same treatment must be used as the antigen control to identify nonspecific reaction possibly existing in serum under test against components in normal tissue. In the test of antigen–antibody titration and complement binding, a proper concentration ratio for antigen and antibody should be chosen through tests. The square matrix method is often used for titration, and the highest dilution (100% non-hemolysis) for the strong positiveness in both antigen and antibody is adopted as the titer for antigen and antibody (univalence).

Antigen with various dilutions is added into a tube and spiked with antiserum with different dilutions. In addition, an antigen control tube not spiked with antigen and an antigen control tube not spiked with antiserum are provided. Complement and indicating system are added according to the test method, and results are observed after incubation. Either 1:64 antigen or 1:32 antigen is adopted as one unit. In the formal test, 2–4 units are generally adopted for the antigen (1:64–1:32) and 4 units for the antibody (1:8).

III. *Neutralization test*

Neutralization test is based on the loss of pathogenicity to susceptible animal post to the combination between virus or toxin to corresponding antibodies. The test is mainly applied to: ① detection of antibodies from serum under test, or detection of viruses from the specimen, so as to diagnose viral contagious diseases; ② identification of toxin of specimen or categories of toxins of bacteria, using toxin in the antitoxin serum specimen; ③ determination of titers of antiviral serum or antitoxin; ④ identification and typing of newly isolated viruses, wherein the neutralization test can be carried out in not only susceptible test animals, but also cell cultures or chicken embryos. This test is a classical method for serum test, featuring not only good specificity and sensitivity but also the capability to determine the content of neutralization antibodies in animals in vivo. Given its tedious and time-consuming operation, however, laboratory manipulation with a higher biosafety level is required in case of a contagious virus, which makes it almost impossible of its application to clinical rapid diagnosis. The test methods include mainly simple qualitative test, viral dilution based on serum, serum dilution based on virus, and plaque reduction.

1. Simple qualitative neutralization test

This test is applied to not only the detection of viruses in a sample but also preliminary identification or typing of viruses. Firstly, test animals (or chicken culture or cell culture) with the inoculation route are chosen based on the susceptibility of viruses. Then the sample is diluted into a certain concentration (about 100LD50-1000LD50 or TCID50). Polluted sample should be added with antibiotics (penicillin 200–1000 units and streptomycin 200–1000 units) or filtrated with a bacterial filter, and mixed with equal volume of known antiserum (diluted properly or non-diluted), with the normal serum spiked with diluted sample as the control. The mixture is kept standing for 1 h under 37 °C and inoculated onto test animals respectively with three animals in each group. The animals are bred separately and observed for onset of disease and deaths. The death in the control without any death in the neutralization group proves the presence of viruses related to the antiserum in the forage. This method is also applicable to the identification and typing of toxins (such as botulin).

2. Viral dilution based on serum

In this method, the virus is often diluted by 10 times and divided into two rows of test tubes. The first row of tubes is added with normal serum (the control), and the second row is added with serum under test (test group). The mixture is kept standing under 37 °C for 1 h. The mixtures of various tubes are inoculated respectively to chosen animals, with 3–5 animals for each dilution, followed by daily observation with the number of deaths recorded. LD_{50} and neutralization index are calculated at the end of the observation. Applicable to a detection for a large sample is often used to detect the neutralization antibody in the serum under test. For virus, the result is usually defined as positiveness for a neutralization index larger than 50, the suspected for the index between10–49 and negativeness for an index lower than 10.

3. Serum dilution based on virus

This method is used to determine the neutralization titer of antiviral serum. The serum under test is diluted two times, added with the equivalent volume of virus solution with known titer (each dosage for inoculation post to mixing with serum contains $100LD_{50}$ virus). The serum is vibrated even, kept under 37 °C for 1 h, and inoculated to the animals.

4. Plaque Reduction Test

Plague reduction test is often adopted during recent years for viral neutralization based on cellular cultures. Firstly, the virus is diluted into a proper concentration (80–100 plaque forming units (PFU) in 0.2 ml) and mixed with an equal volume of serum under test with various dilutions for a reaction for 1–2 h under 37 °C, followed by detection of PFU. The dilution of a serum that achieves a 50% reduction of the plagues is defined as the neutralization titer of this serum.

5.4 Molecular Biological Detection of Viral Nucleic Acids

Along with the continuous development of immune technology and detection methods, molecular biological technology represented by nucleic acid detection has achieved great progress and won wide recognition. It has become the preferred diagnostic method for diagnosing clinically infectious pathogens, due to its advantages including high sensitivity, low missing rate, and the capability to shorten the detection window and monitor viral mutations. In the respect of viral researches, researches on structure and function, replication and expression, and mutual effects between the virus and the host can be realized, using detection technology in molecular biology, thereby laying the foundation for researches on pathogenic mechanism of virus, development of vaccines and development of antiviral drugs.

Detection methods used frequently in clinical practice is the detection of nucleic acids and of proteins. Common methods include nucleic acid hybridization, reverse transcription, polymerase chain reaction, multiple reverse transcription-polymerase chain reaction, enzyme-linked immunosorbent PCR, real-time quantitative PCR, dependent nucleic acid sequence amplification, fluorescent PCR, etc. In recent years, detection and typing of influenza viruses with gene chip is one of the hotspots of the researches, capable of detecting multiple viruses simultaneously, and especially applicable to features of influenza viruses, such as multiple subtypes and vulnerability to mutation. There is a high requirement, however, on experimental conditions by this method. The general advantages of nucleic acid detection include fast detection, high specificity, and easy operation.

I. Detection of nucleic acids, playing a role more and more important in monitoring and diagnosing viral infection in clinical laboratory, as well as prediction of efficacy and prognosis, is the main developing direction in laboratory diagnosis in future. Viral detection can be categorized into two types: the qualitative and the quantitative.

(I) *Qualitative detection*

1. In situ hybridization: an enzyme or a luminescent substrate is used as the labeled probe, and in situ hybridization (ISH) is used to detect directly viral nucleic acid in the samples. It is rarely used however, because it lacks the segment of PCR amplification and its sensitivity is lower than that of PCR.
2. Polymerase chain reaction (PCR): PCR is based on the rationale that denaturation and disentangling may occur in DNA under high temperature, followed by renaturation into double chains when the temperature drops. Its specificity depends upon oligonucleotide primers complementary to both ends of the target sequence. PCR is a molecular biological technology for amplifying specific DNA segments and regarded as a specific biological DNA replication in vitro. The most significant feature of PCR is its capability to amplify greatly the trace amount of DNA. It has been widely used in clinical practice because of its advantages of high specificity, sensitivity, rapidness, and accuracy.
3. Reverse transcription-polymerase chain reaction (RT-PCR): RT-PCR is realized through the application of RNA reverse transcriptase, i.e., viral RNA undergoes reverse transcription into DNA, followed by PCR. It has one more step, the reverse transcription, compared with PCR, and is applied mainly to clinical detection of RNA viruses, besides the test of genetic expression and transcriptional level.

(II) *Quantitative detection*

1. Real-time PCR: it is a technology using the fluorescent signals emitted from the fluorescent probe or fluorescent dye as the parameter during amplification reaction of nucleic acids, based on which the total amount of products post to circulation is calculated. Besides the detection of viral load, it can be used also to monitor viral variation. In addition, it is a common method to evaluate disease course, efficacy of treatment and prognosis. It shows excellent performances in sensitivity, specificity, and repeatability.
2. bDNA: signal amplification of branched DNA (bDNA) is a technology of signal amplification of nucleic acid hybridization nondependent upon PCR amplification. There is no need for extraction and purification of RNA, reverse transcription, or PCR amplification. The results of gene quantification can be obtained as soon as probe hybridization and signal amplification are performed for the sample split by a specific lysate. It has advantages including high sensitivity, wide detection range, accurate quantification, the applicability to the detection of the expression level of genes in the host cell that interact with viruses, besides the test on viral nucleic acids, and the great prospection of its application.
3. NASBA: Nuclear acid sequence-based amplification (NASBA) is a detection capable of performing isothermal nucleic acid amplification with RNA templates and realizing real-time observation of results. Based on amplification of nucleic acid sequence, this technology is an isothermal amplification with a single-strand RNA as the template mediated by a pair of specific primers and catalyzed by three enzymes. Characterized in advantages including simple operation, good specificity, high sensitivity, and resistance to pollution, this technology has been applied widely to the detection of viruses, bacteria, molds, parasites, and cytokines, especially the detection of RNA viruses such as HIV and HCV.
4. TMA: Transcription-mediated amplification (TMA) is a system for amplifying RNA or DNA under an isothermal reactive condition under about 42 °C, using RNA polymerase and reverse transcriptase. The technical principle is roughly the same as NASBA, except for the difference of MMLV reverse transcriptase and T7 RNA polymerase, the two enzymes utilized by TMA. MMLV reverse transcriptase with both reverse transcriptase activity and RNase H activity is a sensitive amplification technology of nucleic acids, characterized in handy operation, suitability for high throughput screening and applicability to rapid test of bacteria and viruses as well as allelic typing of human leukocyte antigens.
5. LCR: Linkase enzymatic chain-promoting reaction (LCR) is a probe amplification based on a target molecule-dependent mutual linkage of oligonucleotide probes, with its amplification proficiency equivalent to that of PCR, and a high sensitivity because of its very high signal–noise ratio. This technology may amplify and detect DNA mutation, and has a good application prospect.
6. Gene chip: It is also called DNA chips or DNA microarray. Its principle is to use methods such as photoconductive in situ synthesis or microprinting to fix intensively and orderly a great amount of probe molecules with specific sequences onto carriers such as silicon slide, glass slide, and nitrocellulose membrane treated correspondingly, to which samples labeled are spiked to undergo multiple hybridization, followed by the analysis of presence/absence of the targeted molecule with its quantity and sequences based on the evaluation of intensity and distribution of hybridized signals, so as to obtain genetic information of sample under test. It has greater and greater application prospects in the respect of analysis of genetic expression, discovery of new genes, and diagnosis of diseases.

5.5 Isolation and Identification of Viruses

I. *Procedures for isolation and operation in chicken embryo culture of viruses*

(I) Experimental rationale for chicken embryo culture. It is one of the common methods for viral cultivation, with simplicity in both operation and management. It is sensitive to respiratory viruses, such as myxovirus, paramyxovirus, poxvirus, and herpesvirus, and applicable to the isolation of these viruses from samples from patients. Methods commonly used for influenza viruses are double-chamber inoculation in the allantoic cavity and amniotic cavity of chicken embryo.

(II) Experimental procedures and determination of results. Avian influenza viruses infecting humans such as H7N9 and H5N1 should be isolated in a biosafety cabinet in a laboratory with the safety level III (BSL-3). The operator who enters the laboratory with safety level III must conform to requirements on individual protection for the biosafety laboratory and biosafety regulations, and implement strictly the standard operating procedures and waste management regulations.

(III) Clinical significance. The death of chicken embryo occurring after 24 h or positiveness in HA test is considered as the presence of viral infection, and an identification should be performed further, using laboratory tests such as complement fixation (CF), immunofluorescence (IF), Enzyme-linked immunosorbent assay (ELISA), HI (hemagglutination inhibition test), and neutralization test (NT) of virus.

(IV) Caution: ① Viral isolate must not be preserved at −20 °C, because influenza virus will be extremely unstable under this temperature. ② Isolation of influenza viruses should conform strictly to biosafety regulations. ③ The unknown clinical sample and the known clinical sample must not be handled simultaneously in the same laboratory; samples obtained from different animals must not be handled simultaneously in the same laboratory; animal samples (such as those from hogs or birds) must be preserved separately with those from human beings.

II. *Procedures for viral cultivation in cells and isolation*

(I) *Apparatus, reagent, and materials*

1. Sample: 0.5 mL of pleural effusion or respiratory secretion.
2. Culture medium: TPCK-treated trypsin (type VIII from bovine pancreas); HEPES buffer solution, and 1 M stock solution; D-MEM medium (high-glucose; containing L-glutamine), and Hank's solution; the stock solution of penicillin G (10,000 IU/mL) and streptomycin (10,000 μg/mL) streptomycin sulfate; component V of bovine serum albumin, and 7.5% solution; 7.5% $NaHCO_3$ (it is unnecessary for most of the commercially available medias for they have been adjusted to the neutral with buffer solution, though it is still needed by some media, which depends on the specific situation. If it is needed, the final concentration obtained should be 1%). Preparation of cell maintenance solution: 500 mL of D-MEM solution is added with 5 mL of stock solution of penicillin and streptomycin (final solution: 100 U/mL for penicillin and 100 g/mL for streptomycin), 12.5 mL of component V of bovine serum albumin (final concentration: 0.2%) and 12.5 mL of HEPES buffer (final concentration: 25 mM). Preparation of virus growth medium: 0.5 mL of TPCK-trypsin is added into every 500 mL of cell maintenance solution (the concentration of the stock solution: 2 mg/mL) to obtain the final concentration of TPCK-trypsin of 2 μg/mL.
3. Cell: dog kidney cells (MDCK)
4. Apparatus and consumables: grade-II biosafety cabinet; high-speed centrifuge; carbon dioxide incubator; inverted biological microscope; disposable plate, cell culture bottles, pipettes, tips with filter element, centrifuge tubes with 1.5-mL screw, culture plates (6-hole and 24-hole plates), disposable filters, and syringes.

(II) *Operational procedures*

1. Treatment of samples

Proper preliminary treatment is required for the sample before it undergoes isolation of viruses.

(1) Nasal/pharyngeal swab sample: ① uncover the tube containing nasal/pharyngeal swabs in the biosafety cabinet and use sterilized tweezers or hemostatic forceps to hold the swab handle to stir gently several times and squeeze out liquid within the cotton swab, in order to prevent from spillage of liquid and production of aerosol. ② Centrifuge the sample under 4 °C and 2000 rpm for 20 min to eliminate most of the impurities. Open the centrifuge tube after centrifugation, and use a 1 mL Tip to pipette 0.5 mL of supernatant and inoculate it onto cells prepared preliminarily.

(2) Sputum: ① If a small amount of mucus is contained in the sputum, the sample can be inoculated to cells according to ② procedure in (1) nasal/pharyngeal swab sample; ② if a great deal of mucus is contained in the sputum, the sputum should be liquidized (added into 1% pH 7.6 trypsin solution with a 1:1 (v/v) ratio and digested for 15–30 min under 25 °C), and a small amount of sample is taken and inoculated to cells according to ② procedure in (1) nasal/pharyngeal swab sample.

(3) The same principle as above is followed, for other samples such as pleural effusion and bronchoalveolar lavage fluid.

(4) If the sample is suspected to be contaminated by bacteria, the sample can be filtrated with a 0.2 μm filter on the basis of centrifuge before the sample is used.

2. Preparation of cells

The MDCK cells were subcultured into a 6-well plate, and the next day when the cells grew to 75–90%, they were used for virus isolation. Volume of the medium involved in the following inoculation procedures should be adjusted properly as required, if culture bottle or culture plates with any other specification are used.

3. Inoculation procedures

(1) Aspirate gently cell growth solution. 2 mL of Hank's Solution is added to cells, using a 10-mL sterile pipette, and shaken gently several times. Then the Hank's Solution for

rinsing cells is removed with a sterile pipette. Repeat the procedures above for rinsing cells three times.

(2) Inoculation into cell culture bottle: ① proper amount of clinical sample (about 0.5 mL) is pipetted onto a cell culture plate, using a sterile pipette, shaken gently for several times, added with 1 mL of Hank's Solution or virus growth solution, and mixed even. Then the culture plate is put into an incubator under 37 °C with 5% CO_2 for adsorption for 1–2 h, during which the plate is shaken twice to improve the even adsorption of the virus. ② The inoculum is sucked out, and Hank's Solution is pipetted with a 10-mL sterile pipette to rinse the cells twice. Then 2 mL of virus growth solution is added into the cell culture bottle, and cultured in an incubator under 37 °C with 5% CO_2. ③ Cytopathy is observed daily. (Cytopathy is characterized in swelling and rounding of cells, increased intercellular space, pyknosis or rupture of nucleus, and in the severe case, partial or complete shedding of cells). The cytopathic effect (CPE) of 0–25%, 26–50%, 51–75%, and 76–100% is expressed respectively as "+," "++," "+++," and "++++," while the normal cell is indicated as "–".

(3) Harvest of cell culture

Cells are harvested when cytopathy is manifested in 76–100% of them. The cells can be preserved in a −70 °C refrigerator and undergo the freeze–thaw cycles twice prior to harvest, in order to improve viral titer in the harvested sample. The cell bottle is shaken gently several times at first. Then a 10-mL sterile pipette is used to pipette virus solution into a 15-mL sterile centrifuge tube, and the virus is mixed evenly. Virus solution harvested may undergo subsequent tests instantly, or be dispensed into cryopreservation tubes and kept in a −70 °C refrigerator until used.

(4) Viral identification can be performed directly when the hemagglutination titer determined from the hemagglutination test (HA) is ≥1:8; if the titer is <1:8, cell passage is continued until the hemagglutination is ≥1:8 when virus identification can be done. Typing and identification can be performed with RT-PCR, if the titer is still <1:8 post to continuous passages. If there is no agglutination of erythrocytes, passages can be continued once or twice, and those that are still negative are considered as negativeness in isolation.

(5) Blind passage

If no cytopathy is observed after 7-day cultivation, cells can be harvested also and inoculated based on the method of cell culture bottle. The final isolation result is considered as negative if there is still no erythrocyte agglutination or cytopathy post to three blind passages, and negative results for both nuclei acid detection and immunological detection.

4. *Issues that should be paid attention to during isolation of virus*

The cells for isolating the virus should be prevented from being contaminated by Mycoplasma. In case of any contamination. The cells should be discarded and the cells stored in liquid nitrogen from the laboratory cell bank should be thawed.

(1) The prepared sample suspension is adsorbed onto a monolayer of cells, and do not add it directly onto cells containing maintenance solution. Cell growth solution should be poured out at first, and the monolayer cells are rinsed with an aseptic serum-free medium. 0.2–0.5 mL of sample is adsorbed firstly onto the monolayer of cells under ambient temperature, while the cells are being shaken gently to prevent peripheral cells from being dried. Then 1 mL of maintenance solution is compensated, which may improve the efficacy of virus isolation, shorten the time to CPE, and decrease the toxicity of the sample.

(2) Toxicity: The rapid aging of cells within 1–2 days after inoculation onto the sample may suggest the presence of nonspecific toxic reaction caused by toxins contained in the sample. The tubes inoculated with the sample should undergo another freeze–thaw cycle under −20 °C before 0.2 mL is inoculated onto a new monolayer of cells to release the present virus. If toxic reaction occurs again, the original sample diluted with PBS can be inoculated again onto the same cells.

(3) Contamination by microorganisms: it is a turbidity of medium or cell death caused by contamination by bacteria, which makes it impossible for the virus to manifest CPE. Original cells should be taken again for inoculation.

(4) Blind passage: during blind passage of virus, cells growing the most vigorously in the logarithmic growth phase is preferred for inoculation. Every time 0.2 mL of viral-cell suspension post to repeated freeze–thaw cycles are inoculated onto fresh cells.

(5) Caution should be taken to avoid cross-contamination of virus during cell inoculation or passages. Do not discard culture solution for cells inoculated with virus. Instead, a pipette should be used to remove the liquid, and the pipette should be replaced with a new one in each step. Intensive vibration should be avoided to prevent the production of aerosol.

5. Viruses isolated successfully should undergo identification through erythrocyte agglutination test, nucleic acid detection, and immunofluorescence detection.

III. *Identification of virus*

(I) Rationale of erythrocyte agglutination test. In 1941, Hirst et al. discovered hemagglutinin (HA) over the surface of influenza virus particles, which had a structure recognizing and combining surface receptor of erythrocytes, and inducing agglutination via a combination of erythrocytes of many mammals and birds to form visible agglutination available for qualification and quantification of virus.

(II) Clinically significant microneutralization has been used successfully to test the increase of systemic virus-specific neutralizing antibodies in individuals infected or artificially immunized, especially for the detection in serum for type H5 antibodies against avian influenza in human. It can be used for adjuvant diagnosis and evaluation of immune effects. When the virus is identified based on known antibodies, the titer of the virus in the test should be $100TCID_{50}$. Also, it can be applied to the identification of antibodies based on known viruses. The detection of a single serum specimen is enough to reflect the status of immune or infection, because of the absence of specific antibodies against influenza in human populations. When diagnosing suspected cases, however, the titer of neutralization antibody should be tested simultaneously for serums of both the acute phase and the recovery phase. The diagnosis can be established if the serum antibody shows a rise for no less than four times in the recovery phase than in the acute phase. For children, especially those aged below 3 years, a 2-time increase of serum antibodies against the influenza virus has the diagnostic value.

5.6 Inoculation onto Animals

I. *Materials and equipment*

① Preparation of Bal/b mice aged 4–6 weeks. ② Specimens treated and dispensed, including pharynx swab, nasal swab, nasopharynx lavage, and nasopharynx aspiration, as well as supernatant of centrifuged lavage from trachea and bronchi; ③ treated and dispensed supernatant of centrifuged tissues including lung, trachea, bronchi and other tissues obtained from autopsy. ④ Sample of serum and plasma; ⑤ The culture separated from harvested samples; ⑥ sterilized PBS; ⑦ Biosafety cabinet; ⑧ quarantine/breeding cages for mice; ⑨ pipette; ⑩ sterilized Tips, electronic balance, and sterilized grinder.

II. *Operational procedures*

1. Dilution of virus: chicken of Specific Pathogen Free (SPF) level is used to titrate virus, in order to determine the content of virus in allantoic fluid. After calculation, sterilized PBS is used for the dilution of certain ratio, and the final content of virus in the dilution is 10^6EID50/50 μL.
2. Anesthesia of mice: peritoneal injection with either 1% (50 mg/kg) pentobarbital or 7% (400 mg/kg) chloral hydrate is performed at 1 cm off the middle line in the right abdominal wall, using a 1-mL disposable syringe, followed by observation of activities of the mouse. The animal in deep anesthesia 30 s after anesthesia is ready to use.
3. Infection of the nasal cavity: 50 μL of diluted virus kept in the biosafety cabinet is transferred with a 100-μL pipette and dropped slowly into the nasal cavity of the mouse during inspiration. The poisoned animal is put into its cage.
4. Measurement of body weight: the bodyweight is measured for mice in every group using an electronic balance in a secondary biosafety cabinet from day 3 prior to the day of poisoning, with the change of body weight documented.

(1) Sanitation system: the frame of individual ventilation cage (IVC) is cleaned up timely according to the actual situation every day. The food box, water box and IVC cages are sealed in pressurized bags in the biosafety cabinet, with their surface disinfected with 75% alcohol, put into the transfer window for 15-min ultraviolet disinfection, and taken out for autoclaving. A breeder wears integrated protective clothing with mask, cap, shoe covers, and anti-bite gloves, which are underneath the positive-pressure protective clothing and reversely worn protective clothing, and he wears finally the exterior gloves. At the end of the work, one should wash and disinfect

hands carefully. All workers bitten or scratched by animals or having any animal-related injury should have their injuries disinfected and treated instantly, with a report delivered to the superintendent of the laboratory, who will take corresponding measures.

(2) Disinfection system: after mobilization or execution of the animal, the surface of IVC cages should be disinfected with 75% alcohol, and the cage sealed a pressurized sterilization bag is put into the transfer window for ultraviolet disinfection for 15 min, taken out for autoclaving under 121 °C for 30 min, followed by a thorough rinse of IVC cages with its all accessories. The laboratory post to one experimental cycle should undergo fumigation disinfection with paraformaldehyde twice, with 48 h for each cycle. The cage cannot return to service until non-occupation for 1–2 weeks.

(3) Observation and documentation system: feeders must observe the animals with detailed documentation in the process of feeding and management, so as to know and grasp the health and dynamics of animals. Main items for observation include operational status of controlling cabinet of IVC cage frame, appetite and food intake (presence/absence of anorexia) and stool (presence/absence of diarrhea, anus prolapse or pus in stool), mentality (presence/absence of phenomenon of mental malaise, or rolling up with head drooped), and skin hair (presence/absence of injury, defect, depilation or bloodstain).

(4) Feeding system: timing and quantitative feeding is provided every day. Access to water ad libitum is guaranteed for animals throughout the day in all weather.

(5) Safety inspection system: personnel engaged in feeding and management should implement strictly the standard operation procedures, and close the door behind themselves when entering or exiting the feeding area. Capture of animal is not permitted unless there is the presence of two persons, who can try their best to help each other if attacked by the animal. After taking up the post, the staff should check firstly the condition of the equipment and animals in the feeding area and frames of IVC cages, and then carry out other work. Personnel should examine thoroughly the intactness of the working area and taming equipment, and they are not allowed to leave unless the safety is confirmed. A special duty system is set up to be responsible for comprehensive safety work.

5. Dissection of mice and collection of disease materials: three mice for each group are taken from biosafety cabinet on day 4 and 6, respectively, post to poisoning, anesthetized deeply and sacrificed using cervical dislocation. The chest cavity and abdominal cavity are cut open, and lungs, spleen, and one kidney are taken out and put into a 15-mL centrifuge tube containing fixative. Finally, the skull is cut open, and all brain tissue are taken out and put into a 15-mL centrifuge tube containing fixative. The surfaces of tubes are disinfected and labeled.
6. Titration of virus in disease materials.

   Disease materials preserved in a −70 °C refrigerator are taken out and put unto ice in a biosafety cabinet, and then put into a grinder added with 1 mL of sterile PBS containing two antibiotics (penicillin and streptomycin) for grinding. Histiocytes suspension in the tissue homogenizer is pipetted carefully to a sterilized microcentrifuge tube kept on ice, with cautions to prevent spillage out of the tube. The centrifuge tube with its surface sterilized and labeled is centrifuged 12,000 g under 4 °C for 15 min, and the supernatant is collected for titrating virus. The grinder disinfected simply is placed in a special vessel, put in a special plastic bag and sealed with the surface disinfected, then taken out of the biosafety cabinet, and placed in another specific plastic bag for autoclaving.

   Virus titration: supernatant obtained from disease materials that have been ground is diluted 10 times with PBS, and 6 dilutions including the original solution are inoculated to 10-day old chicken embryo, with 1 dilution for inoculating 3 embryos. Hemagglutination titer in allantoic fluid is determined after 48 h, with documentation of the number of embryos having hemagglutination titer. Reed–Muench is used to calculate viral content in the sample (expressed with EID50).

III. *The wastes in the experiments need sorting treatment.*

The wastes are generally put into a special container and a plastic bag, sealed, with the surface disinfected through scrubbing, put into another special plastic bag, sealed, and disinfected to undergo autoclaving.

5.7 Inoculation, Cultivation, and Harvest of Chicken Embryos for Animal Experiment

I. *Materials and equipment*

Treated and dispensed specimen, including throat swab, nasopharynx swab, nasopharynx lavage, nasopharynx aspirate and centrifugal supernatant of tracheobronchial lavage fluid. Treated and dispensed supernatant of autopsy tissues, including lungs, trachea, bronchi, and other tissues; SPF chicken embryo aged 10 days; 75% ethanol, egg candler, perforator; 1 mL syringe, needle, adhesive tape; 15-mL centrifuge tube and tube frame, capillary pipette; sterile forceps; biosafety cabinet; ordinary 35 °C incubator; 4 °C or −20 °C refrigerator; centrifuge, etc.

II. *Operational procedures*

Note: all experiments should be done in a biosafety cabinet

1. Preparation: the biosafety cabinet is turned on in advance, and the normal condition of the negative pressure and oriented airflow of the cabinet is confirmed; preparation of wastes' container and disinfectant; preparation of disposable disinfection paper pad containing 75% alcohol, which is spread on the table of biosafety cabinet; experimental materials and samples used in the biosafety cabinet are disinfected with 75% alcohol before they are put into the cabinet.
2. Preparation of chicken embryo

   Preparation of chicken embryo: the chicken embryo is observed with an egg candler. The egg is placed in an egg plate with the chamber side upright, and the boundary of the chamber and fetal position are drawn. The unfertilized eggs, broken eggs, and terminated eggs are removed. A label is made at the injection site, i.e., 1 mm off the borderline between the embryo and the chamber while steering clear of blood vessels. 75% of alcohol is used to disinfect area around the injection site, and a small incision about 2 mm is drilled with a sterilized egg-whisk, with cautions not to hurt shell membrane.
3. Inoculation

   Draw 0.1 mL of treated viral sample with a syringe, use the needle to make a puncture, through which the sample is injected into the allantoic cavity. Withdraw the syringe, and seal the puncture with melt paraffins. Keep the egg in an incubator under 33–35 °C for an incubation for 72 h.
4. Observation and documentation

   Experimental personnel must observe the temperature and humidity of the incubator with proper documentation, during the management procedures, so as to understand and control timely the interior status of the incubator. A timely adjustment is required, and sterile water is added to maintain the interior humidity of the incubator. A thorough examination is required to ensure the incubator is in an operational status.

   The door of the incubator must be closed after the chicken embryo is put into or taken out of the incubator. The extracted chicken embryo is put onto the experimental table. An egg candler is used to observe in darkness the growth and survival of a chicken embryo. All chicken embryos prior to the relocation out of the biosafety cabinet for inoculation and post to observation for chicken embryos with the candler must be disinfected before they are put into the incubator.

   The interior hygiene of the incubator is maintained. The accidentally broken chicken embryo can be covered with a gauze soaked with disinfectant, swiped and sprayed with 5% peracetic acid solution for disinfection. Then the incubator is sprayed thoroughly with 5% peracetic acid solution, and other chicken embryos in the incubator are disinfected by spraying ethanol.

   Daily preventive disinfection is performed, including one disinfection of both interior and exterior of the isolator; the empty incubator should be sprayed thoroughly with 5% peracetic acid solution.
5. Harvest of allantoic fluid of chicken embryos

   Before allantoic fluid of chicken embryos is harvested, the chicken embryos are removed to an environment under 4 °C and kept overnight, or frozen under −20 °C for 1 h. The duration of fast freezing cannot be prolonged, so as to prevent embryos from being frozen which cannot be harvested. Similarly, cold storage under 4 °C should not last too long; otherwise, the yolk will be scattered and the harvest will be affected. Plastic tubes are labeled, based on the labels for the sample. Uncover gently the paraffin sealing the mouth of the tube, and disinfect the surface of chicken embryo with 75% ethanol. Use sterile tweezers to break the eggshell above the gas chamber, take out the fragments, tear the inner shell membrane and chorioallantoic membrane with another pair of sterile tweezers, and suck the allantoic fluid with a sterile capillary pipette. Put the harvested liquid into a 15-mL centrifuge tube and mark it.

Centrifuge under 3000 rpm is performed for 5 min, in order to eliminate blood and cells, followed by hemagglutination test (see hemagglutination (HA) and hemagglutination inhibition (HI) for operation procedures as follows). If allantoic fluid collected has no hemagglutination titer, two passages will be performed in a row. If the result of agglutination is still negative, it is determined that the tested sample does not contain the influenza virus. The centrifuged supernatant is collected, dispensed with a label, and stored in an ultra-low temperature freezer, if the collected allantoic fluid has the titer.

5.8 Requirement on Biosafety

Laboratory biosafety: conditions and status of laboratory biosafety should not be lower than the permissible level, which may avoid unacceptable harms to laboratory staff, visitors, community, and environment and conform to the requirement on responsibility of laboratory biosafety by related laws and standards.

The documents of biosafety management system of the laboratory is formulated, according to related laws and regulations including the Law on Prevention and Control of Infectious Diseases of the People's Republic of China, Regulations on Biosafety Management of Pathogenic Microorganism Laboratories (Order No. 424 of the State Council), and Emergency Regulations for Public Health Emergencies as well as General Requirements for Laboratory Biosafety (GB 19489-2008), General Biosafety Guidelines for Microbiological and Biomedical Laboratories (Ws233-2002), Regulations on Transportation of Highly Pathogenic Microorganism (Bacteria Species/Virus Stains) or Samples Infecting Human Beings (Order No.45 issued by the Ministry of Health), List of Pathogenic Microorganisms with Inter-Human Transmission issued by the Ministry of Health, Administrative Measures on Institutions Responsible for Preserving Pathogenic Microorganisms (Bacteria Species/Virus Strains) with Inter-Human Transmission (Order No.68 issued by Ministry of Health), requirements by national standards, in referencing to WHO Handbook on Laboratory Biosafety (the 3rd Edition, 2004) and materials related to Biosafety Laboratory Management of Developed Foreign Countries, in combination with actuality in this laboratory and specific operational experience in practical work of the personnel.

I. *Biological risks and treatment*
   1. Possible conditions causing biohazards: aerosol may be produced when sample container is uncovered, culture is separated, sample solution is mixed even with the pipette, or the sample is sucked and added onto micro agglutination plate followed by sample dilution. Sample spillage may occur when the container is uncovered after thawing in case of an excessive sample. Leakage of virus solution may take place when a pipette is used to suck samples, and specimen leakage may occur when the hemagglutination plate is overturned or vibrated.
   2. Individual protection and treatment of accidents.
      (1) All experiments are carried out in the biosafety cabinet, with measures to prevent from production and inhalation of aerosol and measures for individual protection, including the gauze containing 75% ethanol spread on the table of the biosafety cabinet in advance, gentle uncovering of sample container in a biosafety cabinet and keeping the sample container in 45 degrees for mixing sample liquid and for sampling; and FS9901-L medical protective masks or 3 M masks worn by experimental personnel during the experiment.
      (2) Measures to prevent sample spillage and individual protection should be taken, including gauze containing 75% ethanol spread on the table of biosafety cabinet in advance, gentle uncovering of sample container by the experimental personnel, detailed operation referencing to the section of Leakage of Virus Solution in volume of Emergent Treatment in Safety Manual, and FS9901-L medical protective masks or 3 M masks worn by experimental personnel during the experiment.
      (3) Measures to prevent from leakage of virus solution and overturn of hemagglutination plate when the pipette is used to suck the sample and the hemagglutination is vibrated include gauze containing 75% ethanol spread on the table of biosafety cabinet in advance, the needle of the pipette should be adhered as far as possible to the liquid surface to suck the sample, minimization of dropping of sample liquid caused by sample adhered to the exterior of Tip of pipette, covering the hemagglutination plate with sticky paper, the prevention from side down of the sample, and FS9901-L medical protective masks or 3 M masks worn by experimental personnel during the experiment.

II. *Disposal of the wastes*
   1. Contaminants such as remnants or wasted culture tubes carrying bacteria are put in autoclaved sterile bags with a certain gap left when the autoclaved sterile indicating belt is used to tie up the bag mouth, so as to ensure air circulation inside and outside the bag and guarantee autoclaving efficacy. In addition, 75% ethanol disinfectant is used to spray the exterior of the sterile bag, before it is removed out of the biosafety cabinet. No disposal or rinsing is permitted, until sterilization with high-pressure steam is performed under 121 °C for 30 min.
   2. Disinfection of working surfaces: working surface is prayed with 75% ethanol with the retention time of disinfection no less than 10 min. Then 75% ethanol is used for wiping and disinfecting exterior walls of the biosafety cabinet.

III. *Clearance and disinfection*

1. Items in the biosafety cabinet should be put in order, have their exterior surfaces wiped with 75% ethanol, removed out of the biosafety cabinet, and put to the designated place;
2. The unused infectious biomaterials shall be disposed or put into the freezer at −80 °C according to the Operation Procedures for Treatment of Wastes and Cultures of Bacteria Species (Virus Strains) in Biosafety Level III Laboratory and operations and treatment shall be documented as appropriate.
3. Contaminated materials in the experimental area shall be treated based on Operation Procedures for Treatment of Wastes and Cultures of Bacteria Species (Virus Strains) in Biosafety Level III Laboratory.
4. 75% ethanol is used to wipe working surfaces, the exterior wall of the biosafety cabinet, and the tables, followed by continuation of operation of the biosafety cabinet for another 10 min before shutting down.
5. Ensure that there are no residue materials from this operation within the experimental area. Check the normality of pressure in the laboratory.

IV. *Exit the laboratory based on Operation Procedures for Experimental Personnel to Enter and Exit Biosafety Level III Laboratory*

References

1. Ge J, Shi L, Yunqing X. Research progress of H7N9 avian influenza in human. J Trop Med. 2016;4:537–40.
2. Gou X, Huang J. Research progress of H7N9 avian influenza and its high pathogenicity. Hainan Med J. 2018;23:3372–5. https://doi.org/10.3969/j.issn.1003-6350.2018.23.037.
3. Li Q, Zhou L, Zhou M, et al. Epidemiology of human infections with avian influenza A(H7N9) virus in China. N Engl J Med. 2014;6(6):520–32.
4. Pham TH, Peter J, Mello F, et al. Performance of the TB-LAMP diagnostic assay in reference laboratories: results from a multicentre study. Int J Infect Dis. 2018;68:44–9. https://doi.org/10.1016/j.ijid.2018.01.005.
5. Xichao O, Qiang L, Hui X, et al. Diagnostic accuracy of the PURE-LAMP test for pulmonary tuberculosis at the county-level laboratory in China. PLoS One. 2014;9(5):e94544. https://doi.org/10.1371/journal.pone.0094544.
6. Adama L, Bojang Francis S, MendyLeopold D, et al. Comparison of TB-LAMP, GeneXpert MTB/RIF and culture for diagnosis of pulmonary tuberculosis in the Gambia. J Infect. 2016;72(3):332–7.

Clinical Diagnosis and Differentiation Diagnosis

6

Shi-pin Wu, Dong-na Su, and Chen Qiu

6.1 Clinical Manifestation

The main subtypes discovered up to now that may infect human beings include H5N1, H5N6, H7N1, H7N2, H7N3, H7N4, H7N7, H7N9, H9N2, and H10N8, among which subtypes H5N1 and H7N9 with high mortality are particularly worthy of much attention. Human infected with different subtypes of influenza viruses differ greatly in clinical manifestations [1], which are correlated mainly to the virulence of these subtypes. Conjunctivitis is the main manifestation of those infected with subtype H7N7. Those infected with H5N1 or H7N9 usually have severe disease with high mortality, in contrast to those infected with H9N2 who manifest milder clinical symptoms of probably upper respiratory infection, or even no symptom in some patients.

Based on statistics from WHO, 861 patients with subtype H5N1 avian influenza virus infection had been reported globally in total from 2003 to May 2019, including 455 deaths with a mortality up to 5.28% [2]. From March 2013 to February 2017, 1258 patients infected with the H7N9 avian influenza virus had been reported in China, with mortality up to 41% [3, 4]. It could be inferred that human infection of subtypes H5N1 and H7N9 avian influenza had the mortality dramatically higher than the mean mortality of 10.9% reported for the SARS outbreak in 2003, and imposed a great threat to human health and life, which is worthy of great attention.

S.-p. Wu (✉) · D.-n. Su
Department of Infectious Diseases, Shenzhen People's Hospital, The Second Clinical Medical College of Jinan University, The First Affiliated Hospital of Southern University of Science and Technology, Shenzhen, Guangdong, China

C. Qiu
Department of Respiratory Diseases, Shenzhen People's Hospital, The Second Clinical Medical College of Jinan University, The First Affiliated Hospital of Southern University of Science and Technology, Shenzhen, Guangdong, China

I. *Incubation period*

The incubation period of human infection with various subtypes of avian influenza virus varies from 1 to 3 days, mostly within 7 days. The length of the incubation period correlates to the subtypes of avian influenza virus, the virulence of the virus, quantity of infected virus, and immune function of infected person.

II. *Epidemiological characteristics*

1. Distribution of populations

   Human avian influenza can be seen in all age groups, mainly in children and young adults. There was no significant difference in incidence rate between men and women. The majority of human avian influenza patients in China have a history of poultry contact or activities in markets with bird slaughter.

2. Seasonality

   In China, this disease occurs often in winter and spring, which correlates probably to the North-South migration of migratory birds. Cases with avian influenza are rarely reported in autumn or summer. Therefore, the incidence of human avian influenza has a significant seasonal distribution.

III. *Clinical manifestations*

1. *Fever.* Almost all patients have fever, with a temperature above 39 °C. The most common heat types include sustained fever, remittent fever, and irregular fever. Patients with mild disease had a short duration of fever (commonly 3–4 days), in contrast to those with severe disease manifesting higher temperature and prolonged duration. The degree of fever with its duration usually correlates to the severity of the disease and the prognosis. A few days after the onset of the disease, the body temperature dropped to normal, and the second heat peak appeared due to secondary bacterial or fungal infection. Respiratory failure and other complications are easy to occur, which should be paid attention to

C. Qiu et al. (eds.), *Avian Influenza in Human*, https://doi.org/10.1007/978-981-16-1429-3_6

2. *Systemic toxemic symptoms*

   Unlike the common cold, most patients with avian influenza have severer systemic toxemic symptoms, manifesting headache, fatigue, general discomfort, and muscle soreness all over the body. The comprehensive analysis of Chinese researches showed that headache and body muscle soreness exist in almost half of the patients with avian influenza.

3. *Respiratory symptoms*

   Compared with the common cold, patients with human avian influenza have milder or absent respiratory catarrhal symptoms such as stuffy nose, runny nose, and sneezing. Most patients have sore throat, cough, and expectoration. However, the amount of sputum is small. It is usually white mucus sputum. Patients with severe disease may have bloody phlegm. Yellow purulent sputum can be observed in those complicated with bacterial infection.

   Chest tightness, shortness of breath, and dyspnea occur often in patients with severe disease on day 5 or so after the onset. Chest X-ray shows large infiltrating opacities in the lungs, which may even develop into the "white lung." Some severe patients manifest hemoptysis, due to diffusive alveolar injuries. Pleurisy and pleural effusion may develop in some patients in the middle or advanced stages of the disease course.

   Pneumonia as one of the complications of avian influenza in humans can be categorized into primary viral pneumonia, secondary bacterial pneumonia, and mixed pneumonia. The disease may aggravate about 5 days after the onset in patients with primary viral pneumonia. Besides manifestations above, symptoms observed in the patients complicated with bacterial infection may include purulent sputum, significant increase of peripheral blood leukocytes and neutrophils, and increase of inflammatory parameters such as C-reactive protein.

4. *Other systemic symptoms*

   Some patients with avian influenza have anorexia, nausea, vomiting, abdominal pain, abdominal distension, and diarrhea in the early stage of the disease and other digestive system symptoms, especially diarrhea. Diarrhea is usually loose stool or watery stool, and tenesmus is not complicated in most of the patients. There is usually no obvious abnormality in microscopic stool examination.

   Myocardial damage is common in patients with human avian influenza. According to statistics, almost 100% of patients in China have myocardia enzymes such as lactate dehydrogenase and phosphocreatine kinase increased significantly. Severe patients may have hypotension or even septic shock, and very few are admitted to the hospital due to hypotension or shock.

   Some of the patients may have symptoms of the nervous system, such as headache, irritability, and convulsion. Injuries in the nervous system include encephalitis, meningitis, myelitis, and Guillain Barre Syndrome. A few patients with severe disease may even manifest convulsion and coma that result in death. Two cases of avian influenza in humans were reported in Vietnam in 2005, manifesting clinically diarrhea, coma, and death, but lacking respiratory symptoms. H5N1 avian influenza viruses were isolated from cerebrospinal fluid, feces, pharynx, and serum, suggesting the probability of invasion by the H5N1 virus into the central nervous system.

5. *Multiple organ failure*

   Severe cytokine storm may be induced by avian influenza virus, causing ARDS and multiple organ failure [5, 6] and becoming the main cause of death in patients with severe human avian influenza. Organs commonly involved include lungs, kidneys, liver, heart, gastrointestinal tract, blood system, and nervous system, manifesting septic shock and multiple organ failure.

IV. *Laboratory examinations and other auxiliary examinations*

1. Blood routine examination: in the early stage of the disease, the total number of peripheral blood leukocytes is generally not high or even may decrease. In addition to severe patients, peripheral blood lymphocytes and platelets are often reduced, which is related to the severity of the disease and prognosis.
2. Blood biochemical examination: The levels of C-reactive protein, lactate dehydrogenase, creatine phosphate kinase, aspartate aminotransferase and alanine aminotransferase increased, and myoglobin in some patients also increased. As mentioned above, almost 100% of the patients in China showed a significant increase in myocardial enzymes such as lactate dehydrogenase and creatine kinase.
3. Etiology and related detections

   If human infection with avian influenza virus is suspected, respiratory tract samples should be collected actively (such as nasopharynx secretion, deep throat secretion, sputum, airway aspirates, bronchoalveolar lavage fluid, etc.) for examination. The detection rate from lower respiratory tract specimens is far higher than from the upper respiratory tract.

   (1) Nucleic acid detection of avian influenza virus: Nucleic acid detection of avian influenza virus is the first choice for laboratory diagnosis. For severe cases, it is suggested that the viral nucleic acid of respiratory secretions be detected regularly until

the result of the viral nucleic acid test turns negative. The results showed that the RT-PCR method had high specificity and sensitivity, which was helpful for early diagnosis and establishment of type and subtype of avian influenza virus.

(2) Detection of avian influenza virus antigen (rapid reagent detection): colloidal gold and immunofluorescence can be used, and the sensitivity is lower than that of the detection of viral nucleic acid. The interpretation of the results should be considered comprehensively in combination with epidemic history and clinical symptoms.

(3) Isolation of virus: avian influenza virus can be isolated from a respiratory specimen from patients, mainly used in laboratory research.

(4) Detection of antibody: It is helpful to establish the diagnosis if the specific antibody IgM of avian influenza virus is positive in serum, or the IgG titer is more than four times higher in the early stage and recovery stage. Serological detection methods include hemagglutinin inhibition test, microneutralization antibody test, direct immunofluorescence method, enzyme-linked immunosorbent assay, single radioimmunoassay hemolysis technology.

4. Chest imaging

The chest imaging findings of pneumonia in patients with avian influenza were patchy shadows and ground glass density. The lesions were diffuse and multilobular. In severe cases, the lesions progressed rapidly, often showing multiple ground-glass opacity in both lungs. And lung consolidation shadow may be complicated with pleural effusion. When the chest imaging findings meet one of the following, it indicates that the lesion is serious.

① Patchy images were found in more than three lung fields; ② Lung imaging lesions are progressing rapidly, which increase more than 50% in 1–2 days.

ARDS is suggested by findings as follows in chest imaging: ① The range of imaging lesions was more than 60% of the whole lung field, or the consolidation of the lung increased significantly; ② "white lung" shown by X-ray is the typical sign of ARDS; ③ Conventional position CT examination showed that the lesions in the dorsal lung were mainly consolidation, while those in the ventral lung were mainly ground-glass opacity.

Because of the rapid progress of lung lesions in severe patients, chest X-ray examination should be performed every 1–2 days according to clinical needs. If possible, a CT scan of the chest at the bedside is feasible.

The absorption of lung shadow and pulmonary fibrosis in patients with human avian influenza is usually slow. We followed up a patient with severe H5N1 avian influenza, who manifested residues of interstitial lesions and fibrosis at discharge. After 5 years of follow-up, the lesions were completely absorbed in the lung.

6.2 Clinical Diagnosis

I. *Basis for clinical diagnosis*

Diagnosis of human avian influenza can be established based on the history of epidemics, clinical manifestations, and laboratory findings. It must be emphasized that epidemiological data are of great significance in the clinical diagnosis of human avian influenza.

(I) Epidemiological history

A large amount of viruses are contained in saliva, nasal secretion, and feces of birds infected with avian influenza. Direct exposure to birds or their excretions is the main route of transmission. The epidemiological data of human infection with avian influenza mainly refers to one of the following situations within 10 days before the onset of the disease: ① exposure to poultry and their secretions and excreta; ② previous visits to the market of live poultry; and ③ history of close contact with humans infected with avian influenza.

(II) Clinical manifestations

The incubation period lasts usually 1–7 days. It is characterized by mild catarrhal symptoms in contrast to severe systemic toxemic symptoms caused by upper respiratory infection. Severe patients manifest high fever without abatement, and rapid development of the disease progressing rapidly into pneumonia, ARDS, septic shock, and multiple organ dysfunction.

(III) Laboratory examinations

The establishment of the diagnosis is contributed by positiveness in nucleic acid detection for avian influenza virus, positiveness in isolated avian influenza virus, and the rise more than four times of IgG antibody against subtype strain of avian influenza in double sera in both early stage after onset and the recovery.

II. *Clinical typing*

Human infected with various subtypes of avian influenza virus differ greatly in clinical manifestations, so it can be categorized into clinical types including the mild type, the typical type, the severe type, the untypical type, and the covert infection.

1. The mild type: it is commonly observed in subtypes H7N7 and H9N2 of the avian influenza virus. These subtypes manifest generally low fever with short duration, mild respiratory symptoms including only mild dry cough without shortness of breath or dys-

pnea. There were few signs of pulmonary inflammation in the imaging examination. The course of the disease is short and the prognosis is good.

2. The typical type: it is also called common avian influenza in humans, characterized by respiratory catarrhal syndromes and typical systemic toxemic symptoms in the early stage, viral pneumonia in the progressive stage, and typical clinical course of convalescence, without severe complications such as ARDS or multiple organ failure. It shows a good prognosis and recovered generally in about 3 weeks.
3. Human avian influenza with subtype H5N1 and H7N9 infection tends to develop into the severe type, manifesting persistent high fever without abatement, rapid progression of disease, and occurrence of viral pneumonia, acute pulmonary injury, ARDS, septic shock, and multiple organ failure. Patients with the severe type have an unfavorable prognosis, with a high mortality.

   We have formulated the diagnostic criteria for severe type of human avian influenza, aiming at the early identification, early diagnosis, early rescue, and determination of prognosis. Those meeting one of the primary criteria or at least three secondary criteria can be diagnosed as the severe type. The primary criteria include: ① endotracheal intubation is needed for mechanical ventilation; and ② vasoactive medication is still needed for those after active fluid resuscitation from septic shock. Secondary criteria: ① respiration rate ≥ 30 per min; ② oxygenation index ≤250 mmH; ③ The imaging findings were multiple lobar infiltration; ④ disturbance of consciousness and/or disorientation; ⑤ blood urine nitrogen ≥7.14 mmol/L;. ⑥ active fluid resuscitation is needed for those with the systolic pressure <90 mmHg.

   The following populations tend to develop into the severe type, and great attention should be paid to them: ① Children under 5 years old; ② elderly people over 65 years old; ③ complications such as chronic respiratory diseases, cardiovascular diseases, kidney diseases, liver diseases, and immune deficiency status; ④ obesity (body mass index larger than 30); and ⑤ pregnant women.
4. Untypical human avian influenza: some of the patients manifest mainly gastrointestinal symptoms such as abdominal pain and diarrhea but without respiratory symptoms. Some manifest mainly symptoms of the central nervous system, such as headache, convulsion, and coma. All these manifestations belong to untypical avian influenza in humans. This type of avian influenza is easy to be misdiagnosed.
5. Covert infection: a few patients do not have any clinical symptoms or signs despite their definite epidemiological history and the positive detection of antibody IgG against subtype of avian influenza virus. The significance of the covert infection as a source of infection is unclear.

III. *Clinical staging*

Human avian influenza can be divided into the following four stages, in order to facilitate clinical observation and formulate a reasonable treatment regimen [7]:

1. Early stage: It is usually the first to the fourth day of the disease. It manifests acute onset, fever complicated with respiratory catarrhal symptoms as well as symptoms of systemic toxemic symptoms such as headache and muscle soreness. The patient may have a dry cough, stomachache, diarrhea, and watery stool. Abnormal findings in imaging examination usually occur about 7 days after fever.
2. Progressive stage: it often takes place from the 5th to the 21st day of the course of the disease. Systemic toxemic symptoms such as fever and muscle soreness may persist or even aggravate. The temperature may rise above 40 °C, and the patients often have obvious respiratory symptoms with significant cough, expectoration of white sputum or bloody sputum, chest tightness, shortness of breath, and dyspnea. X-ray shows the rapid progression of pulmonary opacities and even the "white lung." Most of the patients have ARDS and multiple organ failure. Patients in this stage are vulnerable to secondary infection in multiple sites with multiple pathogens, which is the main predisposing factor for the aggravation of diseases.
3. Recovery period: the disease after the progressive stage ameliorates gradually and enters the recovery period, which usually starts at week 3 during the disease course. The condition is relieved little by little, with gradual disappearance of systemic toxemic symptoms, drop of temperature, and gradual absorption of pulmonary lesions. Most patients meet the criteria of discharge from the hospital after 3–4 weeks of recovery. But the absorption of lung shadow takes a long time. The patients can recover gradually within 2–3 months after discharge, and some patients may have restrictive ventilation dysfunction and pulmonary fibrosis.

According to traditional Chinese medicine scholars, human avian influenza can be divided into four stages, including exterior syndrome stage, high fever stage, wheezing stage, and recovery stage, which is helpful for the treatment based on syndrome differentiation for human avian influenza [8].

6.3 Differential Diagnosis

Human avian influenza should be distinguished from seasonal influenza (including influenza A (H1N1)), community-acquired pneumonia, SARS, novel coronavirus pneumonia, adenovirus pneumonia, chlamydia pneumonia, mycoplasma pneumonia, and legionella pneumonia. The diagnosis mainly depends on etiological examination.

I. *Influenza*

Attention should be paid to the possibility of influenza when a large number of patients with upper respiratory tract infection occurred simultaneously within a certain unit or area during the epidemic season, or the number of patients with upper respiratory tract infection visiting outpatient department increases dramatically. The clinical manifestations of these diseases are hard to differentiate with those of human avian influenza, and epidemiological data is of great reference value. The diagnosis can be confirmed, based on a four times rise of the titer of IgG antibody against influenza virus in early and convalescent period and the presence of influenza virus isolated from nasopharynx secretion of the patient.

II. *SARS*

It is a contagious respiratory disease caused by the SARS coronavirus. It had an epidemic in some regions in China in 2003, and since then no prevalence has been observed. Epidemiological data are very important and clinical manifestations are difficult to differentiate from human avian influenza.

III. *Chlamydia pneumonia*

Chlamydia is a strict intracellular pathogen. Chlamydia pneumonia is characterized by acute respiratory tract infection symptoms such as pharyngitis, laryngitis, and pneumonia. The clinical symptoms include fever, sore throat, and cough, findings in chest X-ray featuring bronchopneumonia changes located mainly in the lower lobes. Teenagers are more common. The diagnosis of a recent infection is based on an increase of more than four times of serum antibody in double sera in complement binding test.

IV. *Mycoplasmal pneumonia*

It is a disease caused by mycoplasma, having a prevalence all year round with autumn and winter as the peak seasons. ① Slow onset in most cases, featuring tracheitis and bronchitis, pneumonia, and tympanitis. ② Fever, headache, sore throat, and muscle soreness at the beginning of the disease. Symptoms also include cough, with a small amount of mucus sputum and sometimes bloody sputum. ③ There is usually a lack of lung signs. ④ The chest X-ray findings are characterized by diversity and rapid change, showing large patches of flocculent opacities or interstitial pneumonitis. ⑤ The leukocyte count was normal and lymphocytes were increased relatively. ⑥ Mycoplasma pneumonia can be cultured from sputum, nose, and throat swabs. Erythrocyte cold agglutination test can be positive. The positive of polymerase chain reaction or positive of specific antibody IgM may contribute to early diagnosis. ⑦ Macrolide and tetracycline antibiotics are effective.

References

1. Cao B. Clinical features of human-avian influenza A(H7N9), A(H5N1) and A(H10N8).Chin Bull Life Sci. 2015(5):549–53. https://doi.org/10.13376/j.cbls/2015072
2. World Health Organization. Cumulative number of confirmed human cases for avian influenza A(H5N1) reported to WHO. 2003–2019. https://www.who.int/influenza/human_animal_interface/2019_05_10_tableH5N1.pdf?ua=1
3. World Health Organization. Antigenic and genetic characteristics of zoonotic influenza viruses and development of candidate vaccine viruses for pandemic preparedness, March 2017.Geneva: World Health Organization; 2017. https://www.who.int/influenza/vaccines/virus/201703_zoonotic_vaccinevirusupdate.pdf?ua=1
4. Xiang NJ, Li XY, Ren RQ, Wang DY, Zhou SZ, Greene CM, Song Y, Zhou L, Yang L, Davis CT, Zhang Y, Wang YL, Zhao J, Li XD, Iuliano AD, Havers F, Olsen SJ, Uyeki TM, Azziz-Baumgartner E, Trock S, Liu B, Sui HT, Huang X, Zhang YP, Ni DX, Feng ZJ, Shu YL, Li Q. Assessing change in avian influenza A(H7N9) virus infections during the fourth epidemic—China, September 2015–August 2016. MMWR Morb Mortal Wkly Rep. 2016;65:1390–4. https://doi.org/10.15585/mmwr.mm6549a2.
5. Newton AH, Cardani A, Braciale TJ. The host immune response in respiratory virus infection: balancing virus clearance and immunopathology. Semin Immunopathol. 2016;38(4):471–82. https://doi.org/10.1007/s00281-016-0558-0.
6. Short KR, Kroeze EJBV, Fouchier RAM, Kuiken T. Pathogenesis of influenza-induced acute respiratory distress syndrome. Lancet Infect Dis. 2014;14(1):57–69. https://doi.org/10.1016/S1473-3099(13)70286-X.
7. Zhou BP, Li YM, Lu PX. Avian influenza in human. 1st ed. Beijing: Science Press; 2007.
8. Infectious Diseases Committee of Chinese Society of Integrated Traditional Chinese Medicine and Western Medicine. Expert consensus on diagnosis and treatment of human avian influenza with integrated Traditional Chinese Medicine and Western Medicine. 2016;34(11):641–7. https://doi.org/10.3760/cma.j.issn.1000-6680.2016.11.001

7 Treatment of Avian Influenza in Human

Shi-pin Wu, Kai Zhou, and Chen Qiu

Patients with mild disease may recover gradually after active symptomatic and supportive treatment, and the prognosis is good. Those with severe diseases feature dangerous and complicated conditions with high mortality, and active rescue is required. To standardize diagnosis and treatment, the National Health Commission of the People's Republic of China [1] has released a Diagnostic and treatment protocol for human infections with avian influenza A (H7N9) (First Edition, 2017).

7.1 Principle of Treatment

(I) "Four-early" principle: The principle of early detection, early report, early diagnosis, and early treatment should be abided by, and antiviral treatment should be initiated as soon as the sample is collected for patients with *human avian* influenza.

(II) "Four-concentration" principle: Centralized treatment should be provided for patients with severe diseases, who should be admitted into designated hospitals with strong comprehensive capacity, based on the principles of concentration of patients, experts, resources, and rescue, combined with local medical resources. The experts should be brought into full play to improve the cure rate in patients with severe diseases.

(III) Principle of comprehensive treatment: Severe human avian influenza may progress fast with a great complexity, and a comprehensive treatment is needed for a series of pathophysiological changes caused by the disease.

(IV) Reasonable usage of glucocorticoids: Glucocorticoids should be used reasonably, emphasizing the principle of individualization and avoiding abuse.

(V) Active control of complications: The patients with severe diseases mostly die of various complications and concurrent diseases, especially infectious complications, which should be controlled actively.

(VI) The importance of intensive care should be emphasized: The patients with critically ill may progress rapidly with great changeability. Close and dynamic observation must be performed, in order to strengthen monitoring, discover various complications and carry out treatment timely.

(VII) Emphasis should be placed on the principle of a treatment integrated with Traditional Chinese Medicine and Western medicine: Traditional Chinese Medicine and Herbs should be brought into full play with differentiated treatment, thereby improving the success rate of rescue.

(VIII) The principle of reasonable medication should be strengthened: The avoidance of abuse of antibiotics; the contradiction of Aspirin or drugs containing aspirin or other salicylic acid preparations in children, so as to avoid Reye Syndrome.

7.2 Isolation

Human avian influenza belongs to Class B contagious disease stipulated by the Law of the People's Republic of China on the Prevention and Treatment of Infectious Diseases, and

S.-p. Wu (✉)
Department of Infectious Diseases, Shenzhen People's Hospital, The Second Clinical Medical College of Jinan University, The First Affiliated Hospital of Southern University of Science and Technology, Shenzhen, Guangdong, China

K. Zhou
Shenzhen Institute of Respiratory Diseases, Shenzhen People's Hospital, The Second Clinical Medical College of Jinan University, The First Affiliated Hospital of Southern University of Science and Technology, Shenzhen, Guangdong, China

C. Qiu
Department of Respiratory Diseases, Shenzhen People's Hospital, The Second Clinical Medical College of Jinan University, The First Affiliated Hospital of Southern University of Science and Technology, Shenzhen, Guangdong, China

C. Qiu et al. (eds.), *Avian Influenza in Human*, https://doi.org/10.1007/978-981-16-1429-3_7

patients should be isolated strictly according to regulations on patients with contagious airway diseases.

In principle, clinically suspected cases and confirmed cases should be admitted to an independent ward with respiratory isolating conditions. Suspected cases and confirmed cases should be admitted to different areas for treatment.

The wards are separated into clean regions, semi-clean regions, and contaminated regions, without overlap between regions. The wards should be provided with good ventilation, and the patients would better be admitted into the negative pressure ward if permitted.

A strict visiting system should be established in the ward, and no chaperonage or visiting is permitted. When leaving the ward for examination and treatment, the patients should wear masks and be accompanied by special personnel.

7.3 Symptomatic Treatment and Supportive Treatment

(I) *Control of hyperthermia*

Physical hypothermy or antipyretic analgesics can be used for patients with a fever above 38.5 °C. Aspirins as an antipyretic are contraindicated in children to lower the temperature, in order to avoid Reye Syndrome.

(II) *Resolving phlegm and relieving cough*

Bedridden patients should turn over regularly and have their back patted regularly to promote the discharge of sputum. The atomized inhalation, expectorants, or drugs expelling phlegm can be used for patients with thick sputum. Secretion in the airway can be eliminated through sputum aspiration in time in patients with bronchial intubation or tracheotomy.

(III) *Oxygen treatment*

1. Indications of oxygen treatment: ① $SpO_2 \leq 93\%$ during natural respiration; ② increased respiratory rate (>24/min), dyspnea or distress in supine position. Generally, oxygen can be given by low flow nasal catheter from 2 L/min to 3 L/min. Higher flow of respiratory inhalation can be provided for the patient with hypoxemia (PaO_2 <70 mmHg or SpO_2 <93%) to maintain SpO_2 in a level no less than 93%, and mask oxygen inhalation should be chosen if necessary.
2. Indications of noninvasive positive pressure ventilation: it can be tried in the early stage, if the respiratory rate is still above 30/min and the respiratory burden is still kept on a high level, despite SpO_2 is still maintained at 93% post to sufficient oxygen treatment, or is still lower than 93% under an oxygen uptake flow ≥5 L/min (or the concentration of inhaled oxygen ≥ 40%). The oral-nasal mask is recommended.
3. Invasive ventilation: the invasive ventilation should be considered as soon as possible for severe patients not responding well to noninvasive ventilation.

   Indication of invasive ventilation: Invasive ventilation should be used instead of standardized noninvasive ventilation, if the latter has been performed for 2 h but any of the following conditions occurs: ① oxygenation index still <150 mmHg; ② unobvious amelioration of dyspnea or distress; ③ rapid progression shown by chest imaging examination.

   Protective ventilation measures for ARDS should be performed to prevent barotrauma: ① low tidal volume: 6–8 ml/kg body weight; ② rationalized level of positive end-expiratory pressure (PEEP), which is generally 10–20 cm H_2O.

   Salvage treatment should be considered as soon as possible if satisfactory oxygenation level (SpO_2 <93%) cannot be achieved through measures above: ① Lung recruitment: Attention should be paid to barotrauma and its effect on circulation; ② Prone-position ventilation: Attention should be paid to effect on circulation by body position; ③ High frequency oscillatory ventilation, which is suitable for patients suffering from barotrauma; ④ extracorporeal membrane oxygenation (ECMO).

(IV) *Maintenance of water, electrolytes, and acid–base balance.*

For critically ill patients, 24-h intake/output should be recorded carefully to maintain the fluid balance. The patient can be kept in a state of slight insufficiency of body fluid to avoid heart failure, pulmonary edema, and ARDS.

Hypokalemia and hyponatremia may occur due to insufficient intake, and cautions should be made to correct them. Metabolic acid–base imbalance often occurs in severe patients, featuring most often respiratory acidosis. Respiratory alkalosis may appear possibly along with the increase of respiratory rate when hypoxemia occurs.

7.4 Antiviral Treatment

Effective antiviral treatment initiated early in sufficient dosage is of great importance to ameliorate the prognosis of patients [1].

Neuraminidase inhibitors used at present include Oseltamivir, Zanamivir, and Peramivir, and the latter can be given by injection in favor of the rescue for the patient in a coma.

(I) *Principle of medication with antivirus drugs*

1. Specimen from the respiratory tract should be collected as far as possible before initiation of antiviral medication, in order to clarify the pathogenic diagnosis.

2. Antiviral medication should be initiated without delay, as soon as the criteria of clinical diagnosis is met, without the need to await the results of the etiology test.
3. The better effect can be achieved by antiviral drugs if used within 48 h after onset. However, antiviral drugs can also be used in patients with more than 48 h of onset.
4. As for patients with severe diseases, the treatment course can be prolonged properly based on results of viral nucleic acid detected from respiratory secretion and the dosage can be increased appropriately considering the disease condition.

(II) Key users of antiviral drugs

1. Patients suffering from H5N1 and H7N9 subtypes of avian influenza
2. Close contacts (including medical practitioners) who manifest influenza-like symptoms, aggregation of influenza-like cases, and influenza-like cases with previous exposure to birds within 1 week
3. Presence of underlying diseases, such as chronic cardiac/pulmonary diseases, juvenile kids, the aged, and the pregnant
4. Influenza-like cases requiring antiviral medications based on clinical consideration and/or the rapid progression of the disease
5. Other cases of pneumonia of unknown origin

(III) Usage of neuraminidase inhibitors

1. Oseltamivir: The dosage for adults is 75 mg bid, successively for 5–7 days. The dosage can be doubled for those with severe disease and the treatment course can be prolonged appropriately. Children aged no less than 1 year can be dosed according to their body weight (dosage form of children is preferred).
2. Peramivir: Peramivir injection can be used for patients with severe diseases or those who cannot take medications orally. The dosage for the adult is 300–600 mg, Qd, intravenously. The conventional course of treatment lasts 5–7 days, which can be adjusted as required clinically.
3. Zanamivir: It is indicated to treat the population aged more than 7 years. The dosage is 10 mg per time divided by two inhalations, twice a day, with an interval of 12 h. It is not recommended for patients with severe disease or those with the complication.

7.5 Usage of Glucocorticoids and Immunomodulator

(I) *Application of glucocorticoids*

Human body under viral stimulation may produce a great amount of cytokines, resulting in the so-called "cytokine storm," causing a variety of cell damages, and inducing extensive pulmonary lesions and exudation [2, 3]. However, corticosteroids are still controversial. In general, we should weigh the advantages and disadvantages to decide whether to use it or not, and the dosage and course of treatment should also be individual. The dosage of methylprednisolone for adults can be 2–4 mg/kg day. The course of treatment should be short, 3–5 days is appropriate. When the clinical manifestations improved, the body temperature is normal for more than 3 days, symptoms improved or chest X-ray showed absorption of lung shadow, the drug can be reduced and stopped as soon as possible. It is not recommended to use it for a long time to avoid superinfection or other complications.

(II) *Application of immunomodulators*

A further investigation is needed for both efficacy and mechanism of immunomodulators in the treatment of avian influenza.

1. Immunoglobulin given intravenously: Incidence and duration of infection can be minimized through medication with intravenous immunoglobulin in patients with severe diseases; its combination with antibiotics may be in favor of the control of infection. An intravenous administration with a high dosage (10–20 g per day for 3–5 days) can be used in patients with severe disease.
2. Thymosin preparation: It can induce and improve differentiation, proliferation, and maturity of T lymphocytes. It can enhance phagocytosis and cytotoxicity of phagocytes. It can increase the activity of NK cells, and raise the activity of Th1 cells and cellular immunity. Preliminary observation showed a significant decrease of CD_4 and CD_8 T lymphocytes in patients infected with avian influenza. Therefore, the usage of thymosin preparation may have certain significance, though further researches are needed to clarify clinical efficacy.

(III) *Passive immunotherapy*

Immunological intervention is an important means to prevent and treat infectious diseases. Based on the different rationales, immunological intervention can be categorized into two types: the active and the passive. Active immunity is defined as the immune response to specific pathogens produced by the human body through vaccination or natural infection. Passive immunity refers to the immune response to specific pathogens through the input of antibodies, antiserum, or T cells. Vaccine is an effective way to prevent highly pathogenic avian influenza infection. A number of H5N1 and H7N9 vaccines, both domestic and abroad, have entered clinical trials, and it will take time for their application to clinical practice. It is noteworthy that the vaccine does not come into effect instantly, instead it usually takes several weeks from vaccination to a specific immune response sufficient in intensity, which makes the vaccine not suitable for clinical treatment of avian influenza in humans.

Unlike vaccination, passive immunization can take effect immediately after adoptive transfer, so it can be used as both an emergent preventive measure and a clinical treatment. Passive immunotherapy products commonly used include convalescent serum and virus-specific monoclonal antibodies. Convalescent serum refers to the serum products containing high-titer specific antibodies post to the recovery of infectious diseases, which can neutralize the virus in patients infected with avian influenza and help the recovery of critically ill patients. There is sufficient scientific experimental basis for the treatment of influenza with convalescent serum [4], and we also have the successful experience of using convalescent serum to rescue patients with severe avian influenza. In clinical practice, convalescent serum targets mainly patients with severe and critical illness. The dosage for adults is usually 200 ml of plasma, once every other day or 2–3 times a week. Due to its complex composition, convalescent serum seems often questionable for its efficacy and safety. In order to eliminate adverse factors, the specific monoclonal antibodies against avian influenza virus obtained by the latest technologies in immunology and genetic recombinant expression are gradually entering clinical application [5]. A number of monoclonal antibodies against H1, H3, H5, and H7 have entered clinical trials, and are anticipated to become a new method for treating severe avian influenza in humans.

7.6 Treatment of Systemic Inflammatory Response Syndrome and Multiple Organ Failure

For systemic inflammatory response syndrome (SIRS) and multiple organ dysfunction (MODS), etiological treatment, mechanism treatment, and symptomatic treatment should be adopted, and prevention should be emphasized and close cooperation among disciplines should be strengthened.

(I) *Active treatment of infectious complications*

Avian influenza patients are prone to secondary bacterial and fungal infections in the course of the disease, which is the initiating factor of SIRS and MODS. In principle, strong antibiotics or antifungal drugs should be used to control the infection in a short time. The selection of antibiotics should adhere to the principles of broad spectrum, sterilization, combination, and low toxicity. In order to achieve the best therapeutic effect, we should pay attention to pharmacokinetics and pharmacodynamics.

(II) *Application of glucocorticoids*

Proper glucocorticoids may be beneficial to the reversal of SIRS and MODS, but overuse of immunosuppressive agents can lead to infection and other complications, which may be life-threatening. Therefore, as mentioned above, the principle of individualization should be emphasized in using glucocorticoids.

(III) *Strict liquid management*

Hypovolemia is an important cause of hypotension and shock in SIRS patients. Correction of hypovolemia with appropriate volume expansion seems very important. Colloidal solutions such as albumin and dextran are often used for volume expansion.

As mentioned above, however, excessive volume loading should be avoided in patients with avian influenza receiving intravenous fluid infusion, lest lung injuries are aggravated. In 2006, a study based on the fluid management strategy in 1000 patients with acute lung injury [4] was published by ARDS Network Working Group, comparing the effects of different strategies of fluid management on the 60-day mortality of patients with acute lung injury in a 7-day treatment cycle. Results showed superiority of conservative liquid management over the free management group, concerning amelioration of pulmonary function, duration of mechanical ventilation, ICU stay, and extrapulmonary organ failure. This research supports the strategy of negative fluid balance implemented for ARDS patients.

(IV) *Protection of integrity of intestinal mucosa*

Ischemia, hypoxia, and injury of intestinal mucosa can lead to the release of a large number of inflammatory factors and promote SIRS and MODS. At the same time, with the decline of intestinal mucosal barrier function, the gut has become the source of endogenous infection, so we should pay attention to the integrity of intestinal mucosa. The most important thing is to restore the gastrointestinal diet as soon as possible and restore the integrity of the gastrointestinal mucosa. Gastric mucosal protectants and antioxidants such as vitamin E and cysteine can also be used.

(V) *Extracorporeal blood purification*

MODS often has endotoxin and inflammatory factor accumulation in the body, acid–base imbalance, water and electrolyte disorder, blood urea nitrogen, and creatinine accumulation. The above-mentioned renal replacement therapy can improve the blood disorder continuously. The mode should be chosen according to the specific situation of patients, e.g., hemodialysis should be considered for hypermetabolism, severe hyperkalemia, and metabolic acidosis; continuous veno-venous hemofiltration should be adopted for patients complicated with hypotension or shock; CRRT may ameliorate gas exchange parameters and myocardial contractility, relieve pulmonary interstitial edema, eliminate multiple inflammatory mediators from plasma, reduce visceral injuries and improve the survival rate of ARDS patients.

(VI) *Treatment of acute respiratory distress syndrome*

The patients infected with the avian influenza virus is easy to develop into acute lung injury (ALI) and acute respiratory distress syndrome (ARDS). Acute respiratory distress syndrome is one of the important causes of death in patients with human avian influenza.

1. Active control of infection and precipitating factors. Active antiviral treatment should be launched for avian influenza in humans. Active treatment of various infections and sepsis and active amelioration of cardiac function for those complicated with cardiac insufficiency should be carried out.
2. Attention should be paid to the control of liquid input and the maintenance of appropriate blood volume. Pulmonary edema both interstitial and alveolar is the main pathological change of ARDS. A slightly negative balance of intake/output is recommended under the prerequisite of ensured blood volume and effective perfusion, lest ARDS be induced. The estimation of the balance of fluid volume can be based on the measurement of central venous pressure.
3. Proper selection of mechanically assisted ventilation

   Two options of ventilation modes are available for ARDS.

   (1) Pressure-control ventilation (PCV): It is the mode commonly recommended now. Fixed maximum suction pressure (peak airway pressure) is set at 30~35 cmH_20. The initial PEEP is set at 8 cmH_20 and increased gradually according to disease situation up to an ideal level.

   (2) Mode of volume-control ventilation (VCV): low tidal volume (5~8 mL/kg) is set, with a lower preset pressure alarm limit (<35~40 cmH_2O) and the close monitoring of the airway platform pressure.
4. The use of vasoactive drugs and diuretics

   Diuretics or CRRT should be used to ameliorate pulmonary edema through ultrafiltration, in case of excessive fluid infusion or pulmonary edema. Swan–Ganz floating catheter of pulmonary artery is recommended for monitoring and evaluating the response.

   Continuous intravenous infusion of vasodilators such as Benazolin can be used. Prostaglandin E_1 and anisodamine can also be used for treatment.

   A research by Cochrane published in 2016 evaluated the influence of inhaled nitric oxide (NO) on mortality of ARDS patients, and the results showed that inhaled nitric oxide ameliorated oxygenation but did not lower the mortality of ARDS patients [5]. Also, the research compared the effects between inhaled Eporostrol and inhaled NO, showing the non-inferiority in inhaled Eporostrol to ameliorate oxygenation compared with inhaled NO, though there was no evidence implying the efficacy of inhaled Epoprostenol in lowering the mortality.
5. Use of corticosteroids

   The effect of corticosteroids seems ambiguous in treating acute respiratory distress syndrome. It has been proved by a rigorously controlled study that corticosteroids have no definite effect on the early treatment of or prevention from ARDS. In 2014, Ruan et al. [6] published a meta-analysis comprising eight randomized controlled trials and 10 cohort studies in evaluating corticosteroids in the treatment of ARDS, showing corticosteroids increased significantly the mortality of ARDS due to avian influenza in human.
6. Pulmonary surfactant

   There were abnormal pulmonary surfactants in ARDS. Surfactant replacement therapy in the treatment of ARDS can improve oxygenation, but meta-analysis showed that it cannot reduce the mortality of patients.
7. Prone-position ventilation

   The efficacy of prone-position ventilation in treating ARDS has been shown by lots of data. In 2013, Guerin et al. [7] published a PROSEVA research evaluating the effect of prone-position ventilation in moderate-severe ARDS patients, which found a lower 28-day mortality in the prone group than in the supine group. In addition, a protective ventilation strategy in combination with prone position might lower significantly 60-day mortality of ARDS patients, as shown by a meta-analysis.

(VII) *Treatment of septic shock*

Septic shock is one of the important causes of death in patients with avian influenza. Active volume expansion is the key measure to improve visceral blood perfusion and organ function, targeting at maintenance of blood perfusion of important organs and mean arterial pressure. The basic principle of capacity expansion is to be timely, sufficient, infusion first fast and then slow, saline first, then glucose solution, crystal and colloid supplement at the same time. Metabolic acidosis is often complicated in case of low volume and should be corrected actively. Sodium bicarbonate and sodium lactate solution are the alkaline drugs commonly used to correct acidosis. CRRT should be considered timely if lactic acidosis is complicated.

Vasoactive drugs, such as norepinephrine or dopamine, should be selected appropriately, in case of difficulty in maintaining or reaching the ideal level of blood pressure after volume expansion. The blood pressure should be monitored during the medication and the dosage should be adjusted in time.

(VIII) *Cardiac function support*

Viral myocarditis and toxic myocarditis are common in patients with avian influenza. When patients with avian influenza develop myocarditis, patients' activities should be strictly limited. In principle, they should rest in bed. It should be emphasized that nursing should be strengthened in order to reduce the burden of heart and oxygen consumption, so as to facilitate the recovery of damaged myocardium. Patients should eat easily digestible food, avoid overfeeding. Intermittent low-flow oxygen inhalation can be provided. Attention should be paid to the supplement of vitamin-energy compounds. Vitamin C and vitamin B can also be given. The use of glucose–insulin–potassium can restore the polarization of the cellular membrane of sick cardiomyocytes, and has a certain effect in protecting ischemic myocardium.

Immunosuppressants can treat acute myocarditis by inhibiting the immune response of T cells, which may be beneficial to some patients. Immunosuppressive agents commonly used include glucocorticoids. A short course of treatment was adopted. Cyclosporine and FK-506 have also been tried in clinic practice. However, the efficacy remains controversial.

Diuretics and vasodilators are the first choices for heart failure. Digitalis preparation should be used with caution. Vasoactive drugs such as dopamine and dobutamine can be given in case of cardiogenic shock. If conventional anti-shock management seems ineffective, mechanical auxiliary circulation should be used, such as intra-aortic balloon counterpulsation and partial or complete cardiopulmonary bypass, so as to help patients get through the dangerous period.

(IX) *Protection and maintenance of renal function*

During the treatment of severe human avian influenza, attention should be paid to the strategy of liquid management, focusing on the maintenance of effective blood volume and perfusion of important organs. Vasoactive drugs such as dopamine are permitted for patients with early damage of renal function, while nephrotoxic drugs should be avoided. Hemodialysis or continuous renal replacement therapy can be performed if renal function deteriorates further.

(X) *Focus on brain protection*

Oxygenotherapy should be given in time, as indicated above, to maintain a satisfactory level of blood oxygen. Attention should be paid to the maintenance of a steady internal environment, especially the steady blood pressure, so as to ensure the provision of blood and oxygen to the brain. Brain edema should be detected and treated in time. The head of the bed should be raised appropriately, and mannitol should be given for dehydration. In addition to the enhancement of symptomatic treatment, ice caps or ice blankets can be given to patients with high fever, and adrenocortical hormone can be given appropriately.

(XI) *Maintenance of coagulation function*

Disseminated intravascular coagulation (DIC) is one of the common complications of avian influenza in humans.

First of all, we should treat the primary disease and eliminate the precipitating factors, which are the key measures to terminate the pathological process of DIC. The treatment includes the active control of all kinds of infections, active correction of shock, amelioration of microcirculation, guarantee of blood perfusion of organs and tissues, especially vital organs, and correction of acid–base disturbance.

Active measures should be taken to supplement coagulation factors when DIC occurs, such as infusion of fresh plasma, platelets, fibrinogens, and prothrombin complexes.

Anticoagulant therapy with heparin can also be used as appropriate. Low molecular weight heparin (LMWH) shows better safety and better anti-DIC efficacy than that of unfractionated heparin. Given the consumption of a great deal of antithrombin III during DIC, the supplement of AT III preparations or blood products containing AT III components aiming to keep the concentration of AT III in plasma above 80% will give full play to the anticoagulation effects of heparin.

In the advanced stage of DIC, secondary fibrinolysis becomes the main cause of bleeding. Antifibrinolytic drugs can be used on the basis of heparinization, such as 6-aminohexanoic acid and antifibrinolytic aromatic acid.

(XII) *Application of extracorporeal membrane oxygenation (ECMO)*

Extracorporeal membrane oxygenation (ECMO), also called extracorporeal life support, is increasingly used in the treatment of severe respiratory failure [8].

Indications of ECMO: ARDS is the most common one. After positive mechanical ventilation treatment, including salvage treatment, satisfactory oxygenation is still not achieved, ECMO could be considered. When the peep was 15–20 cmH_2O, OI $\leq$ 80 mmHg and/or pH $\leq$ 7.2 (caused by respiratory acidosis) for more than 6 h, ECMO could be considered. Initiation of EMCO can be considered when expected mortality exceeds 50% (oxygenation index lower than 150 with Murray Score between 2 and 3, under the condition of concentration of inhaled oxygen higher than 90%). EMCO is generally considered in young patients with reversible respiratory failure, having received mechanical ventilation for less than 7 days.

Contraindications for ECMO include anatomical factors (severe obesity and difficult catheterization) and clinical factors (such as mechanical ventilation for more than 7 days and coagulation dysfunction). Relative contraindications include BMI >45, irreversible cerebral injuries, presence of contraindications for anticoagulation, bacteremia, vasculitis, pulmonary fibrosis, and MOF. Sepsis was considered as a contraindication of ECMO in the past, but it is not considered as a contraindication at present.

ECMO support mode: VV-ECMO is a support tool for respiratory failure, while VA-ECMO is a tool for heart support. When severe hypoxemia leads to acute pulmonary heart disease, patients with respiratory failure will need VA-ECMO support. Evaluation of cardiac function is the basis for determining selected ECMO. Before ECMO treatment, echocardiography is necessary. ARDS patients are often complicated with right heart failure, while echocardiography helps to determine whether the right heart failure is induced by hypoxia or reactive pulmonary hypertension.

Efficacy of ECMO in patients with severe avian influenza: Two groups of data from Italy and Australia showed the survival rates of 68% and 71%, respectively, in patients with ARDS caused by H1N1 influenza treated with ECMO. The exact efficacy needs to be clarified in further study.

References

1. Diagnostic and treatment protocol for human infections with avian influenza A (H7N9). 1st ed. 2017. National Health Commission of the People's Republic of China. http://www.nhc.gov.cn/yzygj/s3593g/201701/2dbdbc6e82dd4fdfa57508499f61cdfc.shtml
2. Short KR, Kroeze EJBV, Fouchier RAM, Kuiken T. Pathogenesis of influenza-induced acute respiratory distress syndrome. Lancet Infect Dis. 2014;14(1):57–69. https://doi.org/10.1016/S1473-3099(13)70286-X.
3. Zhang HX, Xie X, Zhang KJ, Hu J. A research on effect of cytokine storm in infection of influenza virus and its control. Chin J Cell Mol Immunol. 2013;29(5):556–9.
4. Virelizier JL. Rationale for treating human influenza infections by passive transfer of specific antibodies. Influenza Other Respir Viruses. 2007;1(2):61–4. https://doi.org/10.1111/j.1750-2659.2007.00012.x.
5. Salazar G, Zhang NY, Fu TM, An ZQ. Antibody therapies for the prevention and treatment of viral infections. NPJ Vaccines. 2017;2:19. https://doi.org/10.1038/s41541-017-0019-3. eCollection 2017
6. Ruan SY, Lin HH, Huang CT, Kuo PH, Wu HD, Yu CJ. Exploring the heterogeneity of effects of corticosteroids on acute respiratory distress syndrome: a systematic review and meta-analysis. Crit Care. 2014;18(2):R63. https://doi.org/10.1186/cc13819.
7. Guérin C. Prone position: the time of certainty. Réanimation. 2014;23:S394–8. https://doi.org/10.1007/s13546-013-0809-1.
8. Professional Committee of Extracorporeal Life Support of Chinese Medical Association. Expert consensus of adult extracorporeal membrane oxygenation circulation. Natl Med J China. 2018;98(12):886–94.

8 Complications and Image Findings

Yu-xin Shi, Xiu-dong Shi, Ling-wei Wang, Su Zhou, Wei-ya Shi, and Jin-ping Wu

Avian influenza in human, especially the severe type, progresses rapidly and causes multiple complications, such as acute lung injury, acute respiratory distress syndrome (ARDS), pulmonary hemorrhage, pleural effusion, pancytopenia, heart failure, renal failure, multiple organ failure, sepsis, shock, and Reye syndrome. The patients often die from severe pulmonary failure. Compared with adults, children suffering from avian influenza progress more rapidly and are more vulnerable to pneumothorax and secondary infection.

Compared with SARS, avian influenza in humans has faster progression, higher mortality, and easier complications of multiple organs, among which the most common one is respiratory failure.

8.1 Pulmonary Interstitial Fibrosis

Pulmonary fibrosis (PF) is the common complication of viral pneumonia caused by avian influenza in humans. This disease invades mainly pulmonary mesenchyma, and occasionally alveolar epithelial cells and pulmonary blood vessels, with a pathogenic mechanism involving inflammatory injury of pulmonary tissues, structural destruction, and tissue repair with aggregation of pulmonary mesenchymal cells. Viral pneumonia caused by avian influenza in humans is often complicated with respiratory symptoms such as dyspnea, cough, and expectoration. Imaging findings are of great importance in revealing lesions and observing their dynamic changes.

(I) Pathological changes

Hyperemia of capillaries of alveolar wall with significantly increased vascular permeability post to infection results in the entry of fibrin into the alveolar cavity and alveolar septum, with observable connection of cellulose network between adjacent cells. The organization within alveolar cavities and exfoliated cellular components are mixed and wrapped. There is thickening of the alveolar septum, with observable proliferation of fibroblasts and the formation of their clusters in some regions, which can improve the synthesis and deposition of extracellular matrix (ECM), and gradual formation of pulmonary fibrosis.

(II) Pathogenic mechanism

1. Immunology and pulmonary fibrosis

   Disturbance during any of the three stages including pulmonary injury, inflammation, and repair induces pulmonary fibrosis. The inflammation may induce dysfunction of cytokine secretion, whereby a biological healing can be converted to pathological fibrosis [1]. Cells producing the extracellular matrix of the fibroblasts are activated when pulmonary tissues are injured or subjected to harmful stimuli, and therefore excrete a great amount of extracellular matrix. The activation of fibroblasts continues, which excrete more ECM. Cytokines constantly cause inflammation in tissues and collagen overexpression with continuous ECM deposition, which gradually form PF, and finally lead to the loss of pulmonary function at the idiopathic site.

2. Cytokines and pulmonary fibrosis

   Interaction between cytokines and pulmonary tissue/cells, between inflammatory cells and

Y.-x. Shi (✉) · X.-d. Shi · W.-y. Shi
Department of Radiology, Shanghai Public Health Clinical Center, Shanghai, China

L.-w. Wang
Department of Respiratory and Critical Care Medicine, Shenzhen People's Hospital (The Second Clinical Medical College, Jinan University; The First Affiliated Hospital, Southern University of Science and Technology), Shenzhen Institute of Respiratory Diseases, Shenzhen, Guangdong, China

S. Zhou
Intervention Section, Shanghai Public Health Clinical Center, Shanghai, China

J.-p. Wu
Department of Radiology, Third People's Hospital of Changzhou, Changzhou, Jiangsu, China

C. Qiu et al. (eds.), *Avian Influenza in Human*, https://doi.org/10.1007/978-981-16-1429-3_8

between cytokines [2] can induce a series of complicated reactions, aggravates inflammations or immune injuries of pulmonary tissues, and stimulates further division and proliferation of fibroblasts, thereby improving the production and deposit of ECM. TGF-β, the most important factor inducing pulmonary fibrosis, plays its effect through Smads protein pathway. Other factors include IL, platelet-derived growth factor (PDGF), NF-KB, and MAPK, all of which are also factors inducing pulmonary fibrosis.

3. Some proteins correlate to the occurrence of PF, such as heat shock protein 47 (HSP47), epithelial transglutaminase 2 (TG2), Insulin-like growth factor binding protein-5 (IGFBP-5), etc.

(III) Clinical manifestation

The respiratory symptoms caused by PF are mainly shortness of breath and cough, in addition to chest tightness, fatigue, and palpitation observed in some of the patients, and dyspnea, dry cough and chest tightness in some patients with severe diseases. Absorption of pulmonary lesions is mostly slow, and fibrotic changes still remain in the lungs post to clinical cure [3]. In addition, it is common that clinical symptoms and findings in chest CT do not agree fully with each other, manifesting often relatively slow absorption of lesions, with only a trace of absorption of pulmonary lesions shown by chest CT scans post to significant amelioration of clinical symptoms. Fibrous hyperplasia happens possibly with various degrees in the lungs of patients who have not fully recovered post to clinical treatment, thereby forming chronic interstitial pneumonia. Moreover, follow-up of pulmonary function and chest imaging for the patients shows gradual absorption of pulmonary fibrosis over time, with obvious amelioration of pulmonary diffusion function and vital capacity.

(IV) Image findings

Pulmonary mesenchymal changes correlate to alveolar mesenchymal edema, obstructed lymphatic reflux in pulmonary septum, and exudation caused by avian influenza in humans. The image findings show the thickening of interlobular septum manifesting grid-like and striped changes [4]. In the early stage of the disease, lesions mainly included ground-glass opacities and consolidation in the lung field zone, mostly in the lower lung field. Findings in CT scans manifest patches or ground-glass opacities with blurred peripherals, and in some patients, mesenchymal changes [5]. During the absorption, the extent of the lesion shrinks, the density gradually dissipates and becomes lighter, and pulmonary consolidation undergoes reexpansion. Early absorption is observed in lesions occurring in the advanced stage as confirmed by some of the researches, in comparison with the delayed absorption of lesions occurring in the early stage or the progression stage.

It has been considered in some researches that some image findings in the early stage of viral infection suggest the mesenchyma of the alveolar sac and alveolar wall are involved by the lesions, manifesting thickened reticular opacities in interlobular and intralobular septa [6]. Similar image findings cannot be equated with pulmonary fibrosis, because they can also be induced by inflammation or edema. The reticular opacities may disappear in case of amelioration of disease.

The possibility of pulmonary fibrosis should be considered if these imaging findings persist. Despite an interval of only several months between rehabilitation and the acute stage, the pulmonary images manifest mainly ground-glass opacities, but the pathological basis for this manifestation might be different. For acute mesenchymal pneumonia, ground-glass opacities correlate to alveolar septal edema and formation of hyaline membrane in the acute exudative stage, and to hyperplasia of alveoli and septum and formation of hyaline membrane in the stage of proliferation and fibrosis. Pathologic changes of the lungs in the middle and advanced stages are characterized by hyperplasia of the alveolar septum and early fibrosis of alveoli. For patients with clinically pulmonary symptoms, chest CT and pulmonary function examination have a certain value in early detection of pulmonary fibrosis.

Pulmonary mesenchymal hyperplasia induced by viral infection occurs often in the middle and advanced stages of the disease course, with findings in chest CT scans including thickening of the interlobular septum, as well as opacities of streaks, networks, and subpleural arcs, which are distributed mostly in the outer zone of lung tissue [7]. The dynamic observation of images shows firstly consolidation as the intrapulmonary lesions, followed by high-density opacities in patches, networks, and streaks in the consolidations along with the progress of the disease. However, these signs cannot be used as reliable indicators for determining PF, as it has been found in some of the studies that the thickening of intralobular mesenchyma and interlobular septum may appear in the acute stage of the disease. Subpleural arc opacities may be the early change of pulmonary mesenchymal fibrosis, and the duration of its presence is related to the degree of pulmonary mesenchymal fibrosis. In patients complicated with pulmonary fibrosis, the main manifestations of chest CT in discharged patients include ground-glass opacities or grid opacities, which are mostly distributed in the subpleural parts or dorsum of both lungs. In addition, subpleural paraseptal emphysema and localized bronchiectasis can be observed in some cases. The degree of pulmonary fibrosis can progress in some discharged patients, which occurs mainly in the elderly or those with severe disease.

Pulmonary mesenchymal hyperplasia induced by viral infection usually occurs in the middle and advanced stages of the disease, and chest CT scans have important value in monitoring and evaluating the occurrence and development of the disease.

8.2 Secondary Pulmonary Infection

I. Secondary bacterial pneumonia

Patients with avian influenza are easily complicated with infection during the development of the disease, especially secondary bacterial pneumonia, which is also one of the main causes of death in avian influenza in humans.

Risk factors of secondary bacterial pneumonia in avian influenza in humans include senility, prolonged hospital stay, underlying diseases, invasive ventilation, and high dosage of glucocorticoids. Due to the low immunity both humoral and cellular in patients with avian influenza, the systemic immune system is in an inhibited or incompetent state, and its resistance to the outside world is significantly undermined. The increased alveolar exudation due to injuries of alveolar epithelium and pulmonary septal capillaries makes it easy for pathogenic bacteria to proliferate. Mechanic ventilation or some invasive procedures are often required for patients with severe diseases and the high dosage of glucocorticoids are the reasons predisposing them to secondary bacterial pneumonia [8].

The most common pathogens are *Streptococcus pneumoniae*, *Staphylococcus aureus* or *Haemophilus influenzae*, *Pseudomonas aeruginosa*, methicillin-resistant *Staphylococcus aureus* (MRSA), methicillin-resistant *Staphylococcus epidermidis* (MRSE), and *Stenotrophomonas maltophilia*, while mixed infection with multiple bacteria may also occur [9].

The clinical manifestations of secondary bacterial pneumonia in patients with avian influenza include gradual aggravation of the disease or repeated aggravation of clinical symptoms post to temporary amelioration [10], with high fever, severe cough, expectoration with purulent sputum, dyspnea, cyanosis, pulmonary moist crackles or signs of pulmonary consolidation, and increase of leukocyte count and neutrophil count [11]. Sputum is purulent, and the growth of pathogenic bacteria can be observed in sputum culture. Secondary bacteria pneumonia caused by avian influenza in humans may enlarge the scope of pulmonary lesions and prolong the course of the disease. The possibility of concurrent bacterial infection should be considered, once the disease aggravates in patients with avian influenza or clinical symptoms deteriorate further post to the ameliorated disease with manifestation of persistent fever, severe cough, and expectoration of purulent sputum. Bacterial culture of sputum and blood should be carried on, together with drug sensitivity test. According to the results of drug sensitivity, appropriate antibiotics were selected for timely treatment.

Image findings include patchy or spotty patches in the lungs, manifesting fusion and enlargement of the lesions with increased intensity. The previous ground-glass opacities are replaced by consolidations, with bronchiectasis. During the recovery of the disease, secondary bacterial pneumonia may make the pulmonary patchy opacities increase again [12].

Bacterial pneumonia can be complicated with pulmonary abscess, i.e., an inflammatory mass in the lungs with liquefactive necrosis in the center. Lung abscess invades often the airway, forming cavities through draining necrotic tissues. Common pathogens of lung abscess include anaerobes (clostridium and bacilli are the most common ones), *Staphylococcus aureus*, *Pseudomonas aeruginosa,* and pneumococcus. The image findings of pulmonary abscess include a single mass or multiple masses in a diameter of 2–6 cm complicated usually with cavities, whose inner walls can be smooth or rough, with commonly observable gas-liquid levels and consolidations of the adjacent lung tissues.

Pulmonary bullae is a thin-walled intrapulmonary air sac, which is a transient change commonly observed in acute pneumonia and probably caused by obstruction of airway due to blockage of check valve after local necrotic pulmonary tissues are drained out, making it impossible to exhale air during exhalation that has been inhaled into parenchymal space. Pulmonary bullae, observed most often in the recovery of pneumonia, show obvious enlargement of the cyst cavity after days or weeks and induces pneumothorax. Pulmonary bullae manifests often single or multiple thin-walled air-containing opacities, which are located often within pulmonary consolidations or ground-glass opacities. Pulmonary bullae often occur after the infection with *Staphylococcus aureus*, also in patients with other infections, such as pneumococcal pneumonia.

The great limitation of X-ray is the postponed finding in images preceded by the appearance of clinical symptoms, and the understanding of it is of great importance in treating the patients, who usually undergo chest X-ray within hours after the occurrence of symptoms, but there is no obvious abnormality in the results. CT scans, especially high-resolution CT scans, have high sensitivity in revealing pulmonary lesions in comparison with X-rays.

It is helpful to confirm the diagnosis of the patient with clinically suspected pneumonia but with chest X-ray seeming normal or not revealing any abnormality, and capable of evaluating complications with insignificant findings in X-rays, such as ground-glass opacities and cavities.

The main effect of images is to confirm the presence of parenchymal abnormalities consistent with clinical diagnosis, though the value of chest X-ray and CT is limited in defining the pathogenic microorganism. The confirmed diagnosis is dependent upon sputum detection, bronchoscopy, and biopsy with fine-needle aspiration.

II. *Secondary Fungi Infection*

Human avian influenza patients often have secondary fungal infections. Common pathogenic fungi inducing secondary fungal infection include *Cryptococcus neoformans*, actinomycetes, Mucor, and *Candida albicans*. Incidence of secondary fungal infection correlates to sex, age, presence/absence of underlying disease, nutrition, hospital stay, and dosage of glucocorticoids. The diagnosis can be established, based on the presence of symptoms and signs of fungal infection, positiveness of blood culture or the identification for at least two times of the same fungus in sputum, airway secretion, spinal fluid, and feces culture or identification by surgical pathology, and clinical and laboratory examination in consistent with the manifestation of fungal infection. Pulmonary pathological changes induced by fungus after entering lungs through the airway, blood circulation, or lymph has the diversity, manifesting mainly inflammation, necrosis, hemorrhage, abscess, and granulation, and it can induce pulmonary fibrosis in the advanced stage. Therefore, X-ray and CT findings are also characterized in the diversity, manifesting scattered small nodules in the lung, or patchy opacities in the middle and lower fields of both lungs, which can be not only intrapulmonary mass and cavitary changes, but also an extensive opacity of patchy fusions [13]. When intracranial fungal infection occurs, lesions in high, low, or mixed density will be observed in brain CT scans with homogeneous or heterogeneous enhancement in brain parenchyma, and sometimes granuloma and cystic changes may occur.

III. *Concurrent infection with Mycobacterium tuberculosis*

The possible recurrent tuberculosis should be paid attention to, in the case of concurrent tuberculosis in patients with avian influenza. Exudative lesions may appear at a site adjacent to the original lesion, forming possibly cavities including thin-wall, thick-wall, and tension cavities, with the thin-wall cavities as the most common ones. It can also form caseous pneumonia, involving one or more lung segments or lobes with one or more non-wall cavities inside, and bronchial dissemination can be seen in the rest of the lungs. Two or more lesions as above may be present simultaneously.

8.3 Pneumothorax and Mediastinal and Subcutaneous Emphysema

I. Pneumothorax

Pneumothorax is defined as the entry of air into the closed pleural cavity, inducing gas accumulation. It is often caused by the rupture of pulmonary tissue and visceral pleura or tiny emphysema adjacent to the surface of the lung due to underlying pulmonary diseases or external factors, which makes the air in the lungs and the bronchi enter into the pleural cavity. Pneumothorax can be also categorized into simple pneumothorax (also known as closed pneumothorax), communicating pneumothorax (also known as open pneumothorax), and high-pressure pneumothorax (also known as tension pneumothorax).

1. *Pathology and pathogenesis*

The rupture of pulmonary bullae or cysts can be caused by many factors, among which the primary ones include localized airway obstruction, mucus embolism, or bronchial stenosis caused by pneumonia. In the case of the intra-alveolar pressure greater than pulmonary mesenchymal pressure, the air will enter the mesenchyma through the ruptured alveoli and reaches to ipsilateral hilum along the bronchovascular bundle. The air may enter the pleural cavity through the mediastinal pleura to form pneumothorax if rupture occurs at the hilum. Another pathogenesis for pneumothorax is the direct access of air into the pleural cavity through ruptured alveoli, because of the necrosis of pulmonary tissues [14].

It has been shown by most studies that iatrogenic factors outnumber any other cause inducing secondary pneumothorax now. With the development of complex medical procedures and technologies for treating critical patients, iatrogenic injury of the chest is becoming more and more common. One of the important factors of iatrogenic pulmonary trauma is the increased use of equipment involved in positive pressure ventilation. Serious complications can be induced by catheterization, endotracheal intubation, thoracic drainage, and nasogastric feeding. Follow-up with chest X-ray, therefore, is very important post to treatment using equipment involved in positive-pressure ventilation. It has been found in some follow-up investigations that iatrogenic pneumothorax has an incidence exceeding that of spontaneous pneumothorax and a much higher mortality.

2. *Clinical manifestations*

   The severity of pneumothorax symptoms is related to the developing speed of pneumothorax, the degree of pulmonary compression, and the underlying lung diseases. The typical symptoms are sudden chest pain, which is persistent or transient, cutting or needle tingling, followed by chest tightness and dyspnea [15]. Some patients may have an irritating cough, which is caused by pleural stimulation by air. Obvious shortness of breath can be observed in most of the patients with sudden onset, large accumulation of air, or underlying pulmonary lesions. Middle-volume pneumothorax seldom induces discomforts in the youth or healthy populations. In the aged with pulmonary emphysema, however, it may cause significant dyspnea even if pulmonary tissue is compressed for less than 10%.

3. *Image findings and differential diagnosis*

   Pleura lines parallel to the chest wall can be observed in chest X-ray, but this sign is hard to differentiate from pulmonary bullae under certain circumstances. There is a certain difficulty in the differential diagnosis based on only chest X-ray between pneumothorax and cystic lung disease. The manifestations of pneumothorax are possibly covered up by complex contours of lungs or partial adhesion between lungs and chest walls caused by other reasons [16]. Chest CT scans are recommended if the presence of pneumothorax cannot be confirmed based on chest X-ray. In case of difficulty in differentiating lung bullae and pneumothorax in the apex of the lung, CT has a higher sensitivity compared with chest X-ray. Air between pulmonary tissue and chest wall observed in pleural cavity is of great importance to differentiate pneumothorax, pulmonary bullae, and cystic lung disease.

II. Mediastinal and subcutaneous emphysema

   Mediastinal emphysema is defined as the entry of air or any other gas into the mediastinal cavity. Air or gas may enter from mediastinal airway, ruptured alveoli, esophagus, or neck, and cases are reported occasionally about the access from abdominal cavity to mediastinal cavity. In rare cases, the gas may be originated from pneumogenic mediastinal infection.

   The most common reason for mediastinal emphysema is alveolar rupture, wherein the air reaches the mesenchyma around blood vessels or bronchi and enters the hilum and mediastinum through the mesenchyma. Alveolar rupture may be spontaneous or related to barotrauma (such as positive-pressure ventilation).

   Diseases related to spontaneous mediastinal emphysema include pneumonia, diabetic ketoacidosis, diffuse mesenchymal pulmonary fibrosis, etc. The trauma caused by Positive End-Expiratory Pressure Ventilation has long been considered to be the traumatic factor resulting in mediastinal emphysema in ICU patients and can induce extensive mediastinal and hypodermic emphysema. Compartment pneumothorax can be caused by mechanical ventilation applied to patients with acute lung injury or acute respiratory distress syndrome (ARDS).

1. *Pathology and pathogenesis*

   The pathophysiological characteristics of mediastinal emphysema vary with clinical conditions. Pathologically, there are communications from the mediastinum to many anatomical structures, including retropharyngeal space, submandibular space, and cervical vascular sheath. A tissue layer of the mediastinum extends forward through the sternal and costal attachment point of the diaphragm to the retroperitoneal space, which continues with the flank and extends to the pelvis. The mediastinum also communicates directly with the retroperitoneal space through the fascia around the aorta and esophagus.

   Spontaneous alveolar rupture is the most common cause of mediastinal emphysema. Sometimes, alveolar rupture is associated with severe underlying disease of the lungs. Air enters the subpleural connective tissue along the lobular septum in the mesenchyma tissue, forming pulmonary bullae on the surface of the lungs, or resulting in mediastinal emphysema when invading toward the mediastinum. Generally, spontaneous mediastinal emphysema occurs more commonly in healthy young men, and the sudden increase of alveolar pressure may result in alveolar rupture in peripheral regions of the lungs.

2. *Clinical manifestations*

   Clinical symptoms and signs of this disease correlate to volume of gas accumulation inside the mediastinum, rapidness of onset, the primary disease, and its complications. The patients with a large volume of mediastinal emphysema or rapid onset usually have manifestations including post-sternal pain, shortness of breath, and dyspnea due to mediastinal compression.

   Typical clinical manifestations of mediastinal emphysema include post-sternal pain, dyspnea, dysphagia, and weakness [17]. 80–90% of patients with spontaneous mediastinal emphysema have chest pain and most of them are youths, characterized in post-sternal pain with aggravation along with breath and posture changes; dyspnea exists in 50% of the patients. Main signs include subcutaneous emphysema of the neck and chest, with crepitus in palpitation. In addition, intra-mediastinal air often enters hypodermic tissue of the neck with a rustling sound when palpated.

However, an etiological differentiation should also be performed.

3. *Image findings and differential diagnosis*

Image findings of mediastinal emphysema are characterized by widened retrosternal space with increased transparency, and also strip opacities in gray-black density strip shadow distinguishing mediastinal pleura from the mediastinum, or focal vesicle or mass gas accumulation outlining the contour of mediastinal structure [18]. The abnormal gas in the mediastinum shows a vertical transparent strip on the side of mediastinal opacity. The parietal pleura is separated from the mediastinum to form a thin line parallel to the contour of the heart and mediastinum. Meanwhile, an air-band separates the heart from the mediastinum. This line is most obvious on the left, but easily ignorable. Besides, the boundary of the heart and contour of the aorta and thymus in the frontal view seems more obvious than the normal contour.

The transparent bands produced by air in the mediastinum seem usually clearer in lateral view. Sometimes, air around the bronchial sheath is shown by a chest X-ray. Various features of mediastinal emphysema shown by chest X-ray include continuous diaphragm sign, periarterial ring sign, and thymic sail sign. Thymic sail sign is defined as a crescent opacity of one lobe of the thyroid, which is moved and displaced by intra-mediastinal air. Continuous diaphragm sign refers to the distribution of intra-mediastinal air along the diaphragm and cardiac bottom, which makes the diaphragm center visible and connected with its lateral sides.

Air in pulmonary mesenchyma (mesenchymal emphysema) may form mediastinal emphysema, which is often caused by alveolar rupture and sometimes associated with severe underlying lung diseases, such as ARDS or pulmonary fibrosis. Abnormal gas accumulation can be revealed by CT scans very easily. The value and indication of CT scans are to evaluate images normal in chest X-ray or images without specific findings in patients suspected clinically of spontaneous barotrauma or appraise suspected complications in patients with ARDS or chest blunt injury.

The obvious displacement of the thymus exists in some cases so that its boundary can reach to chest wall. This finding may be confused with consolidation and atelectasis of the upper lung lobe. Extensive subcutaneous emphysema shown by chest X-ray may mask mediastinal pneumatosis, but it can be clearly shown on CT. The gas in the dilated esophagus on chest X-ray is occasionally similar to mediastinal emphysema, and its diagnosis can be confirmed based on CT scans. When a thin line parallel to the heart and mediastinum is observed at the left heart margin to separate the heart from the mediastinum, it is hard to differentiate between pneumopericardium and mediastinal emphysema based on chest X-ray. Under this circumstance, however, they can be differentiated using lateral-position projection.

8.4 Acute Respiratory Distress Syndrome

Acute respiratory distress syndrome is an acute respiratory failure characterized by progressive dyspnea and refractory hypoxemia. The pathology is mainly characterized by pulmonary edema rich in proteins and the formation of hyaline membrane induced by an increase of pulmonary microvascular permeability, which can be complicated with pulmonary mesenchymal fibrosis. Pathophysiological changes include mainly decreased pulmonary compliance, increased intrapulmonary shunt, and imbalance of ventilation/blood ratio.

I. *Pathological changes*

Congestion, edema, and lymphocyte infiltration of tracheal and bronchial mucosa are observed, with degeneration, necrosis, and exfoliation of fibroepithelial cells. Focal hemorrhage can be found in submucosa with edema and leukocyte infiltration, and there is fibrin exudate in alveoli containing neutrophils and lymphocytes. There is hemorrhage and hyaline membrane in the alveoli. Atelectasis may occur because of the increased tendency of collapsing of small airways caused by pulmonary mesenchymal edema and decrease of mesenchymal negative pressure, and collapsing and shutting of alveoli are observed, which are caused by the decrease of alveolar surfactants [19].

An autopsy report of a patient with a highly pathogenic avian influenza patient complicated with acute respiratory failure and ARDS in Jiangxi Province in China showed obvious congestion and edema in pulmonary sections. Histological findings show necrosis, exfoliation, and proliferation of some of the bronchiole and alveolar epithelium, and clumps of squamous epithelial metaplasia in alveolar cavities. There is a decrease of air contained in the alveoli, which are filled with multiple exudative components including serous, cellulose, erythrocytes, and neutrophils. Some alveolar cavities have obvious formation of hyaline membrane inside, some have exudate organization, and some show collapse and compensatory emphysema. Capillary thrombosis can be observed, together with mixed thrombosis in small blood vessels. There are also diffuse alveolar injuries in both lungs with secondary infection, disseminated intravascular coagulation (DIC), pulmonary hemorrhage, atelectasis, and compensatory pulmonary emphysema [19].

II. *Pathogenesis*

1. Damages induced by oxygen free radicals and reactive oxygen metabolites. A large amount of oxygen free radicals can be released post to infection in humans by highly pathogenic avian influenza. Oxygen-free radicals, one of the important inflammatory mediators, may drive polymorphonuclear neutrophils and alveolar macrophages to aggregate in the inflammatory region, activate them, and let them release lysosomal enzymes, which damage vascular endothelial cell membrane, cause organic damage of endothelial cellular layer and increase vascular permeability, thereby inducing pulmonary edema [20].
2. The effect of nitric oxide. In case of severe hypoxemia due to severe pulmonary injuries caused by highly pathogenic avian influenza in human, endogenous nitric oxide (NO) in pulmonary circulation can selectively antagonize hypoxic pulmonary vasoconstriction and supply blood flow to hypoxic alveoli, which results in the increase of venous admixture/total perfusion (total blood flow) ratio (Qva/Qt) and decrease of arterial oxygen partial pressure (PaO_2), thereby aggravating further hypoxia of tissues and cells [20].
3. Effect of endotoxin. Complement-mediated neutrophil activation and tissue injury can be enhanced by lipopolysaccharide (LPS)—endotoxin on bacterial cellular wall, in case of highly pathogenic avian influenza in humans complicated with Gram-negative bacterial infection. LPS may react with membrane receptors on monocytes and macrophages, i.e., lipopolysaccharide-binding protein (LBP) and CD14, inducing the production of inflammatory cytokines and other important cellular reactions [20].

III. *Clinical manifestations*

Typical symptoms of ARDS are progressive dyspnea and even distress, with a respiratory rate >30/min, which may accelerate progressively up to more than 60/min. There is no abnormal sign in the lungs, or small moist rales can be heard during inhalation. Arterial blood gas analysis shows the decrease of PaO_2 and $PaCO_2$. With the progress of the disease, patients may manifest respiratory distress and cyanosis, complicated often with irritability and anxiety. There is extensive mesenchymal infiltration of both lungs, complicated with azygos vein dilation, pleural reaction, or a small amount of effusion. Due to hyperventilation caused by obvious hypoxemia, $PaCO_2$ may decrease, and there may be respiratory alkalosis. The respiratory distress cannot be alleviated by normal oxygen therapy. If these diseases deteriorate further, respiratory distress and cyanosis go on aggravating, and multiple organ failure may occur [21].

IV. *The occurrence of ARDS in patients infected with highly pathogenic avian influenza*

H5N1 virus appearing in Southeastern Asia has a toxicity much higher than that of avian influenza viruses in other regions. The range of its hosts is extremely extensive, and it may predispose multiple animals to disease or even death, including wild or domestic birds, cats, rodents, and primates. Infection of H5N1 avian influenza in humans, occurring firstly in 1997 in Hongkong, may sicken mice, which is different from other H5 subtypes. Viral strains discovered since 2003 have stronger toxicity against mice and ferrets and are capable of inducing severe pulmonary diseases and infecting multiple organs outside the respiratory tract, including the brain [22].

Most of the patients infected with the H5N1 virus in Southeast Asia and Turkey develop severe lung disease with the exception of a few cases with mild symptoms. The patients are often complicated with fever, cough, and dyspnea. The primary viral pneumonia progresses rapidly, requiring generally mechanical ventilation within 48 h after admission. Unlike seasonal influenza, avian influenza infection in humans has an onset site more common in the lower respiratory tract than in the upper respiratory tract, higher viral titer in the pharynx than in nasal secretions, and faster progression into ARDS and multiple organ failure. ARDS occurred in 40% out of the 20 patients infected with H5N1 avian influenza in Hong Kong from 1997 to 2003. Though ARDS was not mentioned explicitly in clinical practice for 10 cases of H5N1 avian influenza in human occurring in Vietnam from December 2003 to January 2004, 9 out of these 10 cases had severe respiratory failure, with the mortality rate up to 80%, implying the high proportion of patients meeting the standard of ARDS. Cases in Thailand provided clinical data about children infected with the H5N1 virus, suggesting the probable progression of pulmonary infiltration in very few children, who deteriorated subsequently and manifested ARDS, while all patients with ARDS would surely die. It was shown by a retrospective clinical analysis on cases with H5N1 infection that the mean level of plasma tumor necrosis factor-α is about three times of that of healthy control. It was estimated that plasma tumor necrosis factor-α is probably partial reasons for sepsis, ARDS, and multiple organ failure occurring in patients infected with H5N1.

Stronger inflammatory reaction might be induced by H5N1 viral strain than by seasonal influenza virus, as shown by laboratory analysis. Significantly more tumor necrosis factor-α an interferon-β were produced by macrophages infected by virus in Hongkong in 1997 than by cells infected with H3N2or H1N1 seasonal influenza virus. Compared with H1N1, H5N1 viral strain may induce more secretion of interferon-inducible protein-10, interferon-β, interleukin-6, and chemokines by human bronchial epithelial cells and type-II alveolar cells. The opposite results were obtained in knockout mice; however, showing infection with H5N1 virus did not increase the secretion of tumor necrosis factor-α and interleukin-6, thereby not inducing the deaths of mice, or the lack of functional tumor necrosis factor receptor in mice themselves predispose them to milder diseases. No evidence showed that the strong inflammation observed in cases with H5N1 infection was the cause of the disease because glucocorticoid treatment could neither ameliorate the outcome of infection in mice nor change the fatal course in human infection. Therefore, the strong inflammatory response in H5N1 influenza is only the result of severe and extensive viral infection, though it constitutes an immunity imbalance or cytokine storm.

In the spring of 2013, a novel type of avian influenza virus (H7N9) occurred and spread in China. A research by the Chinese researcher [23] on clinical data in 111 patients with H7N9 infection confirmed based on laboratory tests found the new type H7N9 virus might induce severe diseases, such as pneumonia and ARDS; wherein 76.6% of patients were admitted into intensive care units and 27.0% of the patients died within 15 days post to the occurrence of symptoms.

V. *Application of images to ARDS*

1. *Chest X-ray*

Chest X-ray was applied at first to ARDS imaging, showing diffuse patchy opacities in both lungs [1]. X-ray is also very helpful to detect the dislocation of catheterization and complications related to it. Henschke et al. [24] analyzed prospectively the chest X-ray of more than 1100 patients in the intensive care unit (ICU). On average, each patient had 0.7 X-ray chest films per day, showing improper placement in 12% of tracheostomy cannula, and misplacement in 9% of central venous catheters. Significant changes were recorded in 44% of the examinations post to admission, and 65% of the cases showed new findings that affected the subsequent treatment of patients. Therefore, the authors concluded that the use of daily bedside chest X-rays seemed to provide useful information for patients with catheterization, and could detect quickly catheter abnormalities and evaluate disease progression, despite its limitation in technology. However, more meta-analyses and randomized open cross-over studies reported recently have concluded that non-selective routine chest X-rays can be canceled if it does not increase adverse consequences in ICU patients when doing so.

It is certain that chest X-ray is still the key measure for patients with ARDS. It has been shown by studies that digital bedside chest X-ray can predict changes of lung volume at different levels of positive end-expiratory pressure (PEEP) based on intensity changes shown by chest X-ray. Despite the advent of digitization, however, the role of chest X-ray in ARDS is not out of date.

2. *CT scans*

CT scans with their increasing use can monitor more precisely potential causes and complications of ARDS compared with chest X-ray, despite difficulties and risks for patients due to repeated access to ICU as required by CT scans.

In addition, CT scans may reveal the complex interaction among pathophysiology, lung parenchyma, and mechanical ventilation in ARDS, which is the consensus basis for treatment. First of all, CT proves that acute exudative lesions of ARDS are not distributed randomly, and there is a gravity-related gradient, predisposing hypostatic regions to more consolidations. Secondly, pulmonary ventilation can be evaluated based on visual analysis or CT value determination, which may identify four conditions: excessive dilation, normal ventilation, poor ventilation, and no inflation. The examination provides morphological and functional information for evaluating ventilation status, based on which the target positive end-expiratory pressure and tidal volume can be achieved. It is also helpful for setting ventilation parameters. In addition, CT scans can also evaluate the percentage of potential renewable lung, which varies in patients and correlates closely to the response to positive end-expiratory pressure.

3. *Pulmonary ultrasound*

Pulmonary ultrasound has a great advantage when applied to intensive care units. The main advantages of bedside pulmonary ultrasound include prevention from radiation exposure and avoidance of necessity to transport patients to the radiology department. Ultrasound is superior to auscultation and bedside chest X-ray in monitoring pathological changes of ARDS (pleural effusion, pulmonary consolidation, and mesenchymal syndrome). Pulmonary ultrasound detects "interstitial syndrome" accurately, it can be considered as pulmonary edema if some clinical criteria are met. Ultrasound can be used to differentiate cardiogenic edema and osmotic edema. More patchy opacities and Kerley B lines distributed unevenly may appear often in ARDS patients. A simple semi-quantitative method can be used to evaluate the Kerley B line and measure index of extravascular pulmonary edema.

VI. *Image findings of ARDS*

1. *Acute stage or exudative stage: week 1*

During hour 24–48 post to acute lung injury, chest X-ray may remain normal (latency) except for primary lung lesions. In the following 2–3 days, more and more patchy opacities in both lungs develop into diffuse consolidation, i.e., "white lung" observed in severe cases [25]. Pulmonary volume decreases progressively, and an air bronchogram is observable with a small amount of pleural effusion and diffuse "paving stone" sign. It is prone to the distribution in peripheral lungs, compared to cardiac edema. The gravity gradient usually observed in CT scans is helpful to differentiate the concurrent pulmonary infection [26].

In typical ARDS, diffuse ground-glass opacities can be seen on CT scans, and there are more consolidations in dorsal regions (i.e., hypostatic regions) because of the gravity gradient. Pulmonary parenchyma, normal or over dilated, can be observed in the non-hypostatic regions, during mechanic ventilation. Non-typical ARDS is characterized by the consolidation in the anterior pulmonary region in a supine position, which can be observed in about 5% of the patients and caused by the difference between various ventilation regions [27].

2. *Metaphase or proliferative stage: week 2*

The image findings at this stage are quite stable, except for the advent of iatrogenic complications or new pulmonary infections. Reticular opacities may overlap ground-glass opacities, but they are not a reliable marker of fibrosis, as reticular opacities may disappear later. Early fibrosis can be suggested by patchy opacities or ground-glass opacities complicated with bronchiectasis during this stage, or by pulmonary hypertension (dilatation of pulmonary artery and the right ventricle) [28]. Repeated exudation may lead to mixed image findings.

3. *Advanced stage or fibrosis stage: beyond week 2*

The final results in the survivors may be normal lungs or coarse reticular opacities with a reduction of lung volume. More than 70% of the patients during 6-month follow-up manifest abnormal CT findings, with common responses characterized in fibroblast proliferation post to pulmonary injuries. Appropriate fibroproliferative response may have a positive effect on pulmonary repair, while excessive one is obviously harmful. Bronchoscopy, bronchoalveolar lavage, and CT scan can provide useful information for early detection of fibroproliferation [29].

Findings in CT scans are characterized by persistent ground-glass opacities complicated with thick reticular opacities, air sacs, and pulmonary bullae, which are distributed mainly in the central sector of the lungs. Severer pulmonary fibrosis may exist in patients with prolonged mechanical ventilation with high positive end-expiratory pressure. The antedisplacement of fibrosis may be related to ventilator-induced lung injury involving mechanical ventilation injury or oxygen poisoning, while pulmonary fibrosis in the gravity-dependent area is not obvious, with partial reasons for the protection by atelectasis and consolidation. It was reported by the latest study, however, that only one-third of the cases manifested the "typical" distribution, while most cases had diffuse distribution, and very few cases showed mainly dorsal distribution [30].

In addition, the advent of capillary bronchiectasis or bronchiectasis in high-density areas shown by CT scans indicates the transition of pulmonary diffuse injuries from the exudation to fiber proliferation and fibrosis. During this period, the lung parenchyma undergoes remodeling of pulmonary fibrosis. The degrees of changes of thick reticular opacities are closely related to pulmonary fibrosis images of CT scans; the distortion of airway structure and bronchiectasis correlate to the duration of pressure-controlled inverse proportional ventilation. Fiber proliferation shown by high-resolution CT (HRCT) can be used to evaluate prognosis [30]. Changes in extensive fibroproliferative images shown by high-resolution CT are independent predictors of poor prognosis of early ARDS. The precise determination of disease stage by HRCT is helpful to monitor pulmonary injures related to ventilator, and define responses to treatment in ARDS patients.

CT is superior to X-ray in detecting complications. About 40% of pneumothorax and 80% of mediastinal emphysema detectable by CT are missed in findings of chest X-ray. Pleural effusion and lung abscess can be detected more easily by CT than by chest X-ray.

It is easy to differentiate between osmotic pulmonary edema and cardiogenic pulmonary edema both clinically and based on image findings. The most characteristic image findings of osmotic pulmonary edema are patchy exudative opacities dominated with peripheral distribution, accompanied by air bronchogram, possibly interlobular septal thickening, and a small amount of pleural effusion [31]. The image findings of cardiogenic pulmonary edema are characterized in enlargement of heart opacity, redistribution of pulmonary blood vessels (usually the increase and thickening of vessels in the upper lung field, in contrast to thinning of those in the lower field), edema-exudation opacities distributed mainly in hilum appearing "butterfly wing sign," accompanied by thickening of the interlobular septum and pleural effusion [27]. The accuracy is 80% ~ 90% in identifying cardiogenic pulmonary edema, and 60% ~ 90% in identifying osmotic pulmonary edema, based on the combined imaging findings.

8.5 Reye Syndrome

Reye Syndrome (RS), i.e., encephalopathy-liver fatty metamorphosis syndrome, is a disease characterized by severe encephalopathy complicated with acute cerebral edema, and massive fatty infiltration of the liver and its nature is acute mitochondrial injuries. This disease features the acute onset, fast progression, and occurrence of 90% in children younger than 14 years [32, 33]. The etiology of RS remains unknown and is considered by most studies to be related to multiple factors, such as poisoning, viral infection, mitochondrial damage, abnormal lipid metabolism, heredity, etc. Now it is considered that RS is not only a special clinical disease, but also a comprehensive description of a group of different diseases, including poisoning, infection, metabolism, etc., featuring the main clinical symptoms such as liver dysfunction and metabolic encephalopathy, and manifesting mainly acute onset of consciousness disorder and abnormal liver function. Key points in treatment for RS lie in timely reduction of intracranial pressure, elimination of cerebral edema, and symptomatic treatment.

I. *Pathogenic mechanism and pathological change*

Mitochondrial functional injury is the nature of RS, wherein the abnormal systemic lipid metabolism induces acute non-inflammatory cerebral edema and fatty degeneration of multiple tissues and organs [34]. The most characteristic one among all these is ultrastructural changes of hepatocytes, and its nature is mitochondrial functional injury, with the main reasons including disorders in mitochondrial chemical microenvironment and the inhibition of oxidative phosphorylation, which cause multiple clinical manifestations of RS such as important systemic metabolic disorders of lipid acids, amino acids, and glycogen. Cerebral changes include obvious edema of nerve cells and glial cells with vacuolar degeneration of myelin, showing diffuse cerebral edema, without inflammatory changes in meninges and brain parenchyma.

II. *Clinical manifestations*

The onset of RS in most patients is preceded by precursor symptoms for 1 week and even up to 20 days to 4 months, such as infection in the respiratory tract or digestive tract, followed by symptoms in the nervous system such as consciousness disorders and convulsions complicated with abnormal hepatic function and metabolism disorders. The patients manifest mainly severe headache and frequent vomiting, complicated with progressive deterioration of consciousness, without obvious abnormalities concerning meningeal irritation sign and cerebrospinal fluid examination [35]. The liver is swollen and touches tough or hard, accompanied by obvious abnormal liver function, such as the increase of total leukocytes and neutrophils, and the elevation of transaminase, ammonia, and free fatty acid in blood. Degeneration and necrosis of cerebral cells can cause brain edema, followed by secondary brain hernia. Severe hepatocyte injuries and mitochondrial abnormalities may induce also fatty acidemia, organic acidemia, and lactic acidosis as well as hyperammonemia, which will aggravate cerebral edema and induce clinically convulsion, hyperspasmia, consciousness disorder, and coma. Hepatic functional disorders in various degrees occur in all RS patients, including the increase of serum alanine aminotransferase (ALT), aspartate aminotransferase (AST), lactate dehydrogenase (LDH), and blood ammonia. A mild or moderate increase of liver volume may occur, with a texture touching tough or even slightly harder.

Now the clinical diagnosis of RS can be based on the reference to the following four items: ① acute encephalopathy; ② simultaneous transient abnormal liver function; ③ hepatic steatosis; ④ the above clinical manifestations that cannot be explained by other reasons.

III. *Image findings*

Diffuse edema in white matter and ventricular compression can be observed in CT scans. The manifestations of brain white matter should be differentiated with adrenal leukoencephalopathy, multiple sclerosis, progressive multifocal leukoencephalopathy, and hypoxic encephalopathy [36, 37]. CT scans are indispensable for diagnosing Reye Syndrome, because of the non-specificity of its findings.

8.6 Other Complications

I. Cardiovascular complications

Main pathological changes induced by the avian influenza virus invading the myocardium include myocardial hemorrhage, degeneration, and necrosis. The virus may induce myocarditis, the reduction of myocardial contractility and cardiac output, poor tissue perfusion, and slow blood flow, thereby resulting in hypoxia in various tissues and organs and obvious exudation of vascular tissues. The increased concentration of tumor necrosis factor in case of acute myocarditis inhibits myocardial contractibility, decreases blood pressure, and aggravate pulmonary edema, in addition to its effect to injure endothelial cells, enhance expression of tissue factors and stimulate the synthesis [38]. Tumor necrosis factors produced by myocardial cells are sufficient in inducing myocarditis, cardiac insufficiency, heart failure, or fetal death [39]. Strong oxidative damage to cells by superoxide anion due to the increased oxygen free radicals results in the decrease of oxygen uptake capacity by tissues and disturbance in its utilization by cells, disorders in the metabolism of various nutrients including glucose, fat and proteins, accumulation of lactic acid, metabolic acidosis and aggravation of organ dysfunctions.

The main pathological changes in vascular tissues induced by human avian influenza virus infection are mainly the degeneration, necrosis, and even exfoliation of vascular endothelial cells, forming a rough surface locally, which is the pathological basis inducing platelet adhesion [40]. As the result, it causes damages to the endothelial barrier of capillary venules, with the increase of permeability of vascular wall, tissue edema, and even congestion. Blood having returned to both ventricles cannot be output completely post to the damage of heart function by avian influenza virus, thereby increasing significantly the central venous pressure, reducing cardiac output, and predisposing the microcirculation to the tendency to “congestion state” [41]. Meanwhile, arterial blood pressure drops and tissue perfusion decreases due to the dramatic drop in cardiac output. The significantly reduced velocity of blood in microcirculation with increased viscosity, agglutination of erythrocytes, and adhesion of leukocytes onto microvascular wall, especially in the venous vessels, increases further the resistance of the outflow tract of microcirculation and slows down further its velocity. The further decrease of microcirculatory perfusion reduces dramatically blood perfusion for microcirculation of organs and causes even the absence of perfusion, thereby inducing further pathological changes of degeneration and necrosis of organs and tissues [41].

In summary, cardiac function is undermined because of the damage of the myocardium by the avian influenza virus. Meanwhile, virus effecting upon vascular endothelial cells results in extensive hemorrhage and disturbance of microcirculation.

The clinical course of influenza-associated myocarditis differs, varying in severity from the asymptomatic to the severe. Most patients develop acute cardiac dysfunction including chest pain, dyspnea, syncope, hypotension, and arrhythmia on days 4 to 7 post to the initial symptoms of viral infection [42]. Only 8% of the patients manifest symptoms within 10 days post to the initial symptoms induced by the virus [43]. Bradycardia and mild to moderate increase of myocardial enzymes such as CPK and LDH may appear in 20–40% of patients, and those with severe diseases may have increased heart rate and hypotension and progress into shock.

Characteristic changes in histopathology including cell infiltration and myocyte necrosis can be observed in about 30%–50% of the fatal cases of avian influenza in humans [44]. In addition, myocarditis related to influenza occurs often in patients without previous severe respiratory complications.

Complications possibly occurring in myocarditis include heart failure, cardiac arrhythmia, pericardial effusion, and pericardial tamponade. Congestive heart failure is the most common complication, occurring in 84% of patients. Symptoms often appear on day 10–18 during the disease course, including an increase in heart rate, sinus tachycardia, and acute heart failure, and the patient may die from heart failure or peripheral circulation. Right ventricular dysfunction is more common than the left one. More than half of patients need cardiac support, including intra-aortic balloon pump (IABP), percutaneous cardiopulmonary support, extracorporeal membrane oxygenation, and ventricular assist devices.

II. *Complications of nervous system*

Some avian influenza in humans can be complicated with encephalopathy or encephalitis, i.e., rapidly progressive encephalopathy characterized by the progression into impaired consciousness within a few days of infection. There are many different clinical symptoms, including acute necrotizing encephalopathy (ANE), acute encephalopathy with biphasic seizures and late reduced diffusion (AESD), and reversible mild encephalitis/encephalopathy. ANE is a fulminant complication characterized by multiple cerebral lesions, often involving the thalamus. AESD is characterized in biphasic course, high fever with convulsion, and lesions in brain white matter. Influenza encephalopathy and associated neuropsychiatric syndrome are usually characterized in lesions in the splenium of the corpus callosum, a mild course, and a good prognosis [45]. CT findings of acute necrotic encephalopathy in the brain include patchy low-density opacities, focal or diffuse edema, thrombosis in the superior sagittal sinus, and cerebral hematoma. Its MRI findings are the abnormal signals in the cortex, white matter, or brain stem.

III. *Complications in musculoskeletal system*

Some patients with avian influenza may be complicated with myositis. Based on reports, myositis-related symptoms might appear in a week post to the onset of respiratory symptoms in about 90% of patients, manifesting obvious tenderness of the affected muscles, or weakness and inability to stand, with muscle involvement of the lower limbs commonly observed.

Rhabdomyolysis, occurring possibly in severe cases, is an uncommon but very serious complication. Myoglobinuria often occurs and results in renal failure. The diagnosis of rhabdomyolysis depends upon biopsy, which features necrosis, regeneration, and edema in various degrees. Despite the increased level of creatine kinase in all patients, the rise correlates generally to a poor prognosis. The increase of creatine kinase correlates also to mechanical ventilation and prolonged ICU stay [46].

IV. *Ophthalmological complications*

Eye diseases may be caused by the direct conjunctival invasion by the avian influenza virus, and the most common one is conjunctivitis, followed by retinopathy, uveal leakage syndrome, and optic neuritis [47]. These subtypes, especially subtype H7 avian influenza virus besides H7N9, manifest obvious eye susceptibility, compared with other influenza viral stains. In the outbreak of avian influenza (H7N7) in the Netherlands, 91% of patients showed only conjunctivitis, and 6% showed influenza-like conjunctivitis [47]. Conjunctivitis symptoms appeared in two patients during the pandemic of highly pathogenic avian influenza (H7N3) in Mexico and British Columbia, who were diagnosed as avian influenza in humans [48]. A study carried out in 194 subjects during an outbreak of avian influenza H7N7 in humans in the Netherlands concluded that preventive medication with Oseltamivir reduced significantly the risk, implying the possible efficacy of Oseltamivir in treating influenza-related conjunctivitis. Also, researches on mice models suggested that Oseltamivir decreased replication of viruses H7N7 and H7N3 in the eyes and respiratory system [49].

V. *Urinary complications*

Avian influenza in humans may also influence renal functions, and its complications include acute renal injury, acute glomerulonephritis, minimal glomerular lesions, and acute tubulointerstitial nephritis.

A great amount of proteinuria (>3 g/L) may appear in some patients with severe avian influenza in humans at the onset of the disease, and there are no hematuria, oliguria, and urinary tract irritation symptoms, despite the presence of abnormalities of serum creatinine and urea nitrogen. The reduction of urine-specific gravity and polyuria can also appear in the early stage of the disease, with erythrocytes and tube types observable in urine [50].

The potential pathogenesis of kidney injury is likely to be multifactorial. In addition to renal injury mediated by rhabdomyolysis, it may be secondary to sepsis with a reduction of blood volume and renal perfusion, thereby resulting in acute tubular necrosis. Another hypothesis is the direct renal damage by viruses, though there is little evidence supporting this mechanism [51].

VI. *Liver injury*

Abnormal liver function is complicated in 60–70% of avian influenza in humans, as reported by literatures, manifesting the slight increase of ALT and AST. Almost 100% of Chinese patients with avian influenza have abnormalities in hepatic function, manifesting a mild to moderate increase of transaminase, or moderate jaundice in some of the patients. The elevation of transaminase is more common in cases of highly pathogenic avian influenza in humans, as shown by literature [52], occupying 60% and 66% of patients infected with H5N1 and H7N9, respectively. Abnormal liver function appears usually in weeks 2–3 during the course. However, there is no report on liver failure in patients with avian influenza.

Autopsy of virus-induced fatal cases shows the presence of viral particles in endothelial cells, sinusoidal endothelial cells, and hepatic macrophages. The evidence for virus invading liver cells, however, has no reliable confirmation. Hepatitis may be the result of indirect damage to the systemic immune system or a reaction to medication during the treatment. A study on 11 patients with H7N9 virus infection showed that AST level correlated significantly to Th2 cytokines IL-4 and IL-9. Both the lack of influenza virus antigen in liver cells and the correlation between hepatic examination and systemic inflammation markers including CRP suggest that virus-related potential pathogenic mechanism for liver diseases is probably the result of systemic inflammation [53].

References

1. Pan Y, Huang W, Shen Z, et al. Research progression in pathogenic mechanism and treatment of pulmonary fibrosis. Chin J Pharm. 2012;47(23):1873–6.
2. He Y, Deng G, Gao T. Research progression in mechanism of cytokines in pulmonary fibrosis. Chin J Trauma. 2006;22(6):477–80.
3. Sun B, Meng Z, Hong Y, et al. An analysis of images and pulmonary function in follow up of 7 patients with pneumonia of H7N9 avian influenza. J Clin Pulmon Med. 2016;21(5):927–9.
4. Chen X, Li L, Cao J. Value of CT and MRI in diagnosing pulmonary fibrosis. Chin J CT MRI. 2015;13(8):36–9.
5. Lu P, Zheng Z, Zheng P, et al. Profiles of imaging findings and dynamic variation in severe pneumonia induced by H7N9 avian influenza in human. Radiol Pract. 2014;29(7):740–4.
6. Bin Su. A research on mechanism of pulmonary fibrosis during recovery stage of SARS. 2005.
7. Wang Q, Zhang Z, Shi Y, et al. Emerging H7N9 influenza A (novel reassortant avian-origin) pneumonia: radiologic findings. Radiology. 2013;268(3):882–9.
8. Kash JC, Taubenberger JK. The role of viral, host, and secondary bacterial factors in influenza pathogenesis. Am J Pathol. 2015;85(6):1528–36.

9. Morris DE, Cleary DW, Clarke SC. Secondary bacterial infections associated with influenza pandemics. Front Microbiol. 2017;23(8):1041.
10. Song JY, Cheong HJ, Heo JY, et al. Clinical, laboratory and radiologic characteristics of 2009 pandemic influenza A/H1N1 pneumonia: primary influenza pneumonia versus concomitant/ secondary bacterial pneumonia. Influenza Other Respir Viruses. 2011;5(6):e535–43.
11. Puzelli S, Di Trani L, Fabiani C, et al. Serological analysis of serum samples from humans exposed to avian H7 influenza viruses in Italy between 1999 and 2003. J Infect Dis. 2003;192:1318–22.
12. Lee CW, Seo JB, Song JW, et al. Pulmonary complication of novel influenza A (H1N1) infection: imaging features in two patients. Korean J Radiol. 2009;10(6):531–4.
13. Chen X, Wang Q, Ni F, et al. A case of pulmonary cryptococcosis secondary to severe H7N9 avian influenza in human. Chin J Tuberculosis Respirat Dis. 2016;39(7):558–61.
14. Zhao F, Zhang Z. An analysis on 25 cases of subcutaneous emphysema, mediastinal emphysema and pneumothorax. Beijing Med. 1997;1:32–3.
15. Ge L, He J, Qiu Y, et al. Prevention and treatment of SARS complicated with mediastinal emphysema and pneumothorax. Chin J Thorac Vas Surg. 2004;20(3):141.
16. Zheng Y, Deng J, Lu Z, et al. An analysis on 8 cases of plastic bronchitis induced by influenza A H1N1. Chin J Pediat. 2012;50(7):521–4.
17. Gao C, Jin H, Wu L, et al. An analysis on 35 cases of mediastinal emphysema. Chin J Misdiagnost. 2006;6(12):2366.
18. Yin J, Li K, Li S, et al. An analysis on images of thoracic complications of SARS. J Capital Med Univ. 2003;24(4):401–4.
19. Nash G. Pathology of ARDS. West J Med. 1979;130(3):220–2.
20. Short KR, Kroeze EJBV, Fouchier RAM, et al. Pathogenesis of influenza-induced acute respiratory distress syndrome. Lancet Infect Dis. 2014;14(1):57–69.
21. Li H, Weng H, Lan C, et al. Comparison of patients with avian influenza A (H7N9) and influenza A (H1N1) complicated by acute respiratory distress syndrome. Medicine (Baltimore). 2018;97(12):e0194.
22. Carter MJ. A rationale for using steroids in the treatment of severe cases of H5N1 avian influenza. J Med Microbiol. 2007;56(Pt7):875–83.
23. Gao HN, Lu HZ, Cao B, et al. Clinical findings in 111 cases of influenza A (H7N9) virus infection. N Engl J Med. 2013;368(24):2277–85.
24. Henschke C, Pasternack G, Schroeder S, et al. Bedside chest radiography: diagnostic efficacy. Radiology. 1983;149:23–6.
25. Eisenhuber E, Schaefer-Prokop C, Prosch H, et al. Bedside chest radiography. Respir Care. 2012;57:427–43.
26. Winer-Muram HT, Steiner RM, Gurney JW, et al. Ventilator-associated pneumonia in patients with adult respiratory distress syndrome: CT evaluation. Radiology. 1998;208:193–9.
27. Gluecker T, Capasso P, Schnyder P, et al. Clinical and radiologic features of pulmonary edema. Radiographics. 1999;19:1507–31.
28. Chung JH, Kradin RL, Greene RE, et al. CT predictors of mortality in pathology confirmed ARDS. Eur Radiol. 2011;21:730–7.
29. Burnham EL, Janssen WJ, Riches DW, et al. The fibroproliferative response in acute respiratory distress syndrome: mechanisms and clinical significance. Eur Respir J. 2014;43:276–85.
30. Masclans JR, Roca O, Munoz X, et al. Quality of life, pulmonary function, and tomographic scan abnormalities after ARDS. Chest. 2011;139:1340–6.
31. Caironi P, Carlesso E, Gattinoni L. Radiological imaging in acute lung injury and acute respiratory distress syndrome. Semin Respir Crit Care Med. 2006;27(4):404–15.
32. Luo S, Xi W. Reye syndrome. Jiangxi Med J. 1993;28(1):58–60.
33. Liu J, Bao C. What is Reye syndrome? Chin Gen Pract. 2006;9(24):2055.
34. Yao D, Huang F, Meng X. A research on mechanism of Reye syndrome in inducing hepatic and cerebral injuries. J Gastroenterol Hepatol. 2005;14(3):324–6.
35. Mao L, Wang X, Fei G, et al. Reye syndrome: clinical and imaging manifestations. Chin Comput Med Imag. 2009;15(6):580–2.
36. Bai C, Jiao X. CT diagnosis for Reye syndrome. Chin J Radiol. 1997;6:414–5.
37. Ruskin JA, Haughton VM. CT findings in adult Reye syndrome. Am J Neuroradiol. 1985;6(3):446–7.
38. Sun Y, Ma S, Wang L. Determination of concentration of tumor necrosis factor and interleukin-6 in patients with myocarditis and cardiomyopathy. Chin Circ J. 1998;6(13):367–8.
39. Key NS, Vercellotti GM, Winkelmann JC, et al. Infection of vascular EC with herpes virus enhances tissue factor activity and reduces thrombomodulin expression. Proc Natl Acad Sic USA. 1990;87(18):7095–9.
40. Jin H. Specific regulation on microcirculation under normal and pathological condition and its clinical significance. Chin J Pathophysiol. 1987;3(1):43–6.
41. Zhu X, Fusheng G, Shen L, et al. An observational research on microcirculatory function in patients with acute myocardial infarction. J Capital Med Univ. 1996;17(1):44–8.
42. Onitsuka H, Imamura T, Miyamoto N, et al. Clinical manifestations of influenza a myocarditis during the influenza epidemic of winter 1998-1999. J Cardiol. 2001;37:315–24.
43. Dahdouh Z, Roule V, Lognoné T, et al. Atrial septostomy in cardiogenic shock related to H1N1 infection. Acute Card Care. 2012;15:7–9.
44. Paddock CD, Liu L, Denison AM, et al. Myocardial injury and bacterial pneumonia contribute to the pathogenesis of fatal influenza Bvirus infection. J Infect Dis. 2012;205:895–905.
45. Mizuguchi M. Influenza encephalopathy and related neuropsychiatric syndromes. Influenza Other Respir Viruses. 2013;7:67–71.
46. Mansour DE, El-Shazly AA, Elawamry AI, et al. Comparison of ocular findings in patients with H1N1 influenza infection versus patients receiving influenza vaccine during a pandemic. Ophthalmic Res. 2012;48:134–8.
47. Koopmans M, Wilbrink B, Conyn M, et al. Transmission of H7N7 avian influenza A virus to human beings during a large outbreak in commercial poultry farms in the Netherlands. Lancet. 2004;363:587–93.
48. Tweed SA, Skowronski DM, David ST, et al. Human illness from avian influenza H7N3, British Columbia. Emerg Infect Dis. 2004;10:2196–9.
49. Belser JA, Sleeman K, Pearce MB, et al. Oseltamivir inhibits H7 influenza virus replication in mice inoculated by the ocular route. Antimicrob Agents Chemother. 2012;56:1616–8.
50. Bagshaw SM, Sood MM, Long J, Fowler RA, et al. Acute kidney injury among critically ill patients with pandemic H1N1 influenza A in Canada: cohort study. BMC Nephrol. 2013;14:123.
51. Carmona F, Carlotti AP, Ramalho LN, et al. Evidence of renal infection in fatal cases of 2009 pandemic influenza A (H1N1). Am J Clin Pathol. 2011;136:416–23.
52. Gao H-N, Lu H-Z, Cao B, et al. Clinical findings in 111 cases of influenza a (H7N9) virus infection. N Engl J Med. 2013;368:2277–85.
53. Papic N, Pangercic A, Vargovic M, et al. Liver involvement during influenza infection: perspective on the 2009 influenza pandemic. Influenza Other Respir Viruses. 2012;6:e2–5.

9 H7N9 Avian Influenza in Human

Feng Feng, Yu-xin Shi, Yu-zhe Wang, Yi-bo Lu, Shu-yi Yang, and Qin-qin Yan

9.1 Summary

I. Definition and epidemics

H7N9 avian influenza in human is an acute respiratory infectious disease caused by a subtype H7N9 avian influenza virus. This virus is an avian influenza with mutation and genetic rearrangement, and capable of replicating in human cells and infecting human being. Since the first identification of H7N9 avian influenza in human in the Yangtze River Delta in China in February 2013, pandemics of H7N9 avian influenza have happened successively in more than ten provinces and cities in China, and the mortality of this disease in 2013 was nearly 27% in 2013 [1]. The relapse of H7N9 avian influenza in human occurred during years from 2014 to 2017 with a high mortality remaining between 27.6 and 46.9%. Therefore, it is of great importance to understand profoundly pathogens and clinical/imaging profiles of the novel subtype H7N9 avian influenza virus for implementing careful the controlling principle of "being law-abiding, scientific, standardized and unified," practicing actually the controlling strategy of "being powerful, orderly, effective and abstemious" [2] improving effectively cure rate and ameliorating the prognosis.

II. *Epidemiology*

1. Infectious source

It is considered according to researches that the H7N9 avian influenza virus has been derived through two steps of recombination, among which "H7" has originated from domestic ducks in the Yangtze River Delta and "N9" from wild birds in Korea. Ducks are the intermediate hosts and chickens are the main infection source. Live poultry market, based on epidemiology, serology, and molecular virology, has been confirmed to be the source of the H7N9 virus spreading [3]. Researches have revealed that H7N9 avian influenza viruses separated from birds in live poultry markets and their exudates or excrements are highly homologous with the H7N9 avian influenza viruses infecting humans, with a viral genetic homology up to 99.4%.

2. Transmission routes

Respiratory transmission. It includes inhalation of infectious droplets or droplets nucleus. H7N9 infection in humans is caused mainly by inhalation of virulent viral particles. Airborne viral particles attached to the human respiratory tract become instantly pathogenic in patients having inhaled the particles from the polluted environment when exposed directly to sick birds or asymptomatic birds and their exudates or excrements. The virus may also invade the human body via the upper respiratory tract, the mucous membrane of conjunctiva, or skin wound, due to close exposure to exudates or excrements of infected birds, or direct exposure to the virus. Possibility of human-to-human transmission is very low since the avian influenza virus does not carry swine or human gene, and there is no definite evidence of human-to-human transmission. If mutation keeps happening in viruses, however, the possibility of human-to-human transmission cannot be excluded.

F. Feng
Department of Radiology, Nantong Tumor Hospital Affiliated to Nantong University, Nantong, Jiangsu, China

Y.-x. Shi (✉) · S.-y. Yang · Q.-q. Yan
Department of Radiology, Shanghai Public Health Clinical Center, Shanghai, China

Y.-z. Wang
Department of Radiology, Shanghai Fifth People's Hospital, Fudan University, Shanghai, China

Y.-b. Lu
Department of Radiology, The Fourth People's Hospital of Nanning, Nanning, Guangxi, China

C. Qiu et al. (eds.), *Avian Influenza in Human*, https://doi.org/10.1007/978-981-16-1429-3_9

3. High-risk populations

   The susceptible populations include those closely exposed to poultry, children, and patients with underlying diseases, such as the aged population with chronic obstructive pulmonary disease, patients with hypertension, and/or heart disease, though some people without exposure to poultry are also infected. Therefore, the definite susceptible populations should be confirmed based on further researches.

III. *Main clinical manifestations*

The incubation of infection is generally less than 7 days. Patients manifest mainly influenza-like symptoms, such as fever, cough with little expectoration, and possible complications such as headache, muscle soreness, and general discomfort. Patients with severe diseases show rapid progression, and manifest commonly severe pneumonia on day 5–7, with the body temperature sustained commonly above 39 °C, dyspnea, and the possible complication of hemoptysis. It may progress rapidly to acute respiratory distress syndrome (ARDS), sepsis, septic shock, and even multiple organ dysfunction. Some patients may have mediastinal emphysema and pleural effusion. A large-cohort case report by Chen Wang [4] showed a median onset age of 63 years for human infection of H7N9 avian influenza, which was higher obviously than 26 years for H5N1 and 25 years for H1N1, and 71% of the patients were males. The high risk for acute respiratory distress syndrome is the underlying chronic disease. H7N9 was similar to H5N1, but significantly superior to H1N1, concerning leukopenia, thrombocytopenia, and percentage of increase in alanine aminotransferase, creatine kinase, C-reactive protein, and lactate deaminase. Longer hospital stay and shorter time from onset to death were observed in H7N9 avian influenza in human, than in cases of H5N1 or H1N1. It was indicated by other researches that 92.48% of patients needed hospitalization, 97.3% were complicated with pneumonia, 76.6% were complicated with severe pneumonia requiring treatment in ICU, which was related possibly to the strong virulence of virus H7N9 and the presence of underlying diseases in most of the susceptible populations.

IV. *Laboratory examinations*

1. Blood routine

   The total count of white blood cells is generally normal or lowered. Most of the patients with severe diseases have leukopenia, lymphopenia, and thrombocytopenia.

2. Biochemistry

   There is commonly increase in creatine kinase, lactate dehydrogenase, aspartate aminotransferase, alanine aminotransferase, and C-reactive protein, while myoglobin may increase. The levels of procalcitonin and 1-3-β-glucan increase in some the critically sick patients.

3. Etiology and related tests

   Respiratory samples must be collected before anti-viral treatment is launched, such as nasopharynx secretion, oral gargle, tracheal aspirate, or respiratory epithelial cells. The detection should be performed as soon as possible if equipment for etiological detection is available in the medical institutions. If not, the samples collected should be submitted to designated medical institutions for detection.

   (a) Screening of antigen of influenza A virus. It is based on the positiveness of rapid antigen detection for influenza A, but it can be used as only a preliminary screening test.
   (b) Nucleic acid detection. Realtime PCR (or RT-PCR) is used for samples from the respiratory tract to detect nucleic acid of the H7N9 avian influenza virus.
   (c) Separation of virus. H7N9 avian influenza viruses are separated from samples obtained from respiratory tract of patients.
   (d) Dynamic detection for viral antibodies. A rise for at least four times for level of specific antibodies against H7N9 avian influenza virus in double serums.

9.2 Image Findings

H7N9 avian influenza in humans can be categorized into three types including the asymptomatic (the inapparent), the mild, and the severe. The patient with the mild type has only influenza-like symptoms such as fever, without pulmonary abnormality. Manifestations of H7N9 avian influenza pneumonia in human include:

1. Findings in chest X-ray

   In the early stage, it manifests focal or scattered small flaky opacities (Fig. 9.1) or no abnormality. Large flaky blurred opacities can be observed in both lungs in the progression stage, showing heterogenous density and blurred or clear borders, with bronchograms [5] (Fig. 9.2). Changes similar to white lungs are observed in patients with ARDS [6] (Fig. 9.3). The main modality for evaluating responses in follow-up is bedside X-ray in some of the patients who cannot be moved at will, for most of the patients with H7N9 infection have severe pneumonias [7].

2. CT manifestations [8]

   (a) Scope of Diseases: Lesions may be localized within pulmonary lobes or segments in the early stage (within 3 days post to onset), manifesting focal or

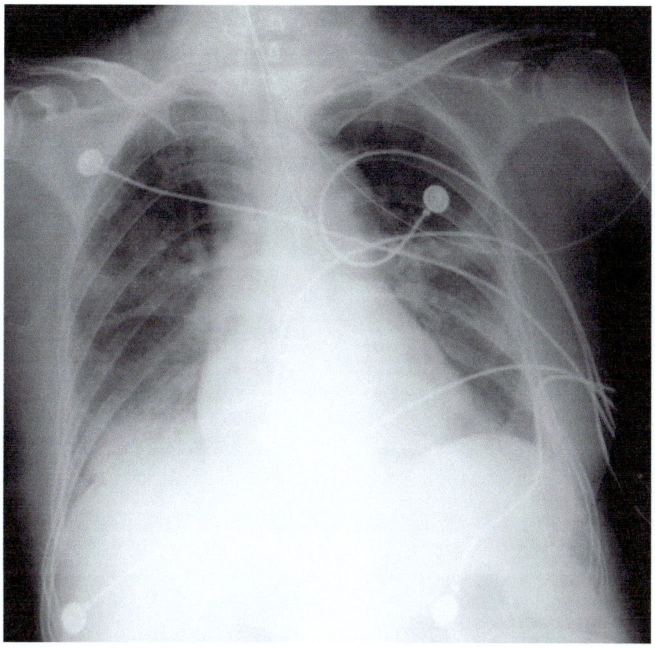

Fig. 9.1 Small flaky opacities in middle fields of both lungs and the lower field of the right lung were shown by chest X-ray in the patient infected with H7N9 avian influenza (early stage)

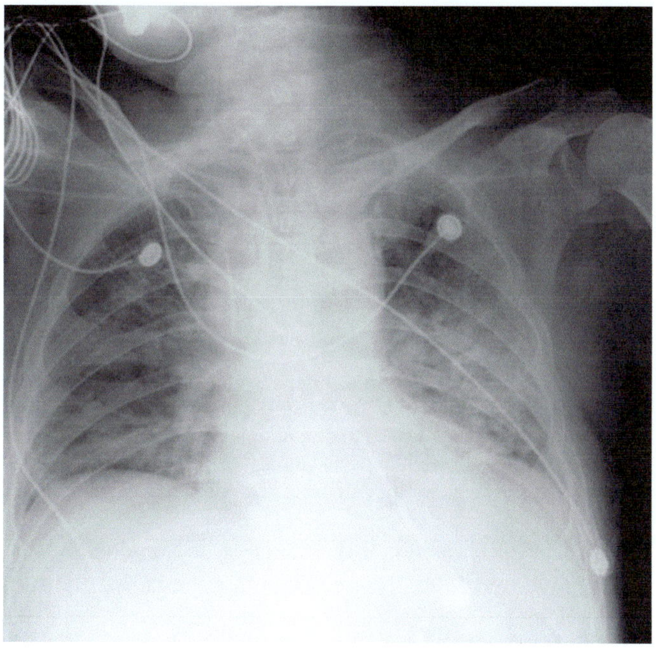

Fig. 9.2 Blurred patchy opacities with unclear borders and bronchogram inside, which were observed in both lungs by chest X-ray in the patient infected with H7N9 avian influenza pneumonia (progression stage)

scattered multiple lesions (Fig. 9.4). The disease progresses rapidly in the progression stage (day 3–6), showing dominantly a distribution in multiple pulmonary segments and lobes. Imaging of patients with

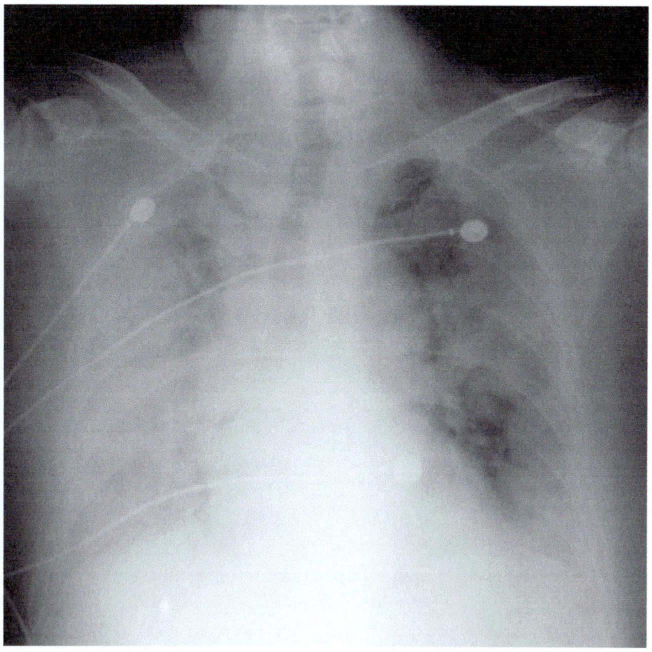

Fig. 9.3 Severe pneumonia induced by H7N9 avian influenza infecting human, with chest X-ray showing large blurred flaky opacities in both lungs, and "white lung" on the right

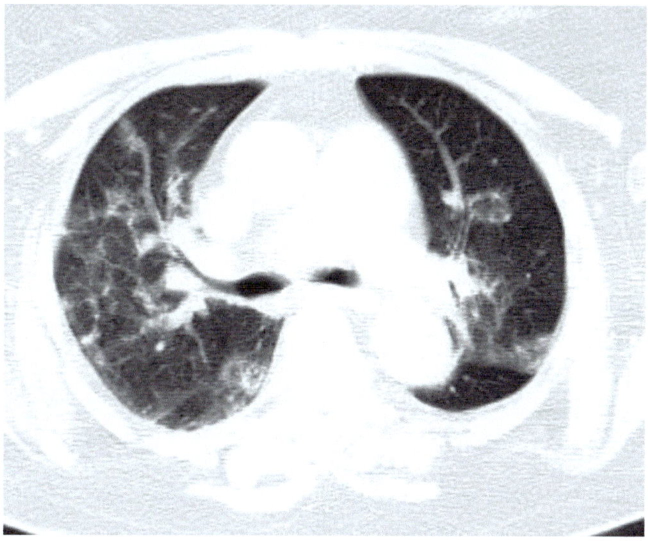

Fig. 9.4 Human pneumonia induced by H7N9 avian influenza (early stage). The pulmonary window of CT scans on day 3 post to the onset showed scattered multiple patchy opacities in both lungs

severe pneumonia, dominated by unilateral lesions in the early stage, shows more extensive bilateral lesions involving usually three or more lobes in the advanced stage, with the highest susceptibility noticed in both lower lobes (Fig. 9.5).

(b) Nature of Lesions: They are dominantly pulmonary parenchymal ones, manifesting mainly ground glass opacities (GGOs) and lung consolidations, with dif-

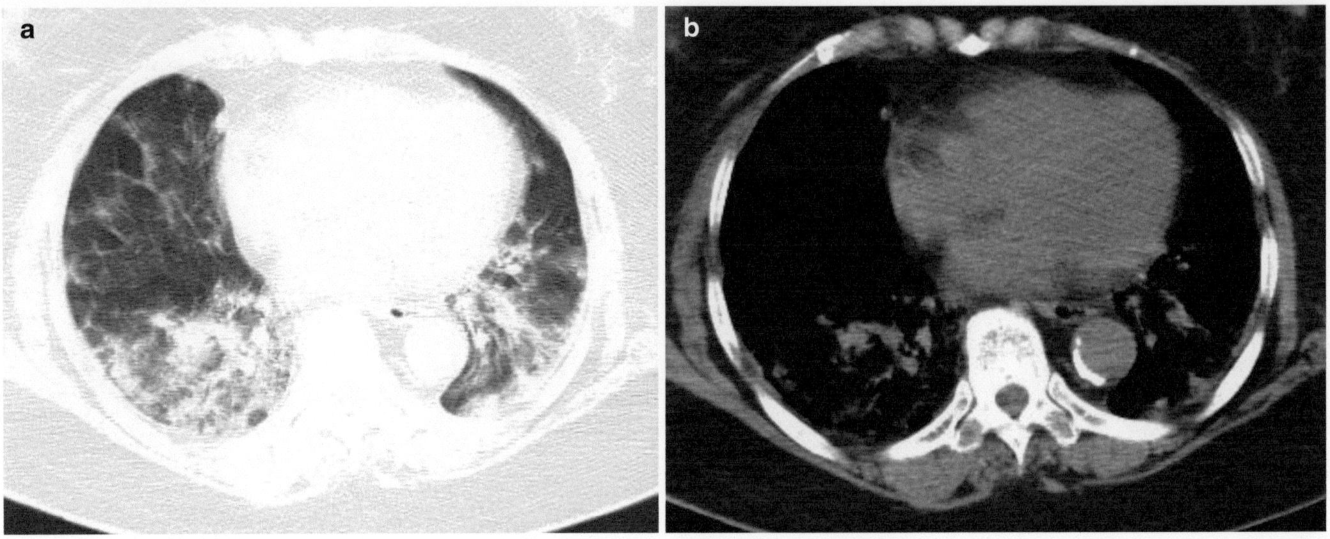

Fig. 9.5 (**a**, **b**) H7N9 avian influenza pneumonia infecting human (progression stage) on day 6 post to the onset. (**a**) (pulmonary windows of CT scans), (**b**) (mediastinal window) show large flaky opacities in both lungs, distributed dominantly in bilateral lower lobes

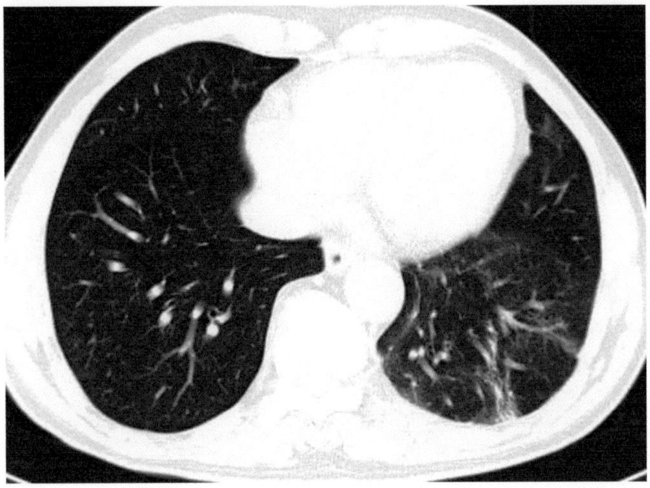

Fig. 9.6 H7N9 avian influenza pneumonia in human (early stage) with mild disease, with the pulmonary window of CT scans showing a small amount of GGOs in the lower lobe of the left lung

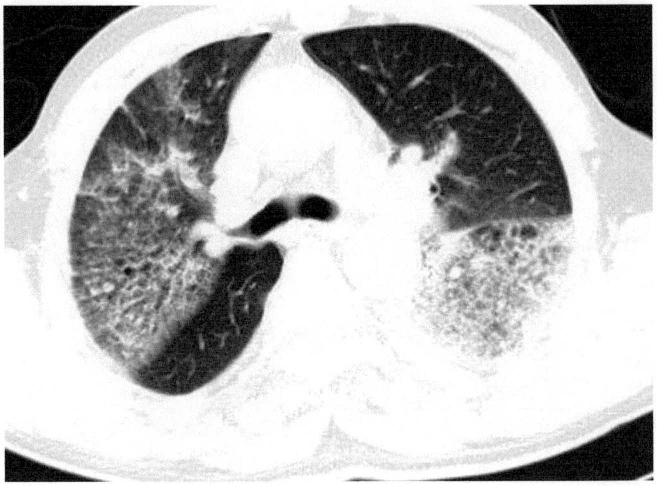

Fig. 9.7 Pneumonia manifesting high severity on day 6 post to the onset in a patient infected with H7N9 avian influenza (progression stage). Pulmonary window of CT scans shows multiple GGOs and grids in the upper lobe of the right lung and the lower lobe of the left lung and consolidations in some areas

ferent ratios between these two signs, which is possibly correlated to severity and course of the disease. Lesions are dominantly GGOs when the disease is mild to a lesser extent, and show an increased ratio of consolidations when lesions involve multiple lobes (Figs. 9.5, 9.6 and 9.7).

(c) Bronchogram is often observed inside GGO and consolidation (Fig. 9.8).

(d) Pulmonary Interstitial Changes: manifestations are dominantly homogenous thickening of the pulmonary alveolar septum, appearing usually grid-like changes. Pulmonary interstitial changes and pulmonary fibrosis seem more obvious in the absorption stage (Fig. 9.9).

(e) Pleural Effusion: It may suggest to some extent the severity of the disease. The infection is usually mild if there is no effusion, and the presence of bilateral effusion often indicates often a severe disease (Fig. 9.10).

(f) Mediastinal lymphadenopathy is rare.

3. Dynamic imaging changes and the clinical significance

No specificity is observed in clinical manifestations in humans infected with H7N9 avian influenza, but pneumonia induced by this virus is characterized by rapid progress of lung lesions, among many others. It is of great significance, therefore, to understand and accurately evaluate the dynamic changes of pulmonary lesions based on

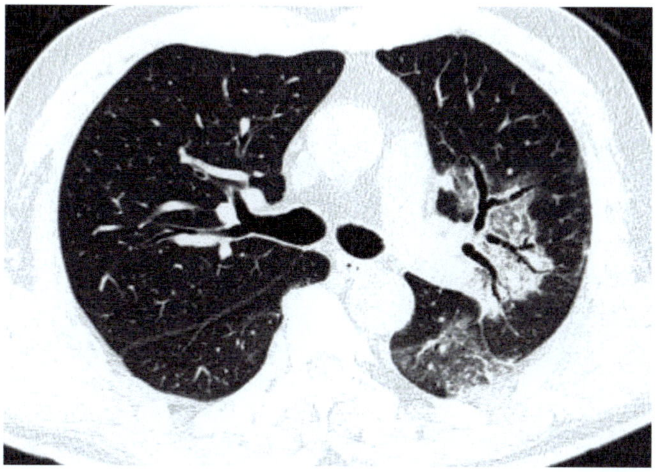

Fig. 9.8 Human pneumonia induced by H7N9 avian influenza (early stage), with the pulmonary window of CT scans showing bronchogram inside the consolidation in the upper lobe of the left lung and small amount of infection in the lower lobe of the left lung

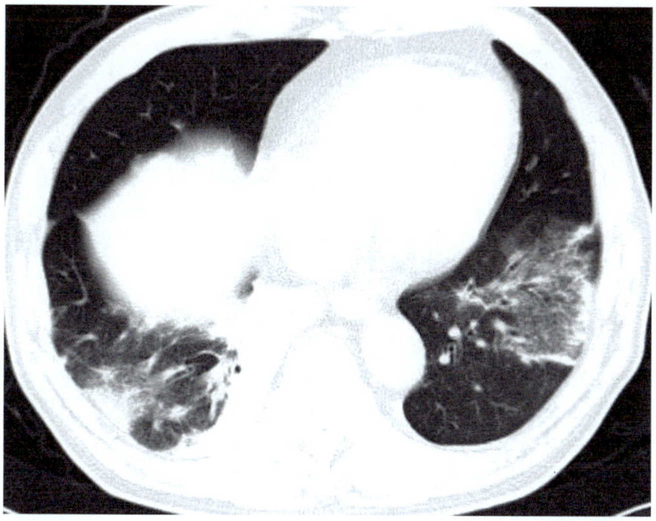

Fig. 9.9 Human pneumonia induced by H7N9 avian influenza (absorption stage), with pulmonary window of CT scans showing local interstitial change in the lower lobe of the left lung in the absorption stage, and small amount of infection in the lower lobe of the right lung

timely chest CT scans for determining diseases and guiding clinical treatment. Lungs under attack post to infection with H7N9 avian influenza virus may manifest instantly signs of pneumonia, showing patchy ground glass opacities (GGOs) in the early stage as shown by CT scans, which progresses rapidly into the progression stage within 48–72 h if it is not diagnosed in early stage and given effective anti-viral treatment in time. The progression stage is characterized by obvious exudates from pulmonary lesions, enlarged pulmonary lesions observed by dynamic CT scans, increased ratio of pulmonary consolidations, the appearance of pleural effusion, and its increase in volume (Figs. 9.11, 9.12, 9.13, 9.14, 9.15 and 9.16). In addition to the estimation of progression of the disease, CT at this timepoint can also be used to evaluate actual response post to anti-viral treatment for cases with confirmed diagnosis, and guide the clinical selection of potentially effective anti-viral medications or revise treatment regimens. Virus in patients with pneumonia of H7N9 influenza can be eradicated generally within 7–10 days with the negative conversion of H7N9 nucleic acid, if the disease is diagnosed in early stage and active anti-viral treatment is launched.

CT findings slightly lag behind the clinical manifestations and results of laboratory tests. CT findings may show the stabilized lesion and its absorption to some extent, decreased proportion of pulmonary consolidation, reduction or disappearance of pleural effusion, and increase of interstitial lesions. The possibility of secondary pneumonia, especially in old patients complicated with underlying diseases (i.e., the high-risk population), is suggested clinically by the inconsistency of dynamic change in image findings in contrast to the foresaid pattern, such as recurrent patchy opacities in lungs in the background of general absorption of pulmonary consolidations and lung lesions dominated by interstitial ones, with the negative conversion of H7N9 nucleic acids (Figs. 9.17, 9.18, 9.19, 9.20, 9.21, 9.22, 9.23 and 9.24).

4. Imaging scores

In the respective sites of lesions, the lateral one third of the lung fields is defined as the peripheral, and the rest as the center. Findings in X-ray and CT scans are scored, using a three-point system, including score 1 (normal), 2 (GGO), and 3 (pulmonary consolidation). CT score for axial images is based on methods described by Grieser et al. [9], to define areas of GGOs and pulmonary consolidations. CT value is determined for the normal lungs, GGOs, and pulmonary consolidations. The two lungs are divided into three parts including the upper, the middle, and the lower. The upper part is the field above the trachea bifurcation, the middle is the field between the trachea bifurcation and the lower pulmonary vein, and the lower is the field below the lower pulmonary vein. The lungs of each patient are divided into six fields. A five-grade system is used to score different CT signs in each field including grade 0 (score 0) standing for normal lungs; stage 1 (score 1) for a lesion <25% of the section, grade 2 (score 2) for the lesion occupying 25–50% of the section, grade 3 (score 3) for a lesion occupying 50–75% of the section and, grade 4 (score 4) for a lesion larger than 75% of the section (Fig. 9.25). Area of the lesion is multiplied by its severity. Products of all fields are accumulated, with the sum in a range from 0 to 72. Researches by Feng et al. [10] show that sum of products of chest X-ray and CT scans at the onset of H7N9 viral pneumonia was 50% higher in the death cohort than in the survivors. Imaging

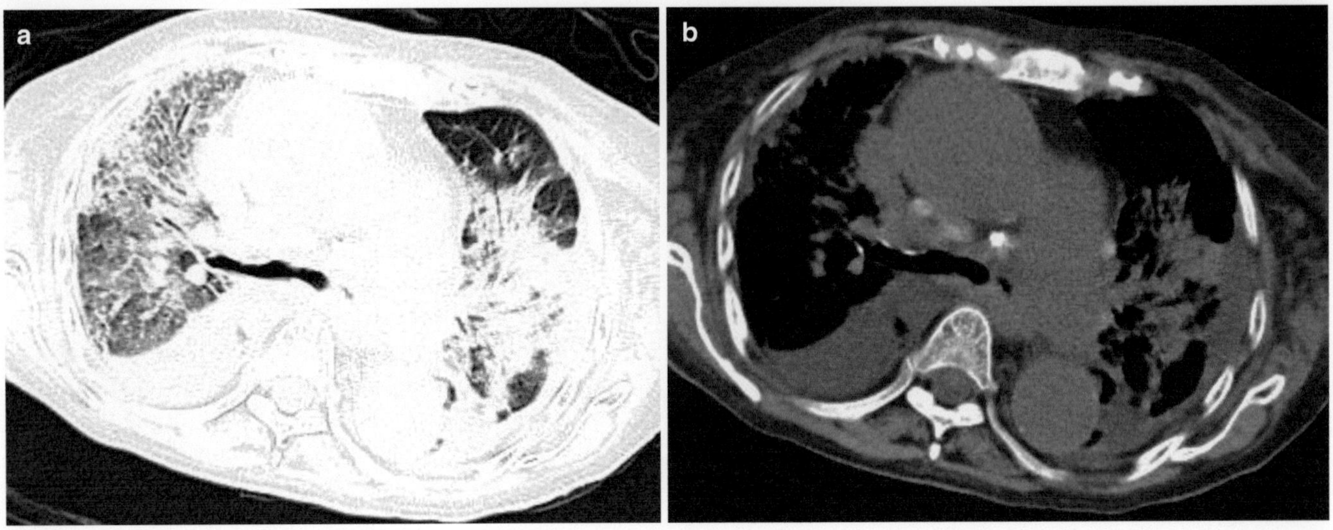

Fig. 9.10 (**a**, **b**) Human pneumonia induced by H7N9 avian influenza. (**a**) Pulmonary window of CT scans shows scattered GGOs and consolidation infection in both lungs; (**b**) Mediastinal window of CT scans shows consolidations in both lungs with a small amount of bilateral pleural effusion

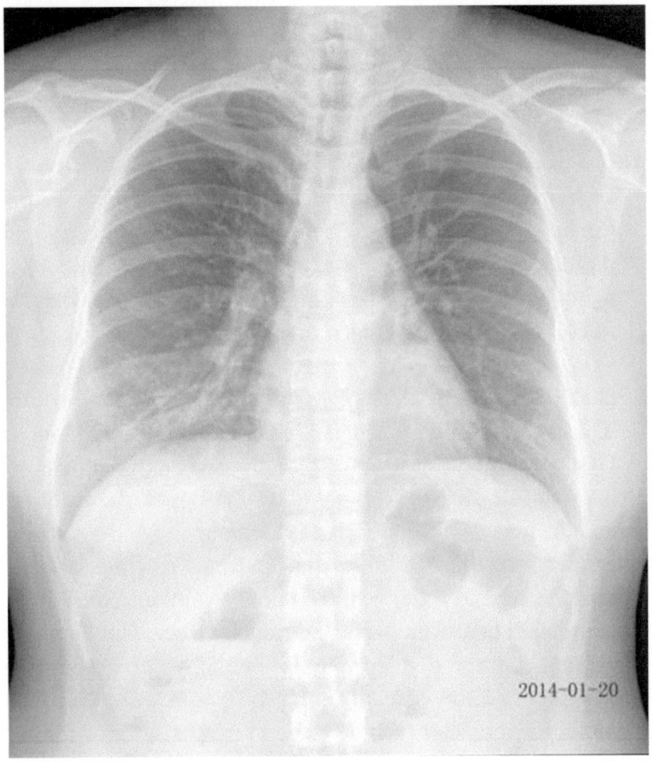

Fig. 9.11 32-year old female, with severe pneumonia induced by H7N9 avian influenza in humans. She manifested fever and cough with expectoration on January 15, 2014, and was admitted on January 23, 2014 (Figs. 9.11, 9.12, 9.13, 9.14, 9.15 and 9.16). January 20th 2014 (day 5 post to the onset). Chest X-ray showed a slightly increased density in the lower lobe of the right lung, suggesting pneumonia in the lower right lung

score is based on respiratory tract disease and the severity in its distribution. The pulmonary parenchymal disease seemed more extensive in the deaths than in the survivors, illustrating a much obviously lower hypoxemia in the former. Severer clinical course, as indicated by previous studies, could be found in viral pneumonia patients manifesting pulmonary consolidations shown by CT scans than in those with GGOs. These abnormalities are correlated to pathologically diffuse alveolar injuries. The deaths usually have more consolidations and asymmetrical diseases, while patients with bilateral consolidations have a much prolonged clinical course. A simple scoring system will be in favor of the triage of patients, so that a more active treatment will be carried out with close monitoring for disease progression for patients with high scores, because H7N9 virus infection is an acute infectious disease with potential fatal risk. Researches in the future are required, however, to confirm the efficacy of this method in lowering mortality. Follow-up with low-dose CT scans can evaluate precisely the variation of the disease, and is especially convenient to perform for wards buildings equipped with the CT machine. Changes in disease can be reflected more precisely by semi-quantification of images and quantification of lesions.

9.3 Diagnosis and Differential Diagnosis

1. Key points in the diagnosis
   (a) Cases suspected of infection with H7N9 avian influenza virus. There are influenza-like symptoms, and

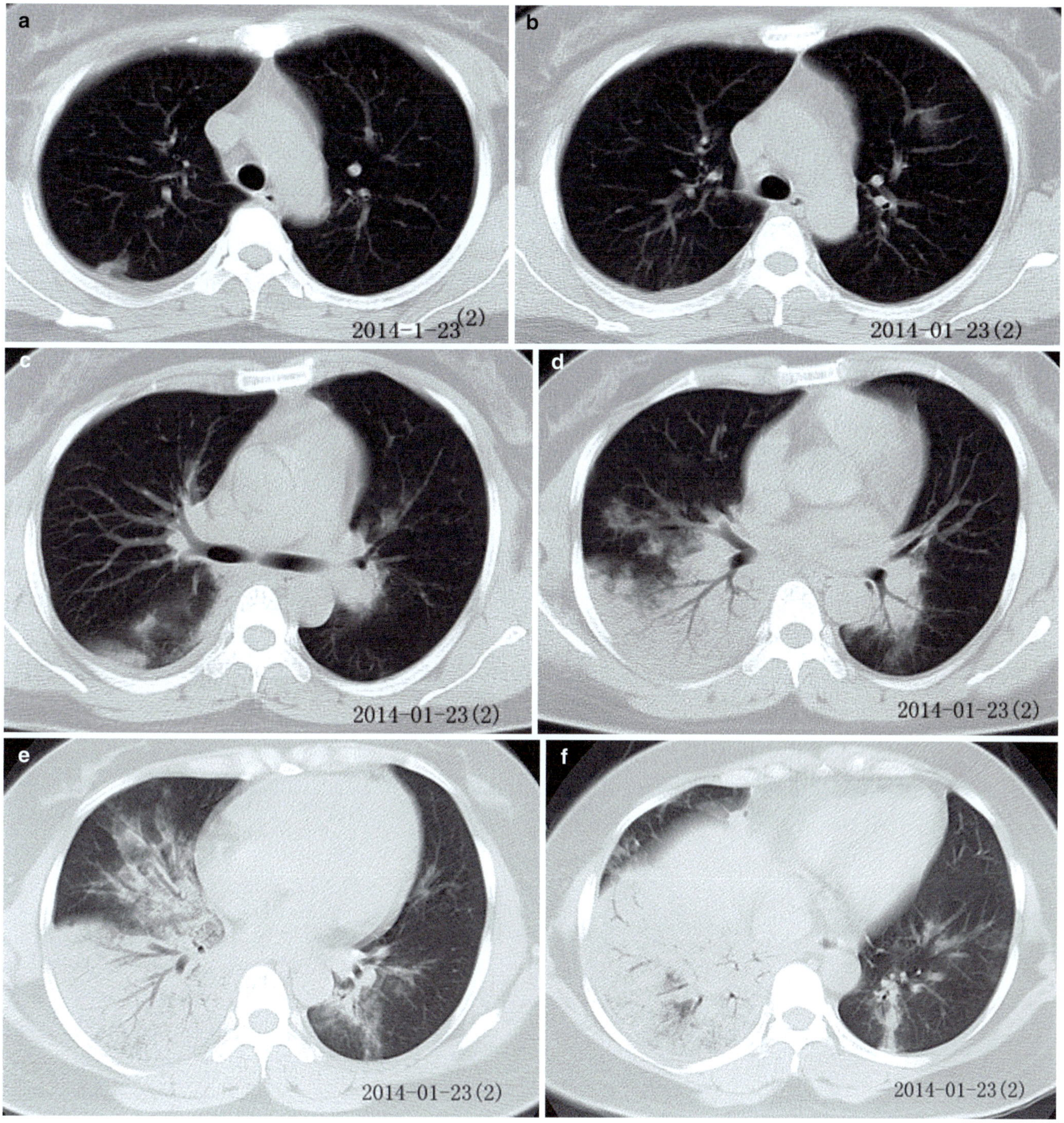

Fig. 9.12 January 23, 2014, (day 8 post to the onset). Chest CT scans (**a**–**f**) showed blurred patchy opacities in both lungs, with bronchogram inside consolidations of both lower lungs, which is significant in the lower right lung. Progression is observed in comparison with chest X-ray on January 20th, 2014

positive antigen against influenza A virus with seasonal influenza excluded, or the presence of epidemiological history (i.e., exposure to domestic poultry and its secretion or excrement within 1 week post to the onset, previous visit to live poultry market or contact epidemiologically with patients infected with H7N9), and results of biochemistry and blood routine meeting changes of H7N9 avian influenza in human.

(b) Cases with confirmed infection with H7N9 avian influenza virus. The case meets the diagnosis criteria

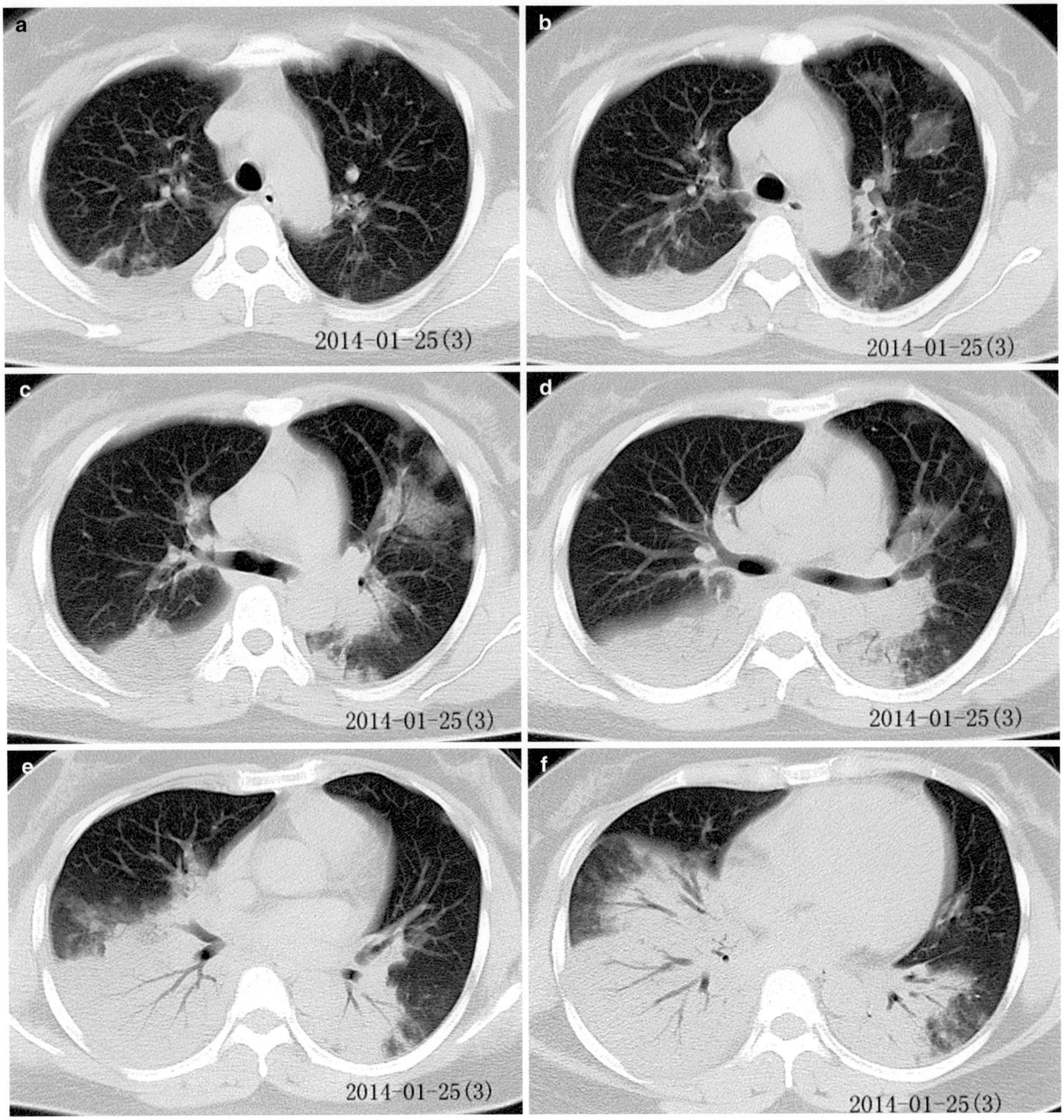

Fig. 9.13 January 25, 2014, (day 10 post to the onset). Chest CT scans (**a**–**g**) showed further progression of bilateral pulmonary lesions with the increase of GGOs in both lungs, and the increase of consolidation in the lower left lung

for suspected cases of the H7N9 virus, and this virus is isolated from the respiratory secretion of the patient, or nucleic acid detection of H7N9 virus is positive.

(c) Pneumonia of H7N9 influenza virus. The case meets the criteria for confirmed diagnosis of infection with H7N9 avian influenza virus, and lesions including GGOs and pulmonary consolidation are observed simultaneously in chest X-ray and CT scans, which are distributed often in multiple pulmonary fields and dominantly in middle and lateral zones of middle and lower fields of both lungs, with bronchogram sign. Involvement of pulmonary parenchyma and mesenchyma may exist concurrently. Severe pneumonia

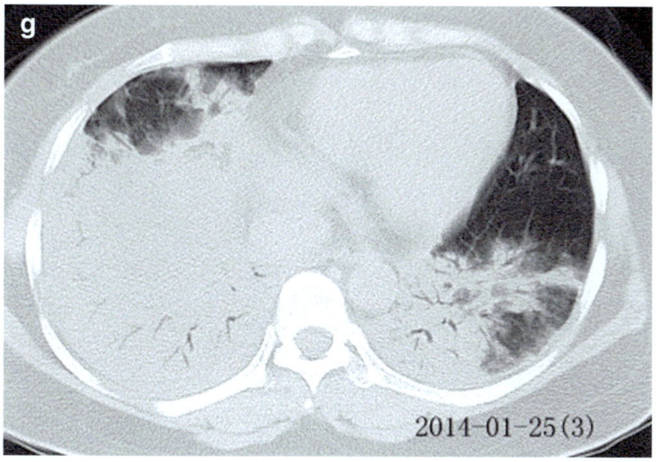

Fig. 9.13 (continued)

induced by H7N9 avian influenza in human is often complicated with respiratory failure or failure of other organs. Patients with severe diseases may have poor immunology and rapid progression of the disease, and most of them have pleural effusion, with vulnerability to ARDS and concurrent secondary infection of bacteria and fungus in advanced stage. Severe pneumonia of H7N9 is common in males older than 60 years.

2. Differential diagnosis
   (a) H1N1, H5N1, and H7N9 all have similar clinical symptoms, and all manifest influenza-like signs. However, they differ in epidemiology. Cases with H1N1 have the epidemiological history of H1N1 with exposure to corresponding patients. Cases of H5N1 and H7N9 have the epidemiological history of avian influenza, and H7N9 patients have the age at the onset greater than patients with H1N1 or H5N1. Image findings of H7N9 patients complicated with viral pneumonia seem similar when compared to those infected with pneumonia due to H1N1 or H5N1, and all of them manifest GGOs and pulmonary consolidations. Moreover, H7N9 progresses faster, more commonly complicated with pleural effusion. Nucleic acid detection should be performed as soon as possible to confirm the diagnosis and treatment should be performed in time, if lesions in multiple pulmonary lobes occur in middle aged or elderly males with the appearance of viral pneumonia in the early stage complicated with pleural effusion, lymphadenopathy and pleural thickening, for whom a diagnosis of H7N9 infection is prioritized when image findings are taken into account.
   (b) Bacterial pneumonia. Patients manifest commonly fever, chills, cough, expectoration, leukocytosis, and neutrocytosis. Image findings include unilateral or bilateral pulmonary consolidation with bronchogram. Partial overlap concerning image findings exists between human H7N9 avian influenza pneumonia and bacterial pneumonia, e.g., both of them may manifest pulmonary consolidation. However, GGOs and pulmonary consolidations start to be absorbed and ameliorate on day 8–14 through active anti-viral treatment in patients diagnosed with pneumonia of H7N9 avian influenza. The probability of concurrent bacterial infection, therefore, is hinted by the absence of obvious absorption of pulmonary consolidations. Certainly, images in Figs. 9.17, 9.18, 9.19, 9.20, 9.21, 9.22, 9.23 and 9.24 needs further confirmed diagnosis based on clinical and laboratory examinations.

9.4 Value of Imaging in Diagnosing H7N9 Avian Influenza Pneumonia in Human

I. Diagnostic significance

H7N9 is a novel virus without specificity in clinical manifestations in patients infected, which brings difficulties to clinical diagnosis. Most patients receive antibiotic therapy in early stage upon the first visit when fever occurs, predisposing themselves to delay in their disease diagnosis. However, the viral pneumonia is hinted probably by the findings dominated by GGO shown by CT scans, if considered in combination with features of viral infection, including influenza-like clinical manifestation with normal or decreased total leukocyte count and drop of lymphocyte percentage. Because most of the influenza viruses have identical medication sites, Tamiflu has an effect in different degrees on various influenzas. Therefore, early diagnosis and timely anti-viral treatment are of great importance to improve the cure rate and prognosis of patients. Early diagnosis of H7N9 virus infection is entirely possible because the examination can be completed within hours, using the rapid virus screening technology. Median time from clinical onset to clinical diagnosis of H7N9 avian influenza in human is 5–7 days, and 76.6% of the cases are severe pneumonia [1]. The low early diagnosis rate may be one of the main reasons for the poor prognosis.

II. Estimation of the disease condition

Infection of H7N9 avian influenza virus occurs firstly in lungs, and severity of pulmonary lesions correlates directly to clinical symptoms. The research by Qingle Wang et al. [8] showed that CT scans could reflect changes of disease of H7N9 avian influenza pneumonia. Qian Ma et al. [11] compared the image findings between H7N9 and H1N1 viral pneumonia and found that the former had a significantly higher probability of consolidation and pleural effusion than the latter, suggesting

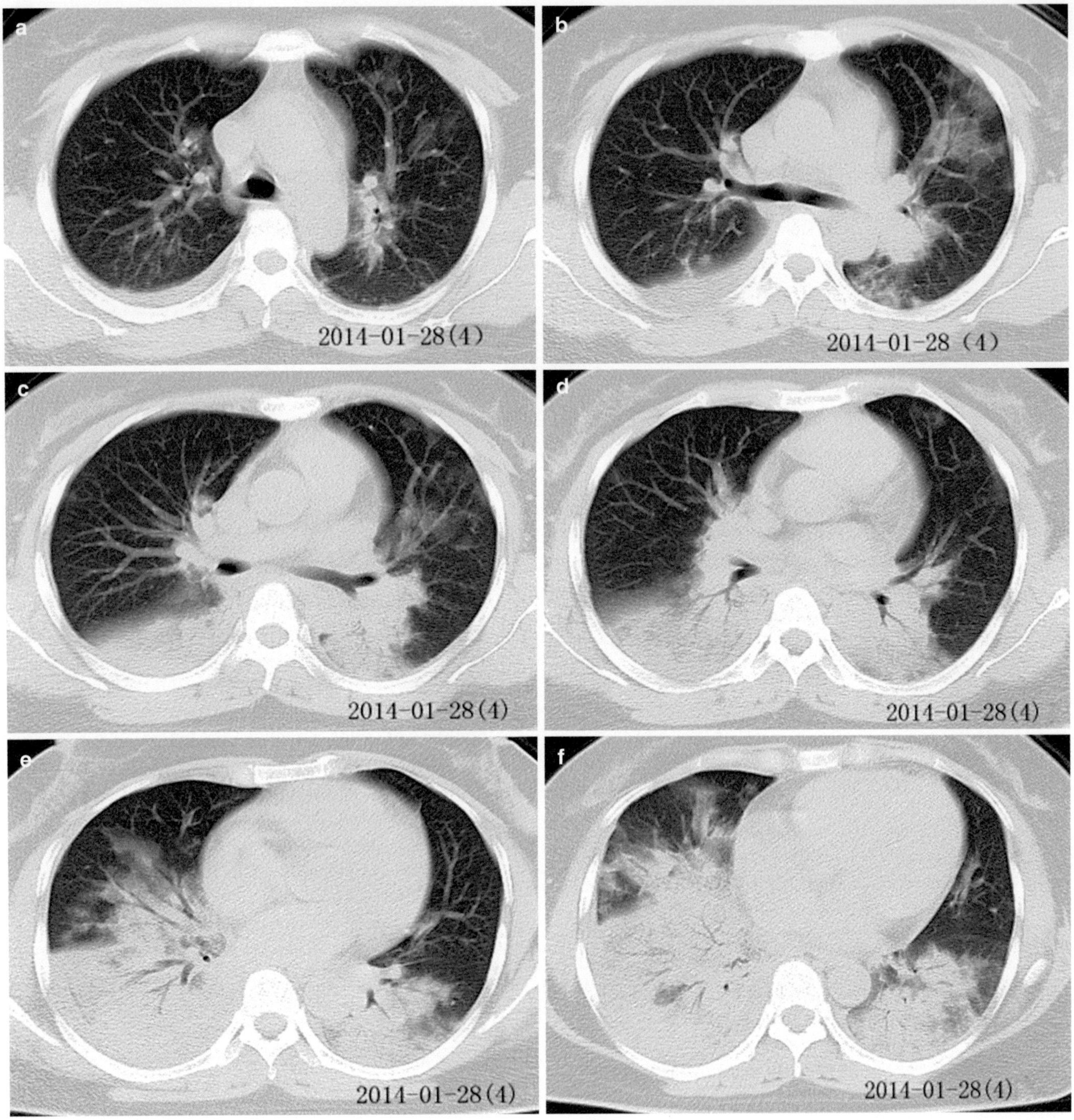

Fig. 9.14 January 28, 2014, (day 13 post to the onset). Chest CT scans (**a–f**) showed absorption and amelioration of bilateral pulmonary lesions, with decreased consolidation

that pulmonary inflammation was more severe in H7N9 than in H1N1. The follow-up research by Ying Zhu et al. [12] revealed that the total area of lesion and degree of consolidations are of great importance for the prognosis of patients, and the drop of C-reactive proteins indicated the amelioration of the disease. Visual or semi-quantitative methods have been often used previously to estimate the extent of lesions, but they are not accurate enough. Pulmonary lesions can be calculated precisely and the volume of GGOs and pulmonary consolidations can be determined, based on settings of CT value, along with continuous development of post-processing technique of CT, thereby providing powerful support for precise diagnosis for H7N9 avian influenza in human.

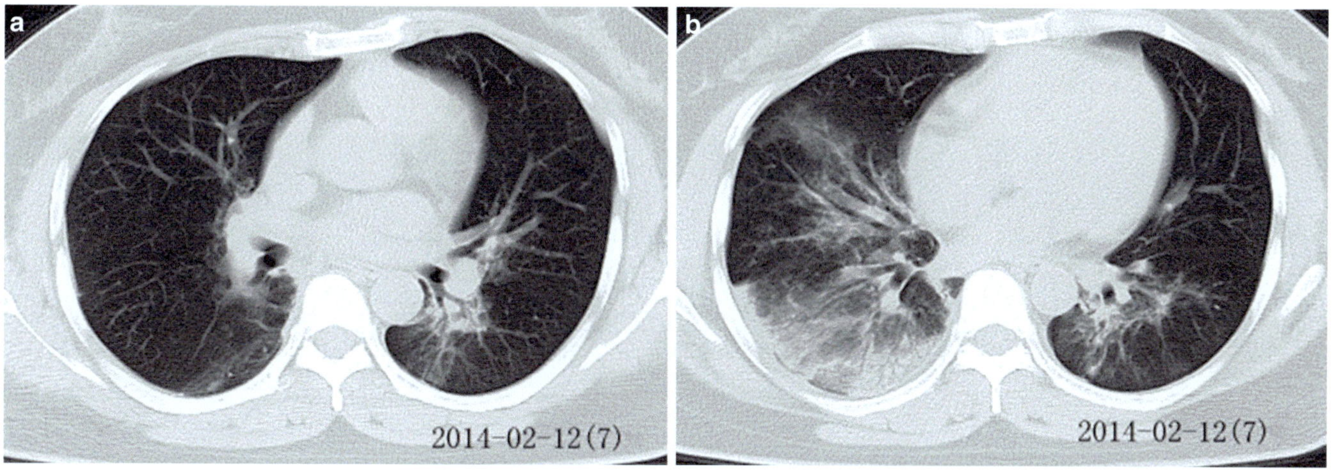

Fig. 9.15 February 12, 2014 (day 28 post to the onset). Chest CT (**a**–**b**) showed obvious amelioration of lesions of both lungs, with small amount of GGOs and fibrous streaks. The patient was cured and discharged later

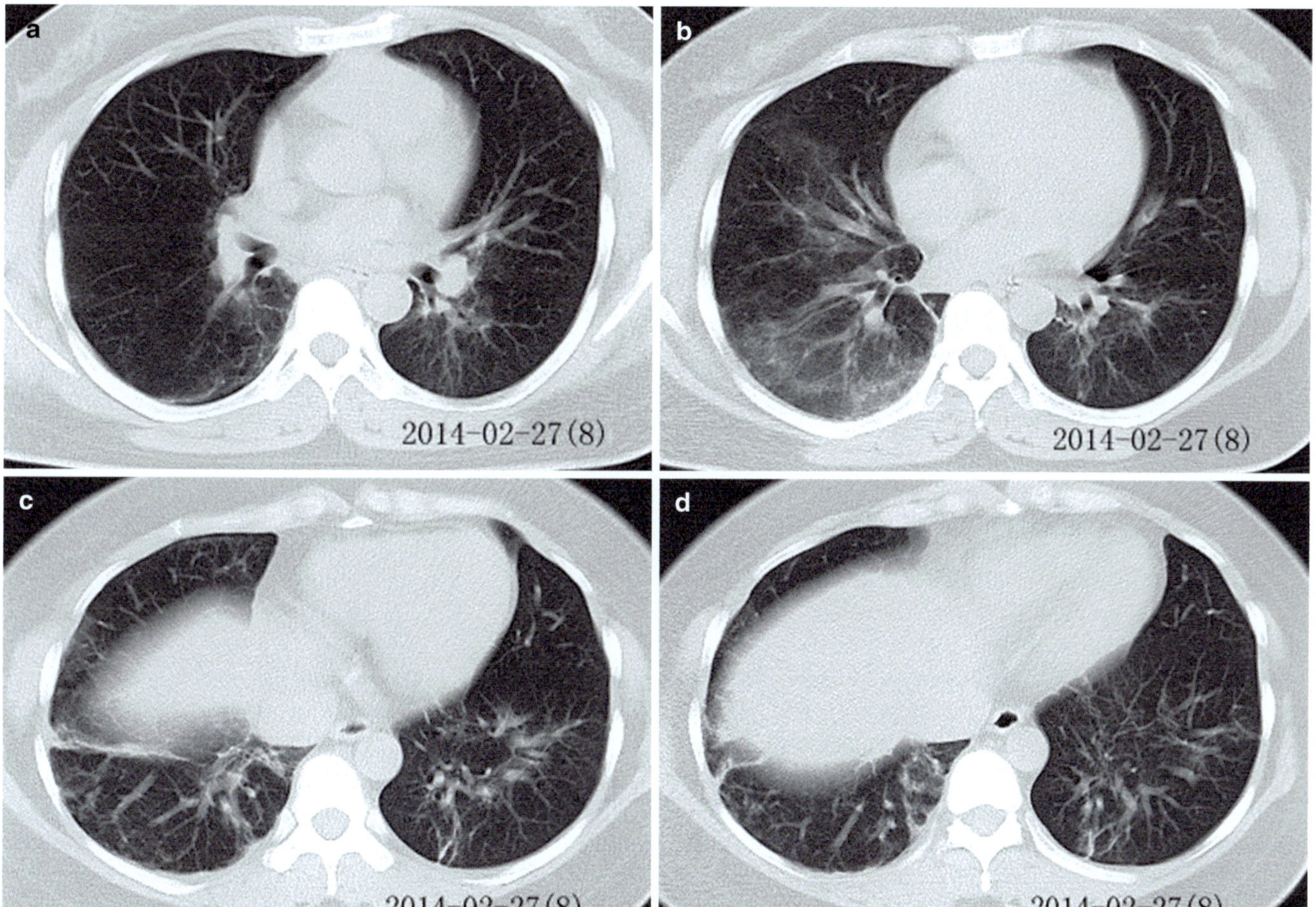

Fig. 9.16 February 27, 2014 (day 43 post to the onset). Reexamination of chest CT (**a**–**d**) post to discharge shows fibrous streaks and pulmonary mesenchymal changes in both lungs, with further absorption of pulmonary lesions compared with CT at discharge

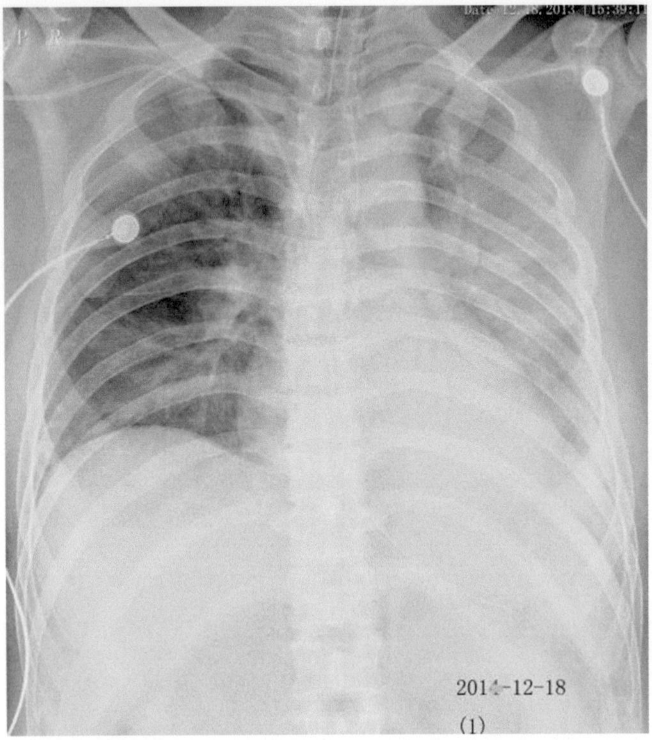

Fig. 9.17 A 38-year-old male, suffering from severe pneumonia induced by H7N9 avian influenza in human complicated with bacterial pneumonitis. He had fever, cough with expectoration since December 9, 2013, and was admitted on December 18, 2013 (Figs. 9.17, 9.18, 9.19, 9.20, 9.21, 9.22, 9.23 and 9.24). December 18, 2013 (day 9 post to the onset). Chest X-ray showed GGOs in the right lung, increased intensity of the left lung, and disappearance of the left costophrenic angle, suggesting the consolidation of the left lung

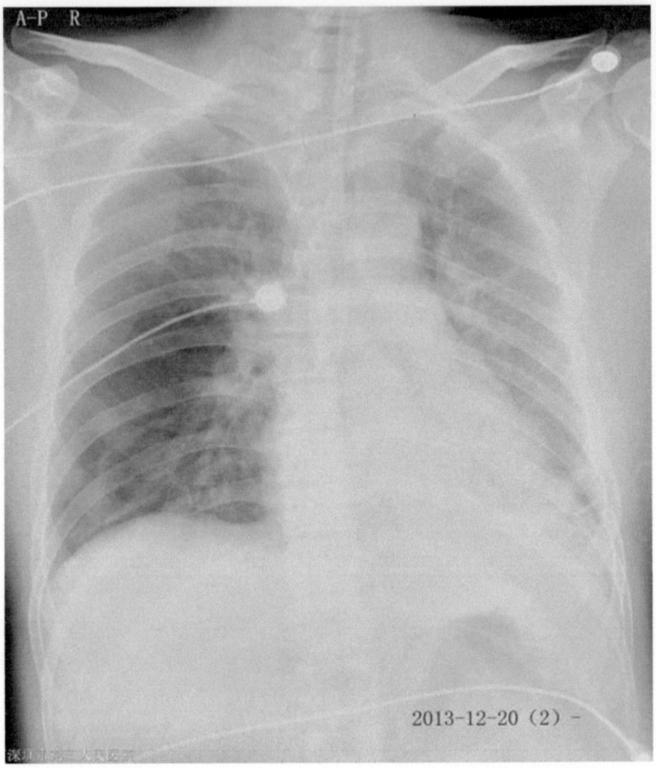

Fig. 9.18 December 20, 2013 (day 11 post to the onset). Chest X-ray showed GGOs in the right lung, partial absorption of lesions in the left lung, and the dimly visible structure at the left hilum

III. Guidance for treatment

H7N9 avian influenza virus replicates in the respiratory tract, pulmonary cells, and blood, inducing infiltration by inflammatory cells in respiratory tract and lungs, acute diffuse alveolar injuries, intra-alveolar bleeding, and fibrous hyperplasia [13]; as well as pulmonary consolidations, disturbed pulmonary ventilation, and even respiratory failure in patients with severe diseases. Some researches pointed out a certain relationship between viral load and the extent of lesions [14]. It is of great importance to calculate precisely the extent of lesions, determine quantitatively viral load, observe closely the disease, estimate its changes accurately and guide active and effective therapeutic measures (drugs and artificially adjuvant ventilation) adopted clinically as soon as possible, for improving outcomes of the treatment.

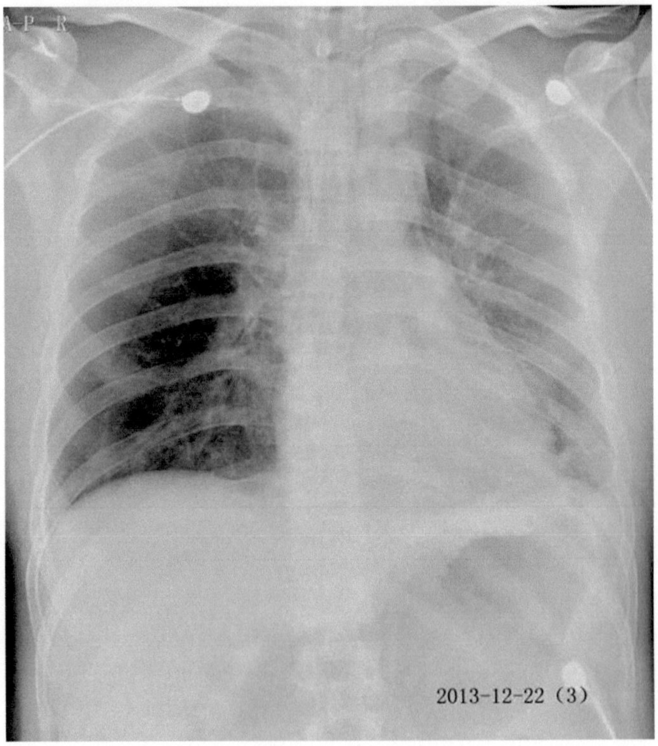

Fig. 9.19 December 22, 2013 (day 13 post to the onset). Chest X-ray showed continued absorption of the lesion in both lungs, and the left hilum and the left costophrenic angle were dimly visible

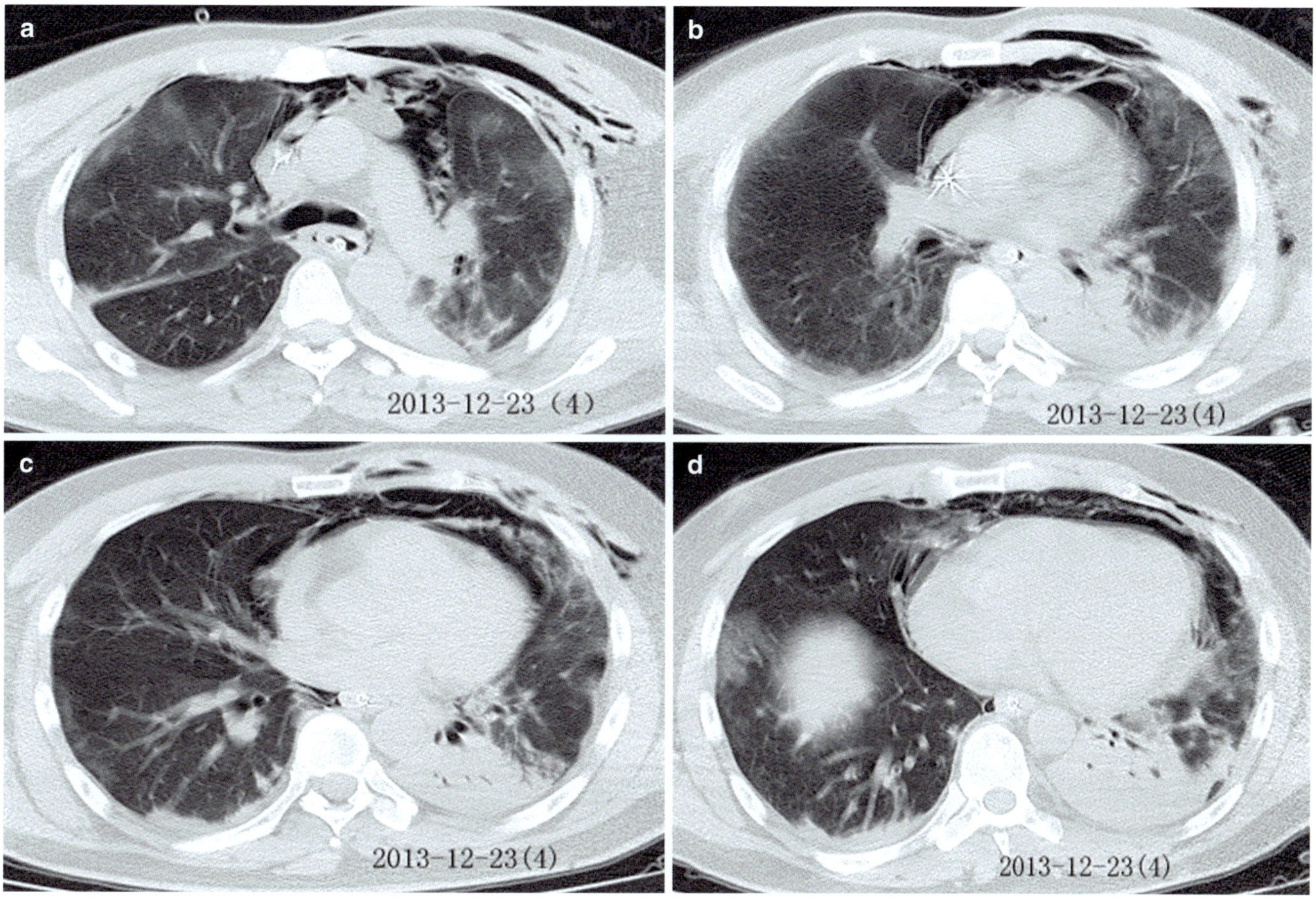

Fig. 9.20 December 23, 2013 (day 14 post to the onset). Chest CT (**a**–**d**) showed emphysemas in the chest wall and mediastinum, flaky GGOs and streaks in both lungs, and a consolidation with bronchogram inside in the lower left lung, which was consistent with signs for bacterial infection. Results of clinical tests showed pan-resistant Acinetobacter Baumannii in blood culture, pleural fluid culture, and sputum culture

9.5 Introduction of the First Case of H7N9 Avian Influenza in Human in the World

I. Summary of disease history

The patient was a 27-year-old male, with the history of chronic hepatitis B, working as a butcher in a farmers' market. He manifested firstly fever and cough with the temperature up to 39 °C on February 27, 2013, and complained that he had a history of exposure to live bird 1 week before the onset. After the onset, he took medicines with details unknown for his cold by himself, but the disease did not ameliorate obviously. His condition worsened on March 2, 2013, and saw a doctor in the respiratory department of a Grade-A Class-Three hospital in Shanghai. Lung CT (Fig. 9.26a, b) showed large consolidation of lung tissue in the lateral segment of the middle lobe of the right lung, with bronchogram inside, and scattered patchy high-density opacities in the medial segment of the middle lobe and the posterior basal segment of the lower lobe, with blurred edges and uneven density. The patient was hospitalized on March 4, 2013, due to unresponsiveness to outpatient treatment, and his condition deteriorated rapidly after admission. He was transferred into ICU on March 5, 2013, and received nucleic acid detection of throat swabs. He underwent mechanical ventilation, anti-infection medication with cefoperazone sulbactam, levofloxacin and linezolid, anti-inflammatory glucocorticoid, anti-viral medication with oseltamivir and amantadine, and intravenous immunoglobulin, but the patient's condition was not improved. Bedside chest X-ray on March 6, 2013, (Fig. 9.27) showed reduced transparency in both lungs with multiple large flaky consolidations dominantly in the right lung with blurred edges and the disappearance of the right costophrenic angle. Compared with the previous image, bedside chest X-ray (Fig. 9.28) on March 8, 2013, showed the increased transparency in the

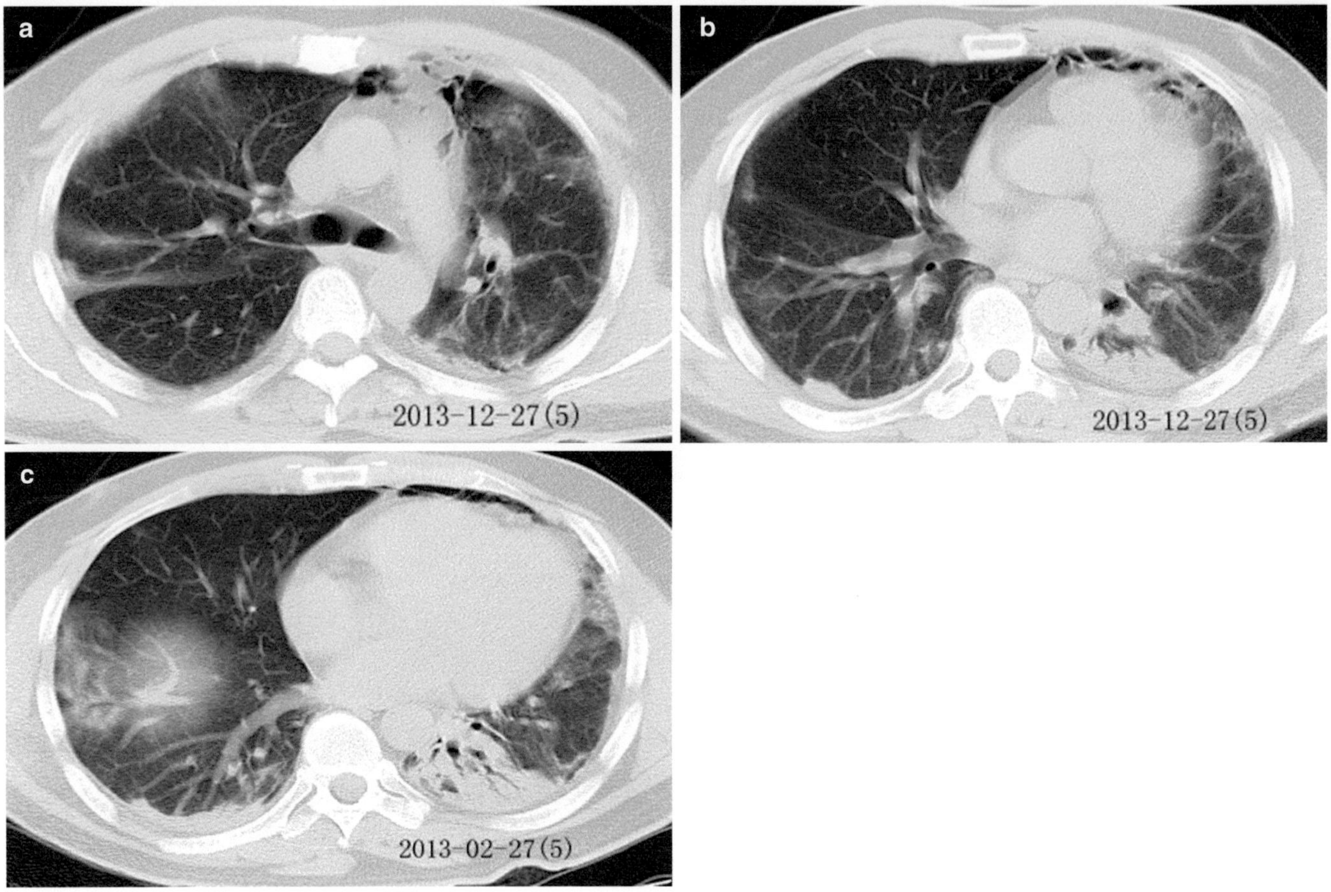

Fig. 9.21 December 27, 2013 (day 18 post to the onset). Chest CT (**a–c**) showed obvious absorption of emphysemas in the chest wall and mediastinum. There was partial absorption of GGOs and streaks in both lungs with obvious absorption of consolidation in the lower left lung post to antibiotic treatment. A small amount of pleural effusion was observed bilaterally.

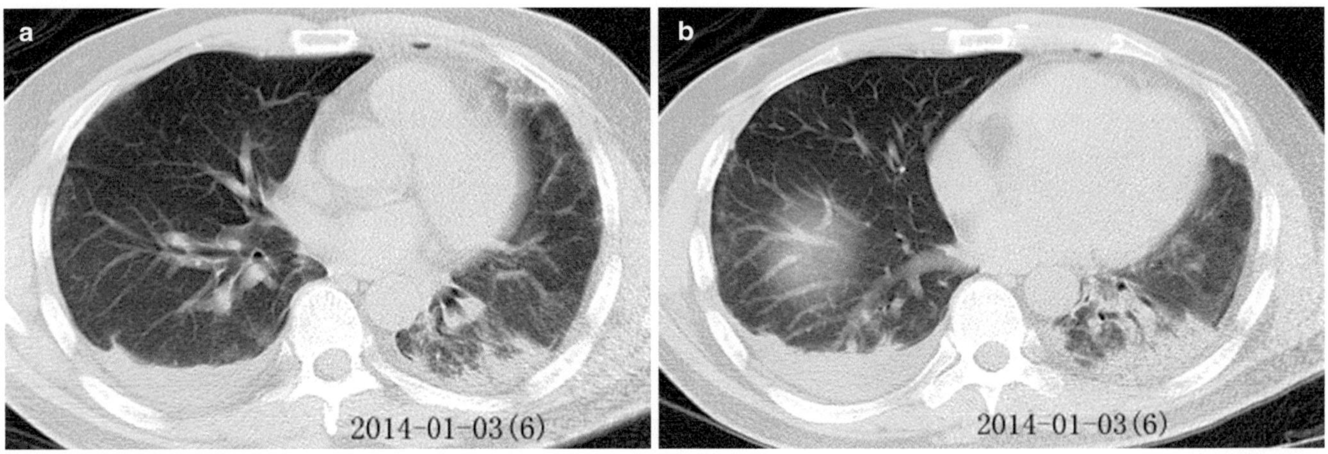

Fig. 9.22 January 3, 2014 (day 24 post to the onset). CT (**a–b**) showed the complete absorption of emphysemas in the chest wall and mediastinum, fundamental absorption of GGOs in both lungs, and continued amelioration of consolidation in the lower left lung. Bilateral pleural effusion increased slightly

right lung, decreased area of the consolidations in the right lung, increased area of consolidations in the left lung and bilateral supraclavicular hypodermic emphysema. Bedside chest X-ray on March 9, 2013, (Fig. 9.29) showed increased area of consolidations in both lungs than before, with extensive hypodermic emphysema in the chest wall and supraclavicular regions. Severe respiratory failure occurred on March 10, 2013, in the patient,

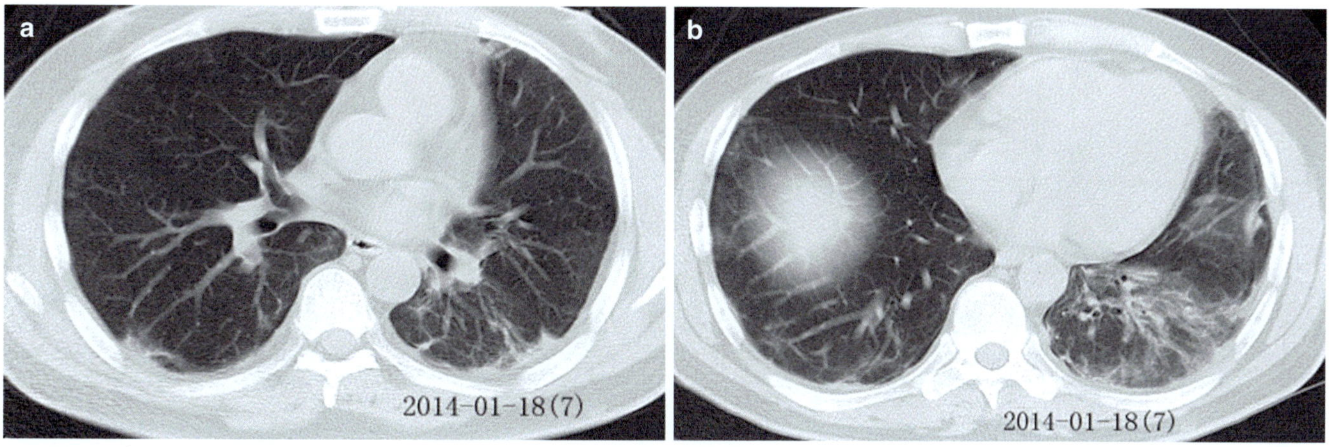

Fig. 9.23 January 18, 2014 (day 39 post to the onset). Chest CT showed fundamental absorption of GGOs in both lungs, and fundamental absorption of consolidation in the lower left lung. Fibrous streaks were seen in bilateral lower lungs, with fundamental absorption of bilateral pleural effusion. The patient was cured and discharged

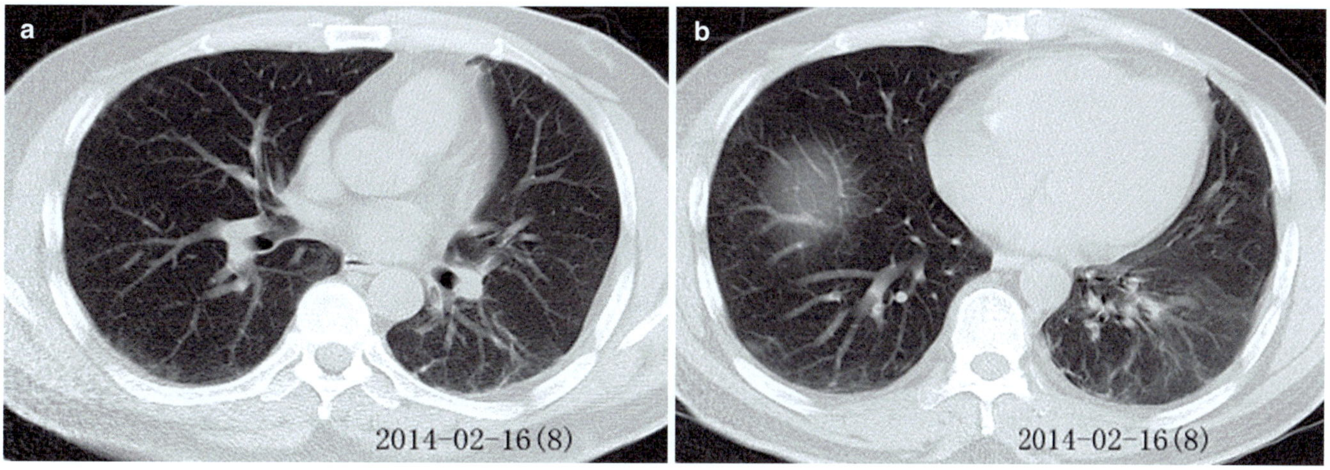

Fig. 9.24 February 16, 2014 (day 67 post to the onset). The first reexamination of Chest CT (**a–b**) showed complete absorption of GGOs in both lungs, and a small amount of fibrous streaks were observed in bilateral lower lungs with bilateral pleural thickening

who died due to unresponsiveness to rescue. Results of the etiological test were obtained on March 30, 2013, concluding the H7N9 virus.

II. *The course of identifying cases of H7N9 avian influenzae in human*

Two cases were identified in Minhang District, Shanghai, China In February 2013, and 1 case was identified in Chuzhou City, Anhui Province, China in March 2013. Their clinical manifestations in all of them included influenza-like respiratory symptoms such as fever and cough in the early stage, which progressed into severe pneumonia and dyspnea, and finally death due to unresponsiveness to rescue. A novel respiratory virus was identified in respiratory secretions from the two cases in Shanghai by researchers in P3 Laboratory of Shanghai Public Health Clinical Center in cooperation with Fudan University and proved deriving through genetic reassortment. The virus was named H7N9 based on International Nomenclature, submitted to and confirmed by Shanghai Municipal Health and Family Planning Commission and China National Center for Disease Control. In the afternoon of March 29 China, the virus was isolated from specimens of related cases by National Center for Disease Control and confirmed to be the H7N9 avian influenza virus. The three patients were diagnosed on March 30, 2013, as confirmed infection of H7N9 avian influenza in human based on clinical manifestations, laboratory tests, and results of epidemiological investigations by experts organized by the National Health and Family Planning Commission, which also notified that they were cases of human infection caused by a new subtype of avian influenza virus firstly identified in the world.

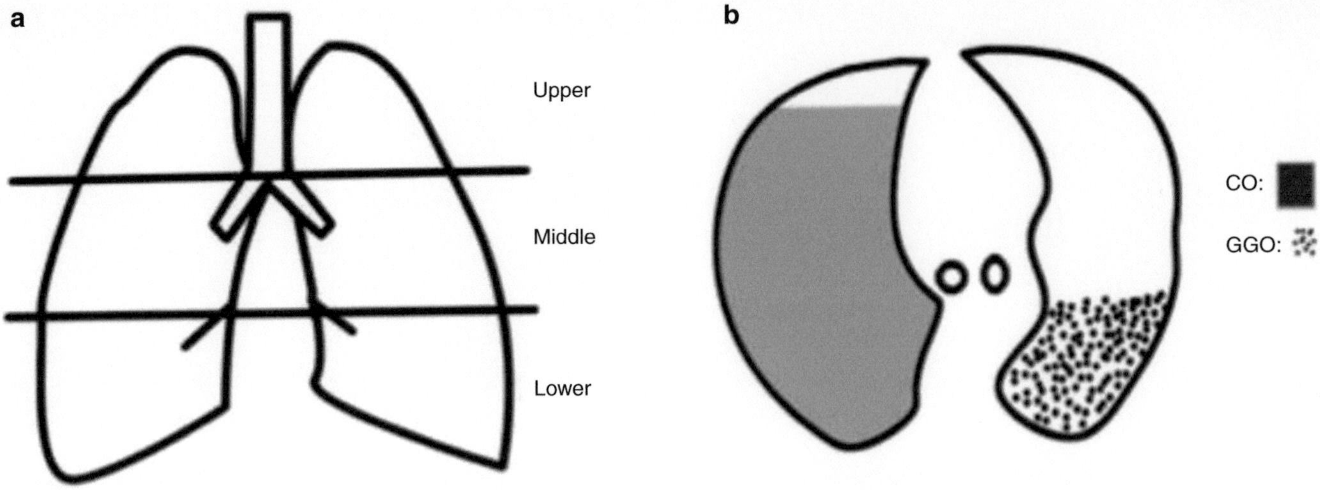

Fig. 9.25 GGOs and consolidations are defined according to methods described by Griese et al. CT value are determined for the normal lungs, GGOs, and pulmonary consolidations. The two lungs are divided into three parts including the upper, the middle, and the lower. The upper part is the field above the trachea bifurcation, the middle part is the field between the trachea bifurcation and the lower pulmonary vein, and the lower part is the field below the lower pulmonary vein. The lungs of each patient are divided into 6 fields. A five-grade system is used to score different CT signs in each field including grade 0 (score 0) standing for normal lungs; stage 1 (score 1) for a lesion size <25% of the section, grade 2 (score 2) for the lesion size occupying 25–50% of the section, grade 3 (score 3) for a lesion occupying 50–75% of the section and, grade 4 (score 4) for a lesion larger than 75% of the section

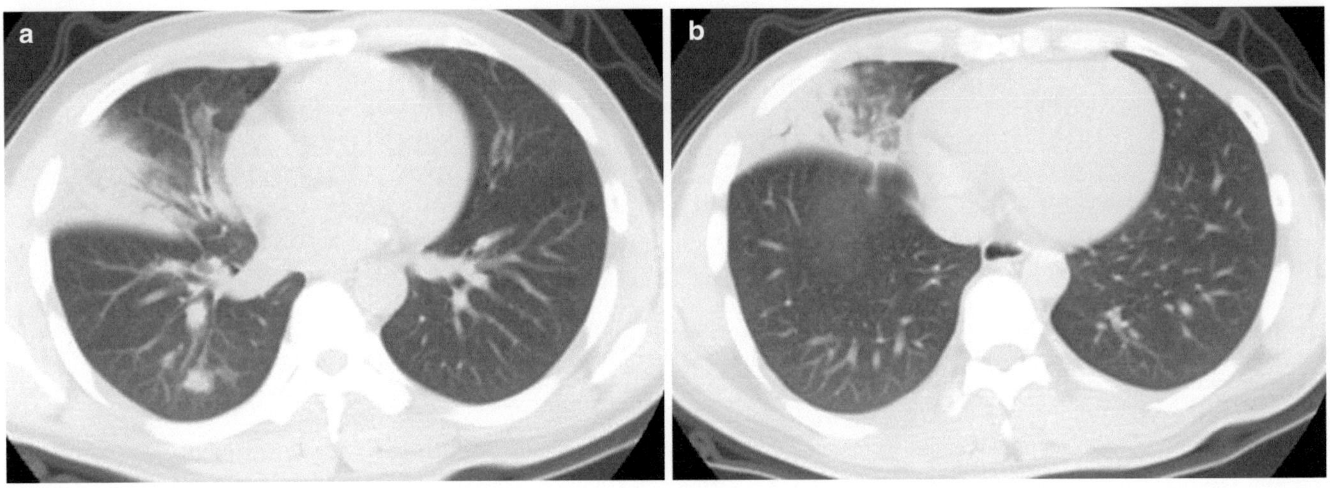

Fig. 9.26 (**a**, **b**) On March 2, 2013, day 3 post to the onset. (**a**) a large flaky consolidation and a flaky exudation in the middle lobe of the right lung were shown by chest CT scans, air bronchogram was contained by the lesions, with a patchy high-density opacity in the posterior basal segment of the lower lobe. (**b**) a large flaky consolidation and a patchy high-density opacity were observed in the middle right lobe

III. *Discussion*

Pathogen for H7N9 pneumonia is a subtype of influenza A virus [15]. H and N refer to two kinds of proteins on viral surface that may become targets attacked by the human immune system. H is the hemagglutinin capable of aggregating erythrocytes, and N is the neuraminidase which can decompose neuraminic acid [16, 17]. Bird sialic acid specifically binding to H7N9 virus is distributed mainly in the lower respiratory tract of human, predisposing human infected with H7N9 virus to main symptoms of lower respiratory tract infection, while common influenza virus causes firstly upper respiratory tract infection first followed by secondary pulmonary infection [18, 19].

Pulmonary lesions in this patient were characterized by multiple lobular and multiple focal distribution, dominantly large flaky consolidations in the lateral segment of the right middle lobe, and patchy high-density opacities in the medial segment of the right middle lobe and the basal posterior segment of the right lower lobe. It is hard to differentiate from ordinary lobar pneumonia based on image findings of lesions including morphology, density,

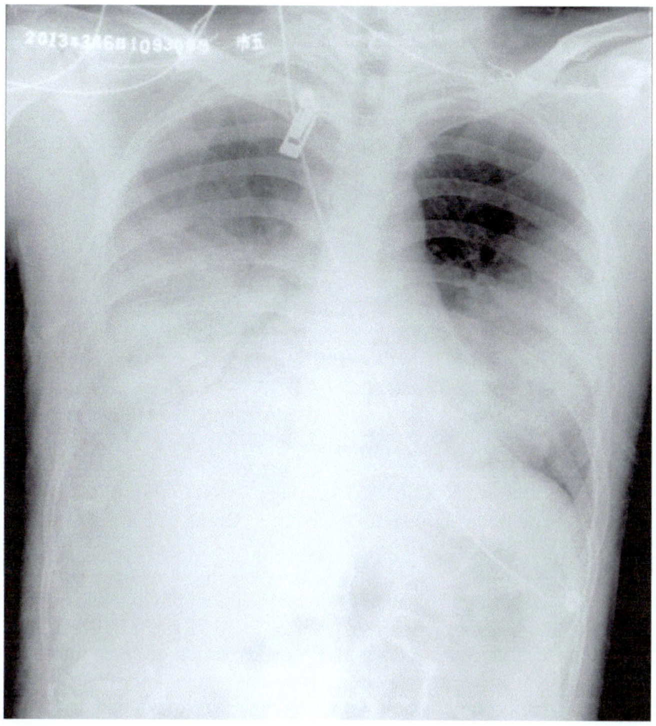

Fig. 9.27 On March 6, 2013, day 7 post to the onset. Bedside chest X-ray showed large flaky consolidations in both lungs with blurred edges, which was more obvious in the right lung, with the disappearance of the right costophrenic angle

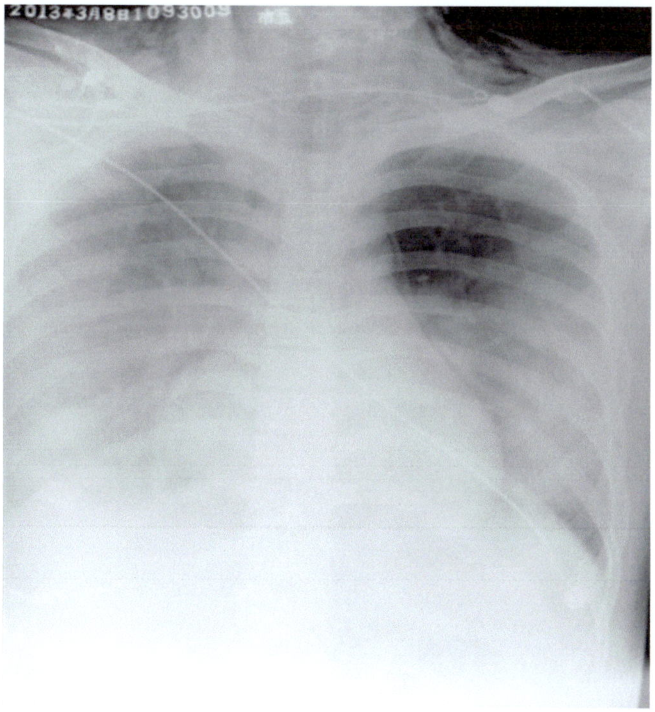

Fig. 9.28 On March 8, 2013, day 9 post to the onset. Bedside chest X-ray showed partial absorption of the lesions in the right lung and increased area of the lesions in the left lung on day 4 of hospital stay compared with the previous image. There were bilateral supraclavicular hypodermic emphysemas

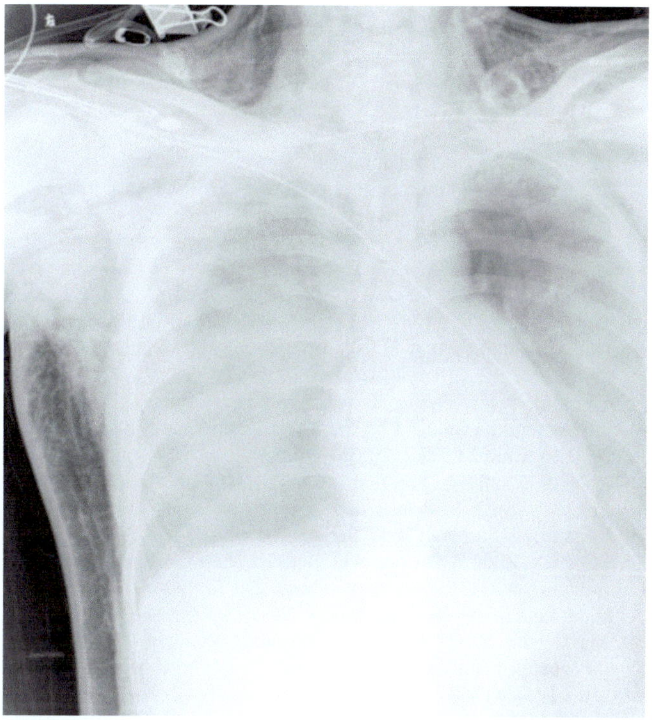

Fig. 9.29 On March 9, 2013, day 10 post to the onset, and day 5 of hospital stay. Bedside chest X-ray showed obvious progression of bilateral pulmonary lesions and chest wall emphysemas

and distribution. The rapid progression of pulmonary lesions shown by reexaminations with bedside chest X-ray in a row on 3 days (day 2, 4, and 5) instead of absorption. Its reason might be the diffuse inflammation induced by a great amount of inflammatory mediators and cytokines produced by immune cells recruited increasingly and rapidly in a cytokine storm triggered by cellular immunity through the release of cytokines by macrophages post to its phagocytosis of H7N9 viruses, which accumulate mainly in lungs and combine with sialic acid receptors on alveolar and bronchiolar epithelial cells after infecting human. A large number of inflammatory exudates enter the alveoli within a short period of time leads to impaired gas exchange, resulting in severe hypoxemia and respiratory failure [20, 21]. The pleural effusion might be caused by the systemic inflammatory response due to cellular immunity triggered by direct viral infiltration to pleura or by viral infection.

Imaging for H7N9 avian influenza in humans, showing a high sensitivity but no specificity, is characterized mainly in the fast progression of lesions. Viral specimen should be obtained as soon as possible, in case of a history of exposure to birds in patients manifesting influenza-like symptoms, in order to determine the type of the virus and avoid missing the best opportunity for treatment [22, 23].

References

1. Gao HN, Lu HZ, Cao B, et al. Clinical findings in 111 cases of influenza A (H7N9) virus infection. N Engl J Med. 2013;368:2277–85.
2. Li L, Liu K. Interpretation of therapeutic regimens for H7N9 avian influenza in human (version 2, 2013). Chin J Clin Infect Dis. 2013;6(2):68–9.
3. Wang D, Yang L, Zhu W, et al. Two outbreak sources of influenza A (H7N9) viruses have been established in China. J Virol. 2016;90(12):5561–73.
4. Wang C, Yu H, Horby PW, et al. Comparison of patients hospitalized with influenza A H7N9, H5N1, and 2009 Pandemic H1N1. Clin Infect Dis. 2014;58(8):1095–103.
5. Wang Q, Shi Y, Zhang Z, et al. Preliminary imaging observation for pneumonia induced by the novel recombinant influenza virus (H7N9). Chin J Radiol. 2013;47(6):505–8.
6. Zhou S, Zhang Z, Shi Y, et al. Clinical manifestation and chest image findings in deaths due to severe diseases of H7N9 avian influenza in human. Chin J Radiol. 2013;47(9):832–3.
7. Song FX, Zhou J, Shi YX, et al. Bedside chest radiography of novel influenza A (H7N9) virus infections and follow-up findings after short-time treatment. Chin Med J. 2013;126(23):4440–3.
8. Ma Q, Shi Y. H7N9 viral pneumonia: asymmetric and irregular changes on computed tomography. Chin Med J (Engl). 2013;126(24):4813.
9. Grieser C, Goldmann A, Steffen IG, et al. Computed tomography findings from patients with ARDS due to influenza A (H1N1) virus-associated pneumonia. Eur J Radiol. 2012;81:389–94.
10. Feng F, Jiang Y, Yuan M, et al. Association of radiologic findings with mortality in patients with avian influenza H7N9 pneumonia. PLoS One. 2014;9(4):e93885.
11. Ma Q, Zhang Z, Shi Y, et al. Comparison of CT imaging between H7N9 avian influenza in human and H1N1 severe viral pneumonia. Chin J Radiol. 2013;47(9):830–1.
12. Zhu Y, Zhang Z, Shi Y. Follow-up researches for discharged patients with H7N9 avian influenza. Chin J Radiol. 2013;47(9):786–9.
13. Yu L, Wang Z, Chen Y, et al. Clinical, virological, and histopathological manifestations of fatal human infections by avian influenza (H7N9). Clin Infect Dis. 2013;57(10):1449–57.
14. Huang X, Huang H, Lu P, et al. CT findings in correlation to viral load and CD4+ T-lymphocytes in H7N9 avian influenza pneumonia in human. Radiol Pract. 2014;29(7):751–4.
15. Wong CK, Zhu H, Li OT, et al. Molecular detection of human H7N9 influenza a virus causing outbreaks in China. Clin Chem. 2013;59(7):1062–7.
16. Liu W, Zhu Y, Qi X, et al. Risk assessment on the epidemics of human infection with a novel avian influenza A (H7N9) virus in Jiangsu Province, China. J Biomed Res. 2013;27(3):163–6.
17. Dai J, Zhou X, Dong D, et al. Human infection with a novel avian-origin influenza A (H7N9) virus: serial chest radiographic and CT findings. Chin Med J. 2014;127(12):2206–11.
18. Chang X, Chang Y, Sun X, et al. Chest image findings of pneumonia induced by H7N9 of type A virus. J Med Imaging. 2015;4:637–40.
19. Bai T, Zhou J, Shu Y. Serologic study for influenza A (H7N9) among high-risk groups in China. N Engl J Med. 2013;368(24):2339–40.
20. Liu D, Shi W, Shi Y, et al. Origin and diversity of novel avian influenza A H7N9 viruses causing human infection: phylogenetic, structural, and coalescent analyses. Lancet. 2013;381(9881):1926–32.
21. Yang PF, Yan QL, Liu C, et al. Characterization of avian influenza A (H7N9) virus prevalence in humans and poultry in Huai'an, China: molecular epidemiology, phylogenetic, and dynamics analyses. Biomed Environ Sci. 2016;29(10):742–53.
22. Ma Q, Zhang Z, Yuan M, et al. Image findings in a cured adult infected with H7N9 avian influenza: the first case in Shanghai City. Chin J Radiol. 2013;47(9):854.
23. Hou Y. Strategy and outcomes of controlling major new occurrence of infectious diseases. Electro J Emerging Infect Dis. 2019;4(3):129–32.

H5N1 Avian Influenza in Human

10

Qian-qian Zhang, He-ping Xu, Yong Sun, Bu-dong Chen, Fei Shi, Guang-ping Zheng, and Pu-xuan Lu

10.1 Summary

Virus H5N1 was first isolated and identified in a domestic goose in Guangdong Province, China in 1996 [1]. The virus may induce zoonosis. The first case of H5N1 avian influenza in humans occurred in a 3-year-old child on May 5, 1997, who was admitted due to common cold and fever unresponsive to prolonged treatment, and died from Reye Syndrome and multiple organ failure 10 days post to the onset [2]. On May 9, 1997, a strain of H5N1 avian influenza virus (AIV) was separated from the tracheal secretion of this 3-year-old boy by WHO National Influenza Center Laboratory in Rotterdam, the Netherlands and USA CDC, and named as A/Hongkong/157/97. The etiology was confirmed to be the infection of H5N1 avian influenza, and this child was the first patient infected with highly pathogenic subtype H5N1 avian influenza in the world.

The infection of the H5N1 virus in humans manifests severe disease with high mortality, so it is called highly pathogenic avian influenza (PHAI). H5N1 avian influenza virus has spread all over the world during recent years, causing continuously infectious diseases in humans. It is speculated that this virus may evolve into a virus capable of causing a pandemic of human influenza through gene rearrangement or mutation, which becomes the focus of global attention. It is classified as class B infectious diseases based on the Law on the Prevention and Control of Infectious Diseases in China, but class A management is implemented for it. Once an epidemic occurs, prevention and control measures for class A infectious diseases will be taken place [3].

Six hundred and twenty-two cases of highly pathogenic H5N1 avian influenza have been reported globally as of March 2013 since the first occurrence of subtype H5N1 avian influenza in humans in Hongkong 1997; these patients have been distributed in 15 countries including 371 deaths. As of December 2019, 54 cases have been reported in China, including 35 deaths.

H5N1 avian influenza in humans is an acute respiratory infectious disease caused by the H5N1 virus, involving simultaneously systemic symptoms, and symptoms in the nervous system and digestive system. The main clinical manifestations of H5N1 avian influenza in humans in the early stage are similar to those of common influenza, including mainly fever, mostly persisting above 39 °C, accompanied by a runny nose, nasal congestion, cough, sore throat, headache, muscle soreness, and general discomfort. Some patients may have gastrointestinal symptoms such as nausea, abdominal pain, diarrhea, and watery stool. Severe patients may have persistent high fever and rapid progression of the disease, manifesting obvious pneumonia, with multiple severe complications such as acute lung injury (ALI), acute respiratory distress syndrome (ARDS), pulmonary hemorrhage, multiple organ failure, disseminated intravascular coagulation (DIC), shock, and Reye syndrome. Secondary

Q.-q. Zhang
Magnetic Resonance Room, Zhoukou Central Hospital, Zhoukou, Henan Province, China

H.-p. Xu
Department of Radiology, The Children's Hospital of Hunan Province, Changsha, Hunan, China

Y. Sun
The Second Affiliated Hospital of Kunming Medical University, Kunming, Yunnan, China

B.-d. Chen (✉)
Department of Radiology, Beijing Ditan Hospital, Capital Medical University, Beijing, China

F. Shi
Emergency Department, Institute of Shenzhen Respiratory Diseases, Shenzhen People's Hospital, The Second Clinical Medical College of Jinan University, The First Affiliated Hospital of Southern University of Science and Technology, Shenzhen, Guangdong, China

G.-p. Zheng
Department of Radiology, The Third People's Hospital of Shenzhen, Shenzhen, Guangdong, China

P.-x. Lu
Department of Medical Imaging, Shenzhen Center for Chronic Disease Control, Shenzhen, Guangdong, China

C. Qiu et al. (eds.), *Avian Influenza in Human*, https://doi.org/10.1007/978-981-16-1429-3_10

bacterial infection may occur, with sepsis and a mortality above 50%. Laboratory findings are mainly a decrease of peripheral leukocyte count and the drop of the absolute value of lymphocytes [4–6].

The studies showed that pandemic of H5N1 avian influenza in humans occurred mainly in countries in East Asia, Southeast Asia, and North Africa. H5N1 avian influenza in humans seems seasonal, and the incidence is higher from every December to March of the next year in the Northern Hemisphere, which may be related to the migration pattern and virus activity of wild birds. In addition, the temperature is relatively lower in this season in Asia and North Africa, which increases the incidence of H5N1 infection. This seems consistent with the outbreak and increased transmission of the H5N1 virus in domestic poultries under cold and dry conditions, and overlaps with epidemics such as human seasonal influenza [7, 8].

10.2 Image Findings

It has been found in studies on replication of H5N1 virus infecting mice [9] that the presence and replication of virus can be detected in pulmonary tissues post to H5N1 virus infection in humans. In the autopsied lung tissues of human cases infected with highly pathogenic subtype H5N1 avian influenza, diffuse alveolar injury is found in the lung tissues, exudative changes in early stage, alveolar epithelial necrosis and exfoliation, and a large number of exudates uniformly dyed pink with extensive formation of hyaline membrane in the alveolar cavity. In the middle and late stages, the main changes include hyperplasia and fibrosis, hyperplasia of alveolar epithelium and bronchial epithelium, exudates in the alveolar cavity, and pulmonary mesenchymal fibrosis. Highly pathogenic H5N1 avian influenza virus may cause severe acute viral pneumonia, alveolar edema, bleeding, fibrin exudation, and pulmonary mesenchymal fibrosis, which are the main pathological changes of the lungs [10, 11].

The main manifestation of chest images is the exudation, i.e., ground-glass opacities and pulmonary consolidations, due to viral infiltration in the lungs of patients with H5N1 subtype avian influenza. Patients with severe disease show rapid progressions, manifesting large flaky ground-glass opacities and pulmonary consolidations, followed by the appearance of "white lungs." Multiple severe complications may occur, including acute pulmonary injury, acute respiratory distress syndrome (ARDS), secondary bacterial and/or fungal infection, multiple organ dysfunction, shock, and Reye Syndrome.

I. *Typical image findings of pneumonia induced by H5N1 avian influenza in humans*

Diagnosis of pneumonia induced by H5N1 avian influenza in humans can be confirmed based on epidemiological history, clinical manifestation, imaging, and etiological examination. The presence of infiltration opacity in the lungs shown by image findings is the important component in diagnosing pneumonia caused by avian influenza in humans. Serial chest X-ray may show the dynamic changes of the disease, which is the main approach to evaluate the progress of the disease, observe the response, and estimate the prognosis of patients. CT scans may evaluate the disease more objectively and comprehensively, capable of finding tiny dynamic changes of lesions and their distribution and acquire more information about the disease than X-ray. In the case of human infected with subtype H5N1 avian influenza infiltrating extensively pulmonary tissues, the image may show multi-lobular and multi-segmental diffuse ground-glass opacities and consolidations, which manifest "white lungs" on chest X-ray and CT at the peak of disease progression, i.e., large patches of cloud-like density seen in most of the bilateral pulmonary fields. It is roughly consistent with images at the peak of pulmonary infection induced by subtypes H5N6 and H10N8 avian influenza viruses [12].

1. Early image findings. Focal patches, ground-glass opacities, and flaky consolidations are observed in 90% of patients in the early stage (within 7 days post to the onset). Small flaky opacities, either solitary or multiple, may appear successively, which are distributed frequently in the right lung and the peripherals. Findings in chest X-ray in pneumonia caused by H5N1 avian influenza occurring in Vietnam manifested multiple focal diseases in more than 90% of patients, and involvement of both lungs in 80% of patients. In addition, opacities of lobular central nodules and pulmonary interstitial lesions were also included (Fig. 10.1).
2. The disease aggravates in the progression stage (day 10–14 post to the onset). Small flaky opacities in the early stage may evolve into large flaky, multiple, or diffuse lesions within 3–7 days, with aerial bronchogram within consolidations. Patients with clinically severe diseases show rapid progress of lesions, which develop from unilateral lung to both lungs, from one pulmonary field to multiple fields, or from ground-glass opacities to consolidations within several days or even 1 day, manifesting the simultaneous presence of pulmonary consolidations and ground-glass opacities in lungs as shown by CT scans (Figs. 10.2 and 10.3).
3. Recovery stage (days 22–30 post to onset). The disease is stabilized and pulmonary lesions start to be absorbed, after active treatment. The absorption of alveolar inflammation is relatively faster, with more rapid absorption of the latest infiltrated site and slow absorption of lesions occurring at first. Imaging manifestations include mainly pulmonary parenchymal changes, showing dominantly flaky ground-glass opacities, streaks or grids, thickening of lobular septum, and subpleural arcs.

II. *Profiles of clinical imaging of humans with pneumonia caused by H5N1 avian influenza*

1. Its main imaging profiles include ground-glass opacities and pulmonary consolidations in both lungs. Alveolar cavities are filled with a great deal of cellulose, erythrocytes, and edema fluid, due to exfoliation of necrotic alveolar epithelium and decreased air contained in alveoli. Chest imaging manifests mainly alveolar exudation and pulmonary consolidation. The exudates inside alveoli fill and cover the pulmonary mesenchymal, manifesting consolidations with increased density. After alveolar exudates are absorbed partially, the images manifest grids. Streaks and patches. Thickening of interlobular septum and the sign of subpleural line can be found by high-resolution CT scans (HRCT). Destruction of alveolar epithelial cells and injured basement membrane are the important features of pulmonary mesenchymal fibrosis. Therefore, the evolution of pneumonia should be monitored closely in patients having severe pneumonia.

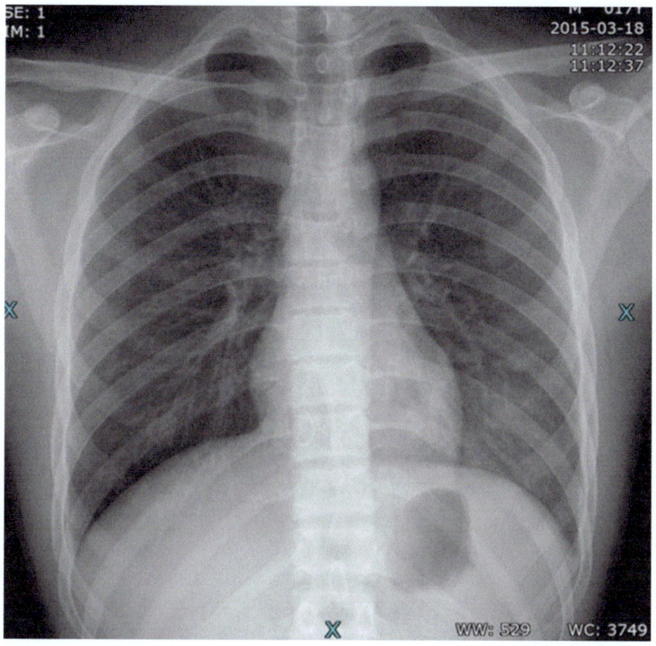

Fig. 10.1 A 17-year-old male, who was admitted due to high fever and dyspnea. He had no dizziness, headache, cough, or expectoration. Laboratory examinations showed a decrease of leukocytes. He denied the history of exposure to deal/alive poultries and the history of traveling to epidemic zones. Pneumonia of H5N1 avian influenza virus infecting humans (the severe case) (Figs. 10.1, 10.2 and 10.3). Chest X-ray on day 4 post to the onset, showing a small flaky high-density opacity with unclear border and uneven density in the lower-left pulmonary field, and images of the upper left lung and the right lung seem normal

2. Rapid progress of lesions. Dynamic observation for images reveals small flaky ground-glass opacities and consolidations in unilateral pulmonary field during the early stage of onset. Within the following 1–2 day(s), the lesions may expand rapidly to upper, middle, and lower fields, involving bilateral lobes, manifesting uneven density and showing ground-glass opacities with unclear borders, which are present concurrently with pulmonary consolidations containing aerial bronchogram. It is significantly different from other viral pneumonias, such as cytomegalovirus pneumonia and pneumocystis jiroveci pneumonia (PJP), which progresses relatively slow. Therefore, reexamination with CT scans as soon as possible is of great importance to understand the outcome of the disease and evaluate the response, for patients with pneumonia of H5N1 avian influenza (Figs. 10.2 and 10.3).
3. Slow Absorption of Lesions

   When the patient shows stable disease and basic indexes recover, such as temperature, respiration, and

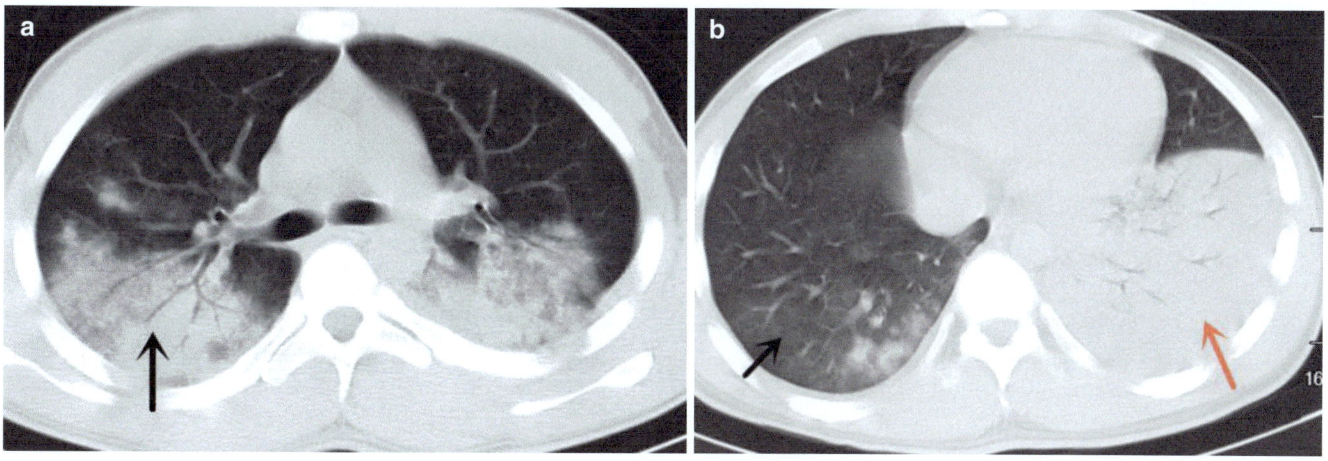

Fig. 10.2 The image on day 6 post to onset. (**a**) pulmonary window of CT shows multiple patchy and flaky high-density opacities in each lobe of both lungs, which have uneven density with aerial bronchogram (indicated by the black arrow); (**b**) ground-glass opacities (indicated by the black arrow) and pulmonary consolidation (indicated by the red arrow) are observed

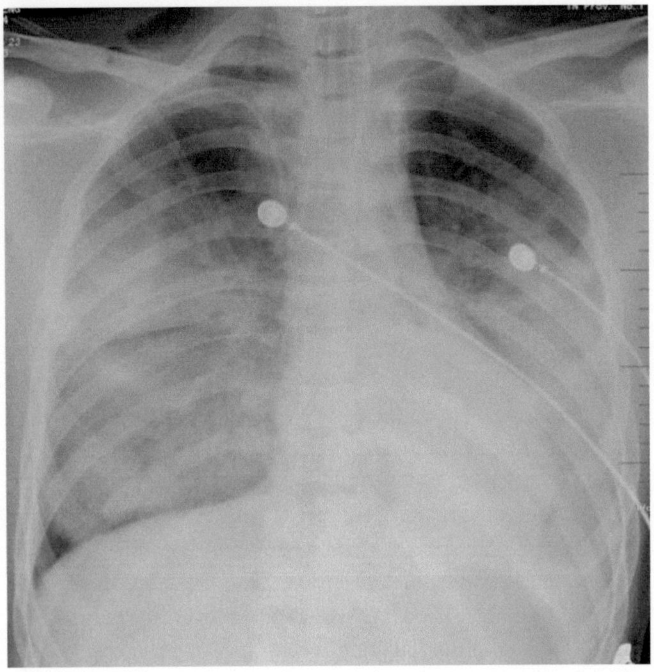

Fig. 10.3 Image on day 9 post to the onset, showing extensive high-density opacities in chest X-ray of both lungs, with the appearance of "white lungs"

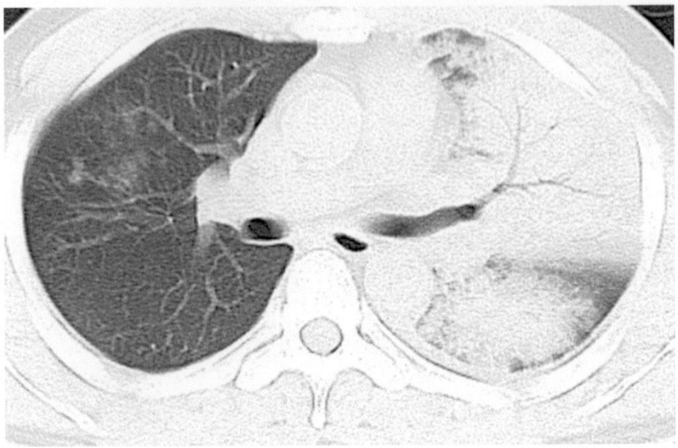

Fig. 10.4 A 31-year-old male had fever, cough, and shortness of breath on June 3, 2006, and was diagnosed as pneumonia induced by H5N1 avian influenza in humans (severe disease). Five-year follow-up for clinical imaging was performed for him after he was cured and discharged. Chest CT after 5 years shows that lesions of both lungs have been absorbed roughly, and only a small amount of fibrous streaks remain with localized bronchiectasis (Figs. 10.4, 10.5, 10.6, 10.7, 10.8, 10.9 and 10.10). Day 6 post to the onset. CT shows small flaky ground-glass opacities in the right lung, and large flaky consolidations containing aerial bronchogram in the left lung

leukocytes, imaging follow-up still reveals opacities in strips, grids, and patches in both lungs. The follow up within 1–5 year(s) for some of the patients post to discharge still shows opacities in fibrous streaks, pale thin opacities in ground glass density, bronchiectasis in honeycombs, beads and twisted, mediastinal and subpleural emphysema, interlobular septal thickening, paraseptal lobular emphysema, etc., but without obvious lymphadenopathy at hilum and mediastinum. This implies the inconsistency between changes of chest images and clinical symptoms/signs in case of prolonged persistence of lesions, i.e., the absorption of pulmonary lesion lags behind clinical symptoms [13–15] (Figs. 10.4, 10.5, 10.6, 10.7, 10.8, 10.9 and 10.10).

4. Complications

Multiple or severe complications may occur clinically in patients with pneumonia induced by subtype H5N1 avian influenza. (1) After the infection of subtype H5N1 avian influenza takes place in humans, significant inflammation occurs in pulmonary tissues, and neutrophils increase and infiltrate into the alveolar cavity during the advanced stage of infection, forming hyaline membrane in alveoli. Extensive high-density consolidations in both lungs are shown by imaging, i.e., the white lungs, implying the complication of ARDS. (2) Secondary pulmonary infections may occur, commonly those induced by *Streptococcus pneumoniae*, *Staphylococcus aureus*, *Pseudomonas aeruginosa*, and fungi including mainly *Candida albicans* and aspergillus fumigatus, as well as secondary infection due to other bacteria, manifesting patchy uneven opacities in the lungs. (3) Pleural effusion: 15% of the 20 patients in Hongkong from 1997 to 2003 had pleural effusion in various degrees. (4) Emphysema, mediastinal emphysema, and pneumothorax. CT scans in the absorption stage show signs of scattered lobular paraseptal emphysema. Mediastinal emphysema, pneumothorax, and subcutaneous pneumatosis are serious complications requiring clinical tracheotomy and tracheal intubation [13]. (5) Reye Syndrome, one of the common complications post to

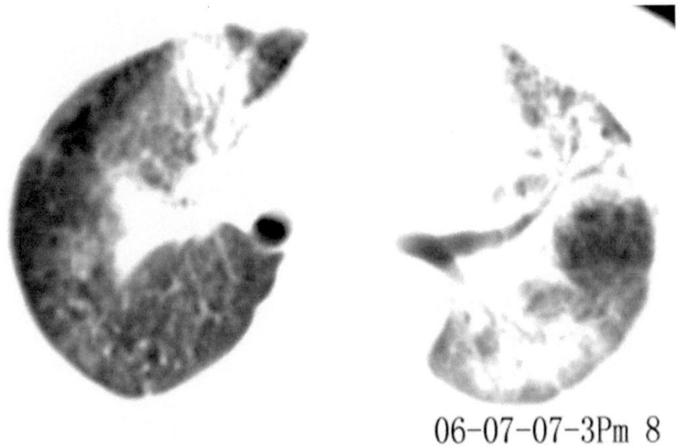

Fig. 10.5 Day 34 post to the onset. CT shows large flaky consolidations and ground-glass opacities in both lungs, with certain absorption of the consolidation in the left lung compared with the image 2 months before

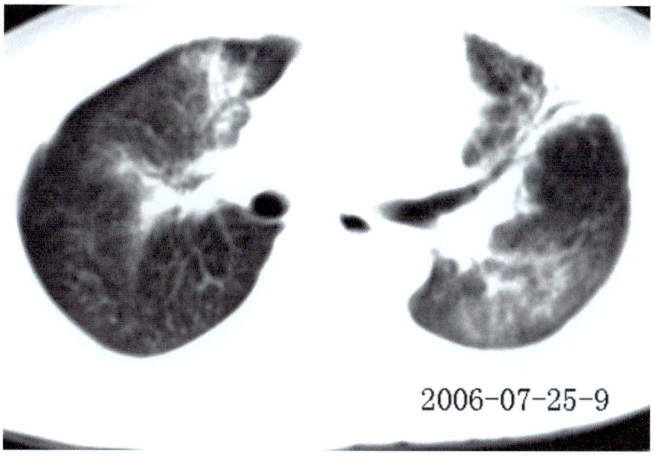

Fig. 10.6 Day 52 post to the onset. CT shows large flaky consolidations and ground-glass opacities in both lungs, with certain absorption of the consolidation in both lungs compared with the image 20 days before

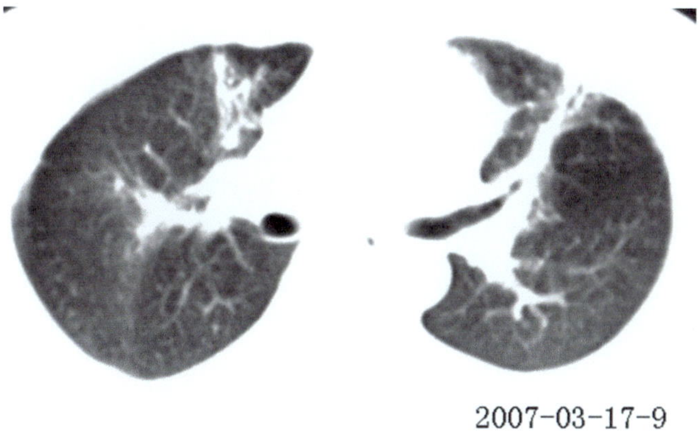

Fig. 10.7 Day 326 post to the onset. CT shows strip consolidations and fibrous opacities, with further absorption of lesions in both lungs compared with the CT scans 8 months before

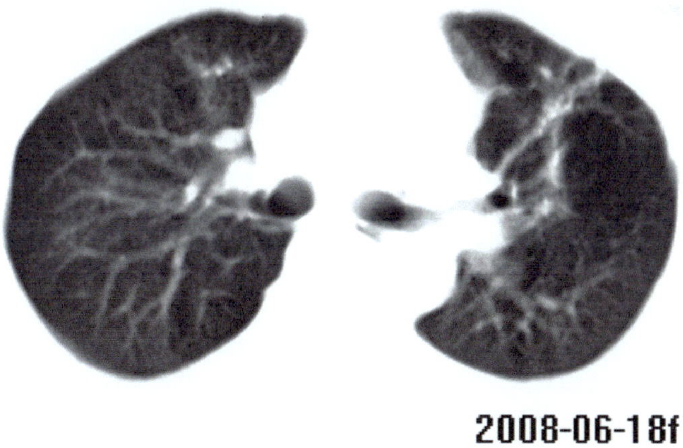

Fig. 10.8 Reexamination nearly 2 years after discharge. Chest CT shows that streaks remain in the lingual segment of the upper lobe of the left lung and the middle lobe of the right lung

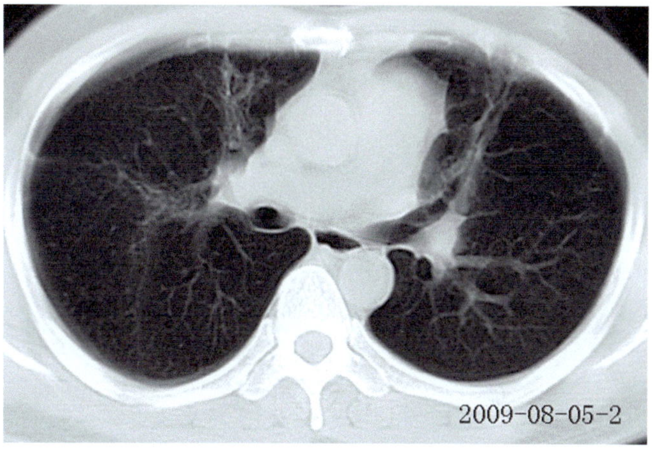

Fig. 10.9 Reexamination more than 3 years after discharge. Chest CT shows that streaks remain in the lingual segment of the upper lobe of the left lung and the middle lobe of the right lung, with certain absorption compared with the previous image

subtype H5N1 avian influenza infecting children, is characterized by acute encephalopathy complicated with liver steatosis. (6) Pulmonary fibrosis. Despite the stable disease, HRCT prior to the discharge shows also irregular grids, fibrous streaks, and patches in both lungs, with concurrent localized pleural thickening. Follow-up of images reveals that pulmonary mesenchymal fibrosis in various degrees can also be observed in lungs within 1–5 years after the patient was cured and discharged [13].

10.3 Clinical Imaging Diagnosis and Differential Diagnosis

Lung images of pneumonia caused by subtype H5N1 avian influenza in humans manifest fast evolution, severe pneumonia, slow absorption, and concurrent presence of pulmonary mesenchymal lesions and consolidation images. Ground-glass opacities and consolidations are characteristic findings in earlier stages post to infection of avian influenza virus in humans. Clinical diagnosis of pneumonia caused by subtype H5N1 avian influenza in humans is mainly based on clinical symptoms and signs, epidemiologic history, and image findings, and its confirmation requires laboratory positiveness in nucleic acid detection for subtype H5N1 virus or virus separation. From the perspective of clinical images, human pneumonia induced by subtype H5N1 avian influenza needs to be differentiated from viral pneumonia, SARS and AIDS complicated with PJP infection.

I. Differentiation with influenza virus pneumonia

Lung markings increase in the early stage of influenza virus pneumonia, with the appearance of small nodules

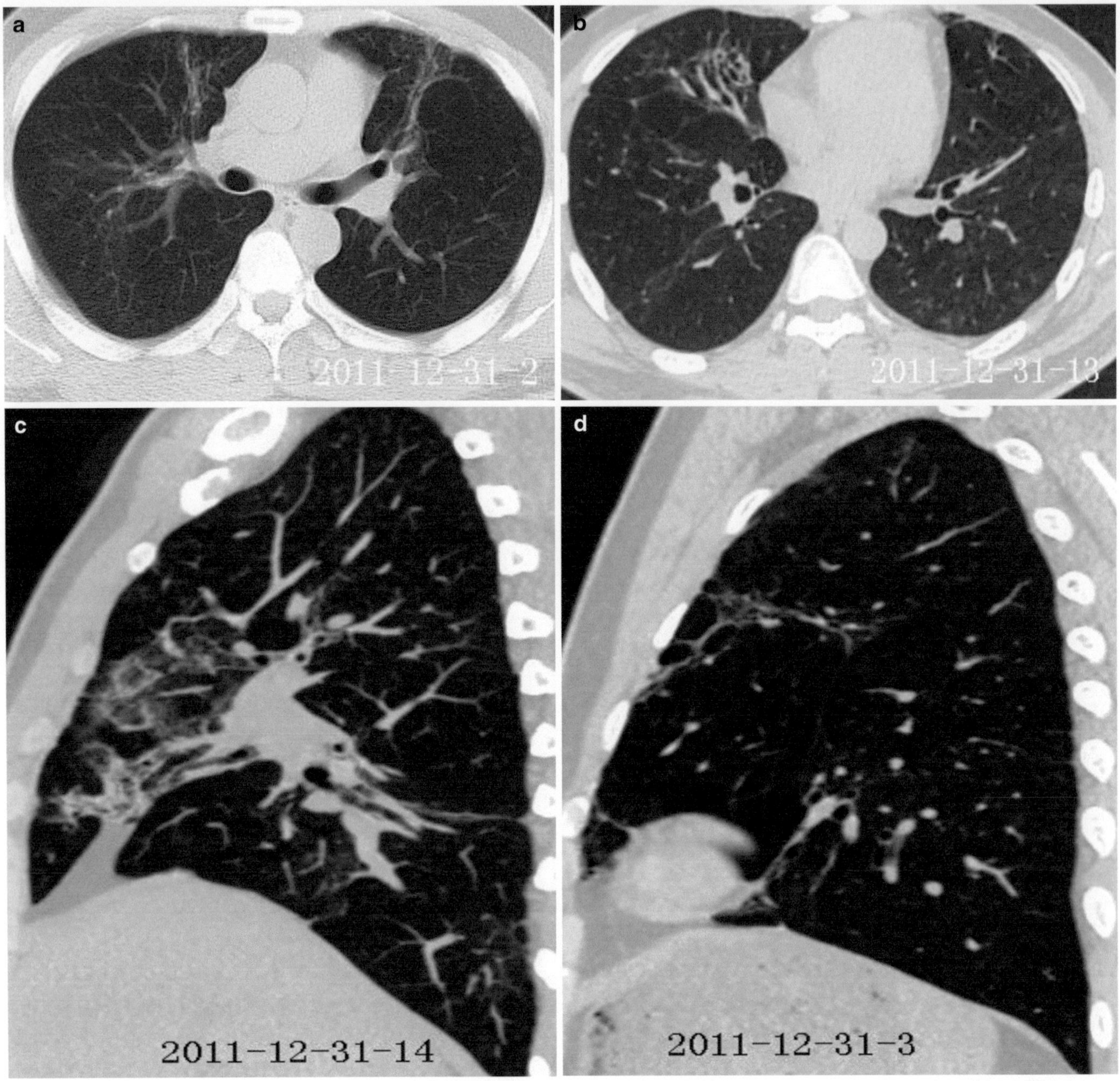

Fig. 10.10 (**a–d**) Reexamination nearly 5 years after discharge. Chest CT shows that lesions in both lungs have been absorbed roughly, and only fibrous streaks remain in the lingual segment of the upper lobe of the left lung and the middle lobe of the right lung, with localized bronchiectasis

along the lung markings. Pathologically, influenza virus pneumonia mainly manifests as interstitial pneumonia involving also alveolar cavities and seeming commonly focal. Patchy or large flaky high-density opacities may appear in the chest, with its dynamic change not so rapid as observed in pneumonia induced by avian influenza virus in humans, and not so severe and extensive as noticed in the pneumonia of subtype H5N1.

II. Differentiation with pneumonia induced by other subtypes of avian influenza in humans

Pneumonia induced by H9N2 avian influenza in humans is relatively mild with its chest manifestations not so serious as subtype H5N1 and generally does not show "white lung" appearance. Pneumonias induced by subtypes H7N9, H5N6, or H10N8 avian influenzas are difficult to differentiate from subtype H5N1 pneumonia if it is based on images alone. Instead, the differentiation depends mainly on epidemiology and etiological diagnosis. Viruses inducing all these avian influenza pneumonias belong to type A virus, all of which may manifest influenza-like symptoms and multiple different-sized ground-glass opacities and pulmonary consolidations shown by CT scans and distributed dominantly in middle or lower lobes of both lungs, and "white lung" may appear. The pneumonia induced by viral subtypes are arranged in descending order as H5N1, H7N9, H10N8, and H5N6 based on the area of pulmonary lesions, and as H5N1, H7N9, H5N6, and H10N8 based on the rate of progression.

Main findings in CT scans of pneumonia induced by H5N1 avian influenza in humans manifest mainly large flaky ground-glass opacities and pulmonary consolidations, with extensive distribution of lesions, fast progress, and slow absorption showing obvious pulmonary interstitial fibrosis and a mortality of about 60%. H7N9 avian influenza pneumonia in humans has an onset originating from the middle and lower lobes of both lungs, dominated by ground-glass opacities and pulmonary consolidations with fast variation and slow absorption. Its mortality is about 36%. Fewer patients with pneumonia induced by H5N6 or H10N8 avian influenza in humans have been reported, and findings in their chest images are dominantly ground-glass opacities and pulmonary consolidations.

III. Differentiation with SARS

SAR is an acute respiratory infectious disease caused by the SARS coronavirus. It broke out all over the world in 2003, and most of the patients had a good prognosis with a mortality of about 9.0%. Findings in chest CT scans include local small patchy ground-glass opacity in the early stage, mostly in solitary and progressing rapidly into diffuse ground-glass opacities alone or combined with consolidations in multiple lobes or both lungs. It is characterized by rapidly dynamic evolution, new lesions alternating with the old, resurgent lesions, and slow absorption in the recovery. It is hard to differentiate SARS from H5N1 avian influenza in humans based on imaging, and the confirmation relies also on epidemiology and etiological tests.

IV. Differentiation from AIDS complicated with PJP infection

AIDS complicated with pneumocystis jiroveci pneumonia (PJP) has diffuse ground-glass opacities with concurrent patchy consolidations in both lungs, as shown by imaging, which is similar to that of pneumonia induced by subtype H5N1. However, changes of pulmonary air sacs exist commonly in addition to the ground-glass opacities, the feature for AIDS complicated with PJP, which is not hard to differentiate if clinical history is taken into account in combination [16].

10.4 Introduction of the First Case in Chinese Mainland

A 9-year-old boy was admitted to Hunan Children's Hospital in China due to "pneumonia with unknown reason" on October 18, 2005, and diagnosed as highly pathogenic avian influenza H5N1 by the Chinese Ministry of Health and World Health Organization. It is the first case of avian influenza in humans rescued successfully both in the Chinese Mainland and in the whole country [17, 18].

I. *Clinical history*

A 9-year-old boy manifesting fever and mild cough on October 10, 2005 sought medical advice in a local primary hospital and was medicated with amoxicillin and cotrimoxazole for 2 days. The symptoms were somehow relieved and no further treatment was given. The boy had a fever again with body temperature unknown on October 15, 2005 after having received an intramuscular injection of Aminopyrine, and then he had frequent cough and underwent subsequent treatment with amoxicillin, compound sulfamethoxazole, and licorice compound. On October 17, 2005, he was admitted to a hospital in Xiangtan City, Hunan Province in China because the symptoms were not relieved. He was lassitude with a fever up to 39 °C at admission, but without vomiting, stomachache, diarrhea, or rash. The disease kept progressing post to admission with body temperature persisting above 39 °C, which was considered to be acute respiratory infectious disease. Therefore, he was transferred to the ICU of Hunan Children's Hospital on October 18, 2005 for isolation therapy.

II. *Symptoms and signs*

Physical examination post to admission: T 40 °C, R 30/min, P 136 beats/min, BP 100/53 mmHg, and bodyweight of 22 kg. He had slight shortness of breath, without obvious anoxia sign, and several soybean-sized lymph nodes were palpable bilaterally in the neck and groin. The pharynx was congested and the tonsils were enlarged in degree II. The breath of both lungs sounded harsh, with fine bubbling rales heard at the bottom of both lungs, without pleural rub. Heart rate was 136 beats/min with a regular rhythm, and the heart sounds were strong. The abdomen touched soft; no enlargement of the liver and spleen; no abnormality in examination of nervous system. Main symptoms: intermittent fever and cough with little expectoration.

III. *Laboratory tests*

Blood routine: leukocyte count 2.8×10^9/L, lymphocyte count 0.75×10^9/L, hemoglobin ICU 111 g/L, and platelet $157 \times 10\ ^9$/L. It is generally normal in blood chemistry, erythrocyte sedimentation rate, and blood gas analysis. H5N1 virus was negative in pharyngeal swabs and serum in laboratory tests. A rise for more than 4 times of H5 specific antibodies was observed in double serums in the advanced stage post to onset and in the recovery stage. It was confirmed to be H5N1 by the World Health Organization and the experts group of the Ministry of Health.

IV. *Epidemiology*

Before the onset of the disease, there were dead ducks in the residential area where the boy was living, and he had a history of eating dead ducks. During this period, the boy ate salted smoked dead chicken many times. The history of direct exposure remained unknown. His elder sister began to have influenza-like symptoms on October 8, 2005, which aggravated on day 5 post to the onset, and she died of "ARDS and respiratory failure" on day 8 (October 17, 2005). The sister of the boy was a suspected case of avian influenza pneumonia in humans, as determined by the World Health Organization and the expert group of the Ministry of health of the country.

V. *Image findings and dynamic changes*

The boy underwent chest X-ray for the first time on day 8 post to onset, showing a large flaky opacity in the upper lobe of the left lung, a large patchy dense opacity in the upper lobe of the left lung, a paramediastinal patchy opacity in the upper lobe of the right lung, and opacities in the upper lobe and lingula lobe of the left lung, with blurred border. The increase of bilateral lung markings was observed, which seemed blurred with disorderly arranged structures at both hila. The left intercostal space was slightly narrowed. Reexamination performed 1 day later showed the obvious progression of lesions in both lungs. The patient underwent subsequently reexamination of chest X-ray on day 12 post to onset until day 55 post to onset, i.e., February 11, 2006, which showed roughly absorption of lesions in both lungs shown by X-ray, with small amount of fibrous streaks. Reexamination of chest CT scans at discharge: subpleural arcs and streaks are observed in bilateral upper lobes and the lower left lobe. The complete absorption of these lesions was shown by reexamination with plain X-ray and CT scans 13 months later (Figs. 10.11, 10.12, 10.13, 10.14, 10.15, 10.16, 10.17, 10.18 and 10.19).

VI. *Treatment*

The patient was treated with broad-spectrum antibiotics, amantadine, ribavirin, gamma globulin, and a low dose of hormone. After a 5-day rescue in Hunan Children's Hospital, his temperature recovered to normal with ameliorate mental state and appetite, the cough was lessened, and pulmonary rales in auscultation were reduced. Rales in pulmonary auscultation disappeared after 8-day treatment, and lesions were absorbed gradually and the disease became stable. He was cured and discharged on November 12, 2005.

VII. *Discussion*

This pediatric patient was the first confirmed case of pneumonia induced by H5N1 avian influenza in humans in the Chinese Mainland. Before the onset of the dis-

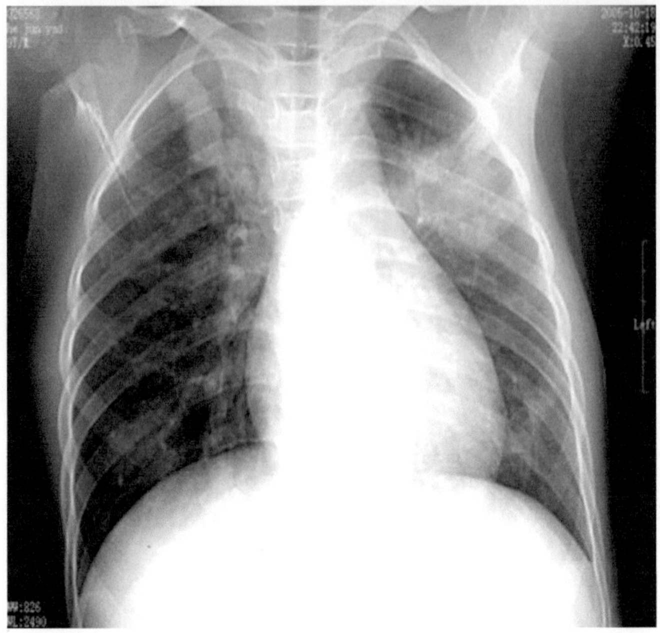

Fig. 10.11 The patient was a 9-year-old boy. He had a fever and mild cough on October 10, 2005. Before the onset of the disease, there were dead ducks in the residential area where the boy was living, and he had a history of eating dead ducks. He was diagnosed with severe pneumonia induced by H5N1 avian influenza in humans (Figs. 10.11, 10.12, 10.13, 10.14, 10.15, 10.16, 10.17, 10.18 and 10.19). On day 1 (October 18, 2005) of hospital stay, i.e., day 8 post to the onset, chest PA showed a large flaky dense opacity in the upper left lobe, and patchy opacities in the left upper lung and paramediastinal upper right lobe, with blurred border. Bilateral lung markings increased and became blurred, and structures of bilateral hila seemed disordered. The left intercostal space became slightly narrow

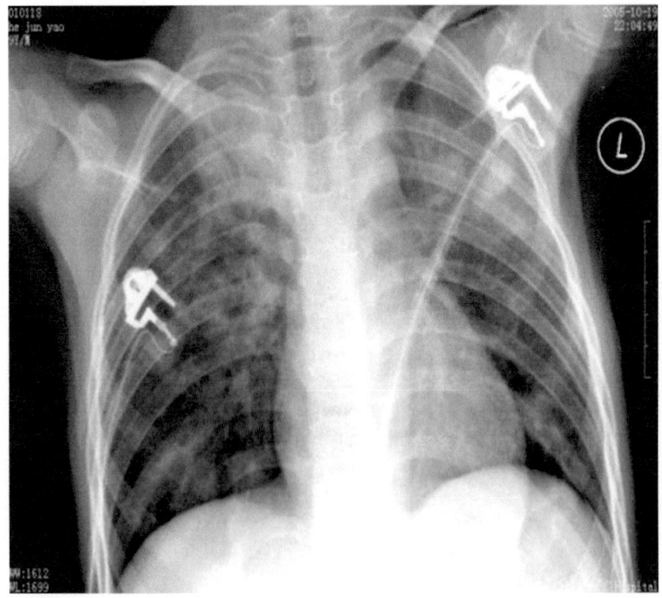

Fig. 10.12 On day 2 (October 19, 2005) of hospital stay, i.e., day 9 post to the onset, chest X-ray showed gradual increase of lesions in both lungs with increased density and enlarged area

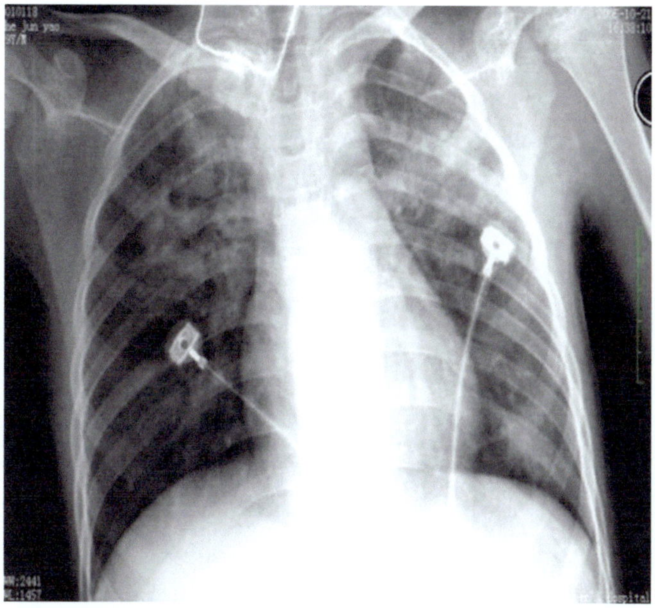

Fig. 10.13 On day 4 (October 21, 2005) of hospital stay, i.e., day 11 post to the onset, chest X-ray showed the enlarged area of flaky high-density opacity in the lower left lobe and starting absorption of lesion in the lower right lung

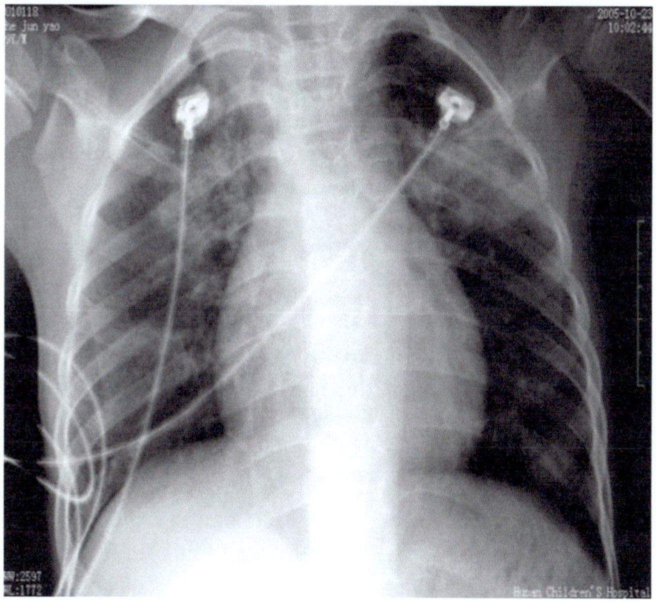

Fig. 10.14 On day 6 (October 23, 2005) of the hospital stay, i.e., day 13 post to the onset, the slight absorption was noticed in lesions in the outer zone of the upper right lung and the lower left lung

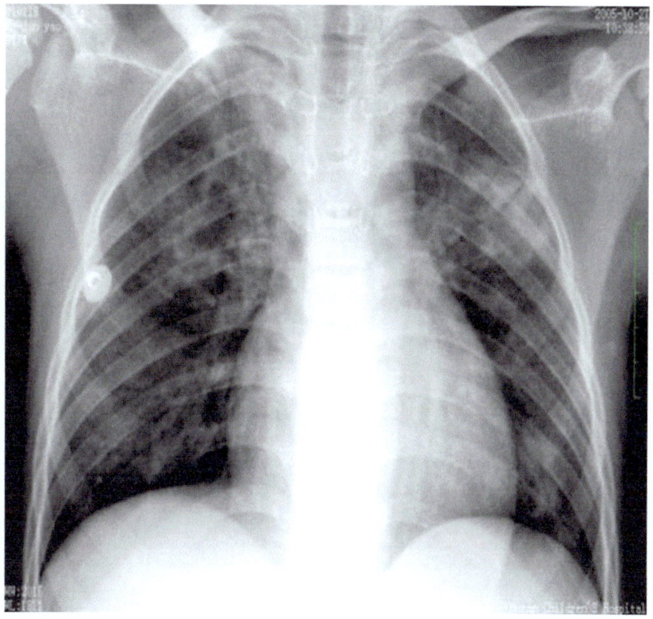

Fig. 10.15 On day 10 (October 27, 2005) of hospital stay, i.e., day 17 post to the onset, lesions in upper lobes of both lungs faded with their areas shrunk, and the area of flaky opacity in the lower right lung increased slightly

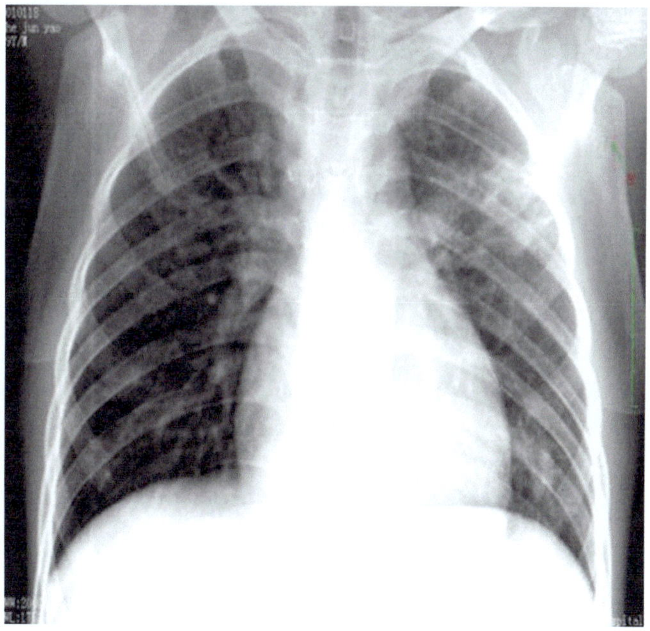

Fig. 10.16 On day 17 (November 3, 2005) of hospital stay, i.e., day 24 post to the onset, obvious absorption of the patchy opacity in the right lung was observed in comparison with previous images, but there was still scattered small patchy opacities. A slight absorption and shrinking of flaky opacities in the upper left lung was found, and lesions in the middle and lower left lung were absorbed slightly

ease, there were dead ducks in the residential area where the boy was living, and he had a history of eating dead ducks. During this period, the boy ate salted smoked dead chicken many times. His elder sister died from ARDS and respiratory failure on day 7 of the onset of the boy. Despite the failure in collecting acute respiratory tract specimen from this pediatric patient and in detecting segments of nucleic acid of H5N1 avian influenza virus or isolating the virus in the laboratory, confirmed H5N1 epidemics of animals did take

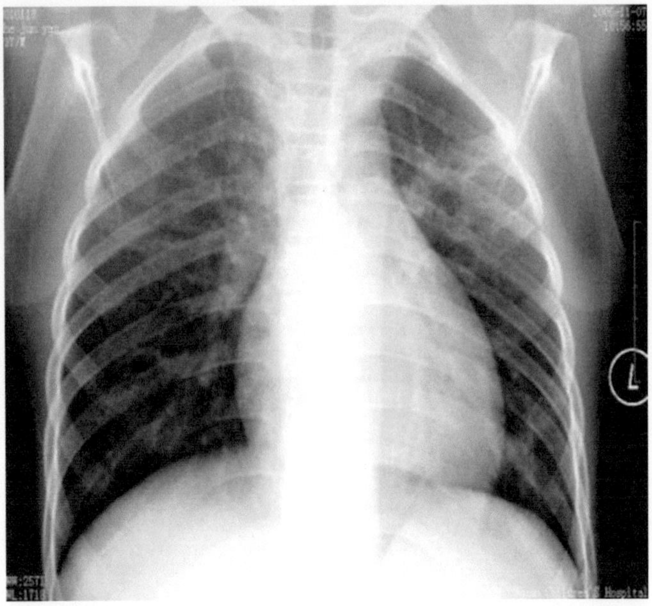

Fig. 10.17 On day 21 (November 7, 2005) of hospital stay, i.e., day 28 post to the onset, there seemed to be an absorption of the patchy opacity in the right lung compared with the previous image but scattered small patchy opacities were still observable. The flaky opacity in the upper left lung was absorbed slightly and shrank, and lesions in the middle and lower left lungs are absorbed slightly

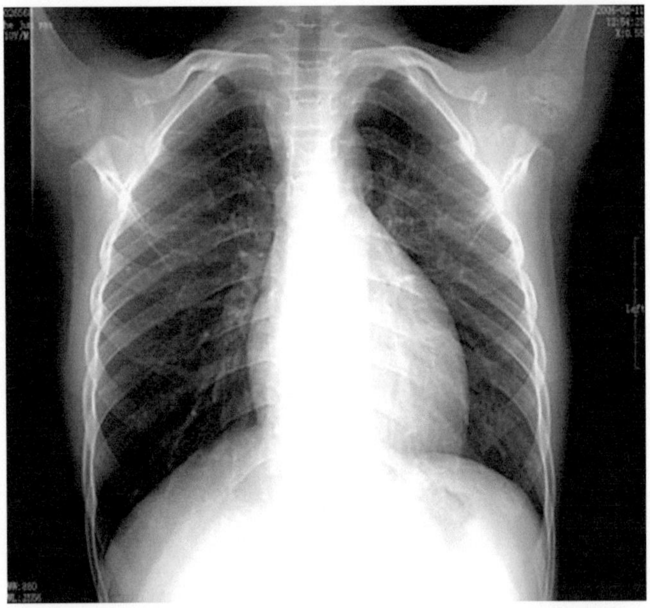

Fig. 10.18 On day 32 post to the onset (February 11, 2006), chest X-ray showed the fundamental absorption of lesions in both lungs

place in the boy's home and he did have an obvious history of exposure to the environment polluted by sick or dead poultries. The diagnosis was established, taking the clinical manifestations into consideration based on more than 4-time rise of HS-specific antibodies in double sera in both the acute stage and the recovery stage.

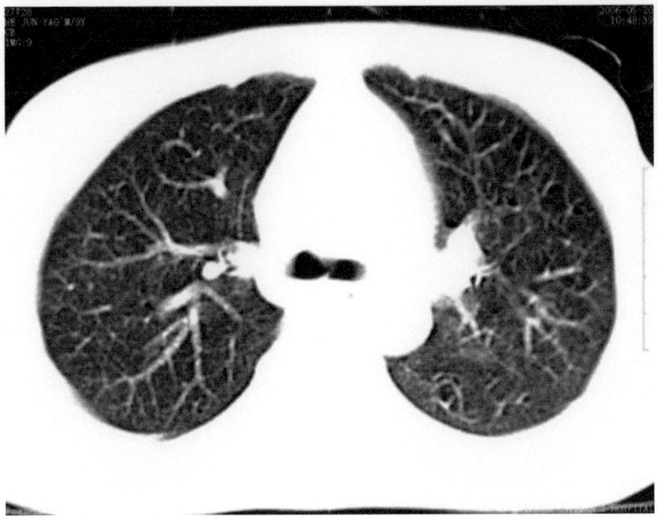

Fig. 10.19 On day 25 of the hospital stay, i.e., day 33 post to the onset, reexamination of CT scans at discharge showed multiple streaks in upper lobes of both lungs and the lower left lung, with thickening of the alveolar septum

His elder sister was diagnosed as a suspected case of pneumonia induced by avian influenza viruses in humans.

Studies have shown that the mortality of children infected with the H5N1 subtype avian influenza virus is high, which is up to 89% in Thailand. The cause of death is respiratory failure [19]. General recovery was achieved in this patient post to active treatment, the temperature was normalized on day 12 post to the onset, and absorption of lesions was shown by reexamination with plain chest X-ray and CT on month 13 post to the onset. In contrast to his sister with a severer disease not treated with antiviral drugs such as amantadine, this patient received antiviral medications including amantadine, which suggested a certain efficacy of Amantadine in treating H5N1 infection. Image findings for the pediatric patient showed a large flaky dense opacity in the upper lobe of the left lung in the early stage, with paramediastinal patchy opacities in the upper lobe of the right lung and patchy opacities in the upper lobe and lingula lobe of the left lung, with blurred border. The markings of both lungs increased and became blurred, and bilateral hilar structures seemed disordered. Thereafter, lesions progressed within a short time, manifesting firstly the enlargement of lesions in both upper lungs, followed by novel lesions appearing in the lower left lung and the right lateral lung, manifesting large flaky flocculent opacities distributed extensively. The area of partial pulmonary lesions (mainly those in the middle and lower fields of the right lung) shrank post to active treatment, manifesting absorption and amelioration. Streaks in the upper left lung were shown by plain chest X-ray on day 21 post to onset, with a small amount of streaks in the upper right lung. Reexamination with plain X-ray and CT showed the complete absorption of lesions 13 months later. The complete absorption of lesions post to active antiviral treatment for subtype H5N1 virus correlated probably to younger age, stronger self-healing, and milder disease of the patient.

The diagnosis was evidenced by symptoms, epidemiological history (history of contacting and eating dead ducks), image findings, and a rise for at least four times of H5 specific antibodies in double sera in the advanced stage post to onset and in the recovery. It also provided evidences for the suspected severe pneumonia of avian influenza virus in his elder sister. Antiviral medication such as Amantadine launched earlier by clinicians won a greater chance of recovery for the patient, suggesting the efficacy of active treatment in achieving complete absorption of pulmonary lesions in children infected with H5N1 avian influenza virus.

References

1. Duan L, Bahl J, Smith GJ, et al. The development and genetic diversity of H5N1 influenza virus in China, 1996–2006. Virology. 2008;380:243–54.
2. Yuen KY, Chan PK, Peiris M, et al. Clinical features and rapid viral diagnosis of human disease associated with avian influenza A H5N1 virus. Lancet. 1998;351:467–71.
3. http://www.chinacdc.cn/jkzt/crb/zl/rgrgzbxqlg/
4. Yang Y, Liu M. An analysis on clinical features of highly pathogenic H5N1 avian influenza in human. Dis Surveillance. 2011;26(04):328–33.
5. Li H, Lu P, Shi Y, editors. Imaging of influenza, vol. 1. Beijing: Science Press; 2016. p. 93.
6. Tao Z, Wang S. One case of a child infected with highly pathogenic avian influenza virus. Chin J Infect Control. 2007;6(2):136–7.
7. Durand LO, Glew P, Gross D, et al. Timing of influenza A (H5N1) in poultry and humans and seasonal influenza activity worldwide, 2004–2013. Emerg Infect Dis. 2015;21(2):202–8.
8. Lai S, Qin Y, Cowling BJ, et al. Global epidemiology of avian influenza A(H5N1) virus infection in humans, 1997–2015: a systematic review. Lancet Infect Dis. 2016;16(7):e108–18.
9. Liu C, Wu X, Zhao G, et al. An analysis of features of mice infected with human H7N9 avian influenza virus, highly pathogenic H5N1 and H1N1 avian influenza virus. Acta Lab Anim Sci Sinica. 2014;22(1):8–11, 4–5.
10. Liu X. Pathological and etiological features of human infected with highly pathogenic avian influenza virus H5N1. New Med Innov China. 2015;12(23):111–2.
11. Lu M, Xie Z, Gao Z, et al. Pathological observation for human infected with highly pathogenic avian influenza virus H5N1. Chin J Pathol. 2008;37(3):145–9.
12. Puxuan L. Epidemiological and clinical imaging characteristics of the globally first case of avian influenza in human occurring in China. Electron J Emerg Infect Dis. 2017;2(2):124–6.
13. Zhu W, Lu P, Zhou B, et al. Imaging evaluation and long-term follow up for severe pneumonia induced by subtype H5N1 avian influenza in adults. Chin J Med Imaging. 2014;22(8):598–601,606.
14. Lu P, Zhou B, Zhu W, et al. Imaging findings characteristics of Pneumonia induced by highly pathogenic subtype H5N1 avian influenza virus in human. Chin Med Imaging Technol. 2007;23(4):532–5.
15. Lu P, Deng Y. Epidemiological features and image findings of lungs of avian influenza in human. Chin J Med Comput Imaging. 2010;16(5):431–4.
16. Lu P, Zhou B, editors. Clinical imaging diagnosis of new infectious diseases, vol. 5. Beijing: People's Medical Publishing House; 2013. p. 239.
17. Luo R, Zhu Y, Xu Z, et al. Report of the first case of H5N1 avian influenza in human in Chinese Mainland. Chin J Pediatr. 2006;44(5):342–5.
18. Yu H, Chen Y, Shu Y, et al. Investigation and confirmation of the first case of human infected with avian influenza virus 1 in Chinese Mainland. Chin J Epidemiol. 2006;27(4):281–7.
19. Beigel GH, Farrar J, Han AM, et al. Avian influenza A (H5N1) infect ion in humans. N Engl J Med. 2005;353:1374–85.

11 H5N6 Avian Influenza in Human

Hua Huang, Yue Zeng, Qing-si Zeng, Jia-fu Lin, Gui-xia Wang, Xiao-yan Huang, and Pu-xuan Lu

11.1 Summary

Human infected with animal-derived influenza has been monitored and reported every year all over the world. This disease occurs commonly in winter and spring, and most of the patients have a history of exposure to live poultry. Influenza viruses can be categorized into four types including A, B, C, and D. Type A is more common in animal infections, such as poultry and livestock. Avian influenza and avian influenza in humans can occur repeatedly and become epidemic. Influenza virus belongs to myxoviridae, which is a single-stranded RNA virus. Avian influenza in human is an acute respiratory infectious disease caused by some strains of some subtypes of avian influenza virus. At present, avian influenza viruses can be divided into 18H subtypes (H1–H18) and 11N subtypes (N1–N11), which means theoretically that there can be 198 subtypes. However, subtypes of avian influenza viruses discovered until now that infect human beings are less than ten. Among all avian viruses in the world, the subtypes occurring firstly in China include H7N9, H5N1, H10N8, H5N6, H9N2, and H7N4. H5 and H7 are highly pathogenic avian influenza (HPAIV) [1–3]. Wild birds are natural hosts of avian influenza virus, and the virus carried by wild birds will not induce symptoms of infection. In most cases, the low pathogenic subtype virus causes mild symptoms when transmitted from wild birds to domestic poultry. Highly pathogenic avian influenza (HPAI) derives from poultry adaptive mutants. If transmitted back to wild birds, some of the viral strains will cause serious infection and even death of them. For example, infection induced by highly pathogenic avian influenza H5N1 in 2006 caused deaths of thousands of wild birds in Qinghai Lake of Western China. There are still many subtypes of viruses that have not surfaced yet. Human beings have no immunity to avian influenza virus. The mortality of infection with avian influenza virus is high and the virus may mutate. This virus is prone to mutation, so the immunity generated after previous infection cannot last, which is why people are so alert to avian influenza. It is commonly considered in the medical field that avian influenza in humans may be the greatest potential threat to human beings, and it can be said now it is just the end of the beginning of a war between human and avian influenza virus.

Subtype H5N6 virus is a novel recombinant virus transmitted mainly through the respiratory tract. Contact with poultry infected by the virus is the high-risk factor of this disease, and this disease correlates to history of occupational exposure, living environment, and the close contacts. In addition to air through which avian influenza virus is transmitted mainly, the infectious route includes also digestive tract and infection at skin wound. Viruses pollute air and environment along with secretion, excrement, and blood, organs, and tissues from corpse of the sick bird. Therefore, the close contact with survival or dead domestic poultry with avian influenza is the main spreading route. The source of H5N6 avian influenza infecting human have been found correlated to the exposure to birds. Human infection is caused mainly through inhaling H5N6 avian influenza virus, in addition to the route of close exposure to secretion or excrement of birds infected with virus (such as feces, feathers, respiratory secretion, and blood), or through the direct contact with the virus. However, no evidence for human-to-human transmission has been found up to now.

H. Huang
Department of Radiology, The Third People's Hospital of Shenzhen, Shenzhen, Guangdong, China

Y. Zeng · J.-f. Lin · G.-x. Wang
Department of Infection, Affiliated Hospital of North Sichuan Medical College, Nanchong, Sichuan, China

Q.-s. Zeng · X.-y. Huang
Department of Radiology, The First Affiliated Hospital of Guangzhou Medical University, Guangzhou, Guangdong, China

P.-x. Lu (✉)
Department of Medical Imaging, Shenzhen Center for Chronic Disease Control, Shenzhen, Guangdong, China

C. Qiu et al. (eds.), *Avian Influenza in Human*, https://doi.org/10.1007/978-981-16-1429-3_11

Experts engaged in long-term researches on infectious diseases in animals point out that subtype H5N6 is an extremely typical avian influenza virus. The possibility of its pandemic in the population is very low, and generally the infection features sporadic cases. The results of genetic sequencing imply that genes of H5N6 virus in specimen from the patients are highly homologous to the virus genes in the external environment. Reducing the chance of close contact between human and live poultry can effectively prevent human infection with H5N6 avian influenza. One of the important measures is to implement centralized slaughtering of live poultry, cold chain distribution, and fresh sales. Employees should try their best in personal protection, e.g., workers engaged in poultry breeding, trafficking, sales, and slaughtering should wear masks, gloves, and work clothes during working. Publicity efforts should be strengthened, so as to change dietary habits of the residents and improve their health literacy. As a novel avian influenza virus, H5N6 has been reported to be transmitted through domestic poultries in Provinces including Jiangxi, Guangdong, and Sichuan since 2013.

H5N6 avian influenza in human has similar symptoms to those observed in H7N9 cases, and both of them manifest symptoms of respiratory infection in the early stage including fever and cough [4]. The disease post to the onset manifests severe pneumonia. Its onset is acute and manifests dyspnea and related signs in 5–7 days post to the onset, followed by progressive aggravation into severe pneumonia. Specimens can be sampled and submitted to the Disease Control Center for detection, using a method of real-time PCR (RT-PCR) and virus isolation using specific pathogen-free (SPF) animals (chick embryo). Categories of specimens have certain influences on the results. In order to improve the detection rate, it is recommended to collect specimens in the lower respiratory tract for patients suspected to be infected with avian influenza virus. Some reports on posterior pharyngeal swab have revealed negativeness in H5N6 avian influenza nucleic acids for the upper respiratory tract, but positiveness for the lower respiratory tract.

H5N6 avian influenza virus, belonging to the family of positive myxoviridae, is a segmented negative-strand RNA virus. Similar to H5N1 and H7N9, H5N6 is one type of avian influenza virus. Positiveness of nucleic acid of H5N6 was detected in the throat swab from a patient with severe pneumonia monitored by Nanchong City on May 9th, 2014, which was confirmed later to be H5N6 avian influenza virus by the Chinese Center for Disease Control. The patient with a history of exposure to dead sick birds was diagnosed as acute severe pneumonia, and died post to unresponsiveness to rescue with all strength by the expert group. This was the first case of H5N6 avian influenza in human in the world. Geese in Shuangcheng District, Harbin City, Heilongjiang Province showed symptoms of suspected avian influenza. Statistics showed that 20,550 geese got sick and 17,790 died. The diagnosis was confirmed to be subtype H5N6 highly pathogenic avian influenza by National Avian Influenza Reference Laboratory. 25 epidemics of bird infection of H5N6 took place in China as of December 31st, 2014, involving Heilongjiang, Zhejiang, Hubei, Guangxi, Anhui, Chongqing, Guizhou, Tibet, Guangdong, Hunan, Hebei, Fujian, and Yunnan (some of the specimen derived from farms, and some from live poultry market or they were environmental specimens). Epidemics of avian influenza with a great risk of mortality in human brings a great threat to human being.

Health and Family Planning Commission of Guangdong Province notified a patient of H5N6 avian influenza virus, which was the first case in Guangdong Province and the second case in the world. A 58-year-old man living in Panyu, Guangzhou, bought a live chicken in the market and went home in the rain. Then he had respiratory symptoms. Chinese Center of Disease Control reexamined this case on December 22nd, 2014, and the result showed positiveness in nucleic acid of H5N6 avian influenza. National Health and Family Planning Commission organized experts to conduct the consultation and study on December 23rd, 2014, and made a diagnosis of H5N6 avian influenza based on clinical manifestations, results of laboratory tests, and epidemic history. Individual cases were diagnosed in provinces in China from April 2014 to September 2018, including 1 case in Sichuan, 5 in Guangdong, 2 in Yunnan, 1 in Hubei, 1 in Huan, 1 Anhui, 1 in Guangxi Zhuang Autonomous Region, and 1 in Jiangsu.

Primarily, diagnosis of avian influenza is mainly based on influenza virus isolated from secretion of respiratory tract of birds, and strains of influenza viruses can be detected through immunohistochemistry staining. Secondly, specimen can be collected with the same method, and RT-PCR is used to detect viral genes, and the diagnosis can be confirmed if the result is H5. Thirdly, the diagnosis can be confirmed based on the detection of viral nucleic acid.

11.2 Image Findings

The disease at the onset is mainly located in the respiratory tract in the patient with avian influenza. Chest imaging (including plain chest X-ray and CT scans) can be used to understand the location, involved range and imaging characteristics of the disease. Evolution of the disease can also be made known by clinical imaging follow-up.

1. Site and area of lesions: The lesion is located within unilateral or bilateral lung(s) at the onset, and expands to multiple segments and lobes of both lungs. The focal lesion at the early stage may involve multiple lobes until

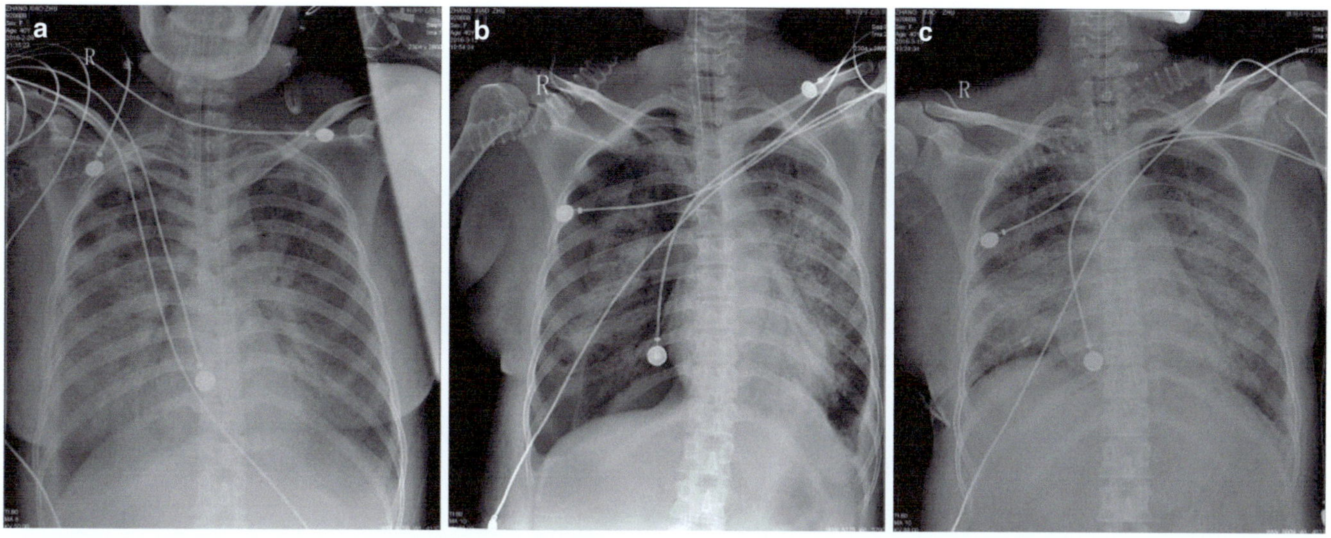

Fig. 11.1 (**a–c**) A 40-year-old female complaining of cough, expectoration, fever, and polypnea for three days was diagnosed as pneumonia of H5N6 avian influenza in human. (**a**) Day 3 post to the onset. Chest X-ray showed ground glass opacities in both lungs. (**b**) The right pneumothorax observed on day 21 post to the onset, with progressive lesions in both lungs. (**c**) Day 23 post to the onset witnessed the aggravation, and the patient died on day 25 due to the severe disease unresponsive to the rescue

all segments/lobes, and even the manifestation of "white lungs" (Fig. 11.1).

2. Morphology of the lesion: It manifests mainly pulmonary consolidations and ground glass opacity (GGO), which are dominated by consolidations with bronchogram inside. The disease in the early stage manifests dominantly mesenchymal lesions, which are switched later to the dominance by parenchymal lesions. Normal pulmonary tissues can be observed among lesions at the onset, and then ground glass opacities develop into consolidations (Fig. 11.2).
3. Progression of the disease. The disease progresses rapidly if there is no effective control of pneumonia of avian influenza in human, and pulmonary lesions are characterized in enlarged area, evolution from the focal into the complete pulmonary or from the unilateral to the bilateral and eventually diffuse distribution in both lungs, and the progression into acute respiratory distress syndrome (ARDS) in patients with severe diseases manifesting diffuse flaky consolidations in both lungs. Chest X-ray shows the appearance of white lung. The lesion may manifest increased density of the lesion, i.e., the evolution from GGOs into pulmonary consolidation, and severe pneumonia exists at the onset in some of the patients (Fig. 11.1).
4. Concurrent signs: Thickening of adjacent pleura, multiple mediastinal lymphadenopathies, pneumothorax, pleural effusion, and pericardial effusion.
5. Absorption stage: After effective treatment is carried out for patients with H5N6 avian influenza pneumonia, the area of the lesion starts to shrink with decreased density, i.e., the conversion from consolidation to GGOs, grids, or fibrous streaks, while some of the patients show the fibrous streaks and thickening of alveolar septum, with amelioration of clinical symptoms.
6. Complications: Extensive consolidations appearing in both lungs in the period with the severest disease, i.e., the "white lung," indicates the complication of ARDS. Patients with avian influenza receiving adjuvant ventilation are vulnerable to pneumothorax. Fewer patients can be complicated with unilateral or bilateral pleural effusion. Avian influenza in human differs from influenza in the secondary bacterial pneumonia, which is seldom observed in the former, but is the main cause of death for the latter during its pandemics.

Relationship between images and clinical manifestations: major features of patients with avian influenza is the rapid deterioration of clinical symptoms and chest images. Patients during the severest clinical manifestations have lassitude, obvious rise of body temperature, significant respiratory symptoms, and leukopenia, when chest images show the severest findings and the most extensive lesions.

However, the clinical manifestations may be severer than the chest image findings, and they don't synchronize with each other. One case of human avian influenza patient reported by de Jong et al. [3] died on the day next to the onset, and there was not any manifestation of human avian influenza pneumonia yet. Fouchier et al. [5] reported a patient manifesting conjunctivitis at the onset, and chest X-ray showed only a flaky opacity in the lower right lung when ARDS occurred clinically.

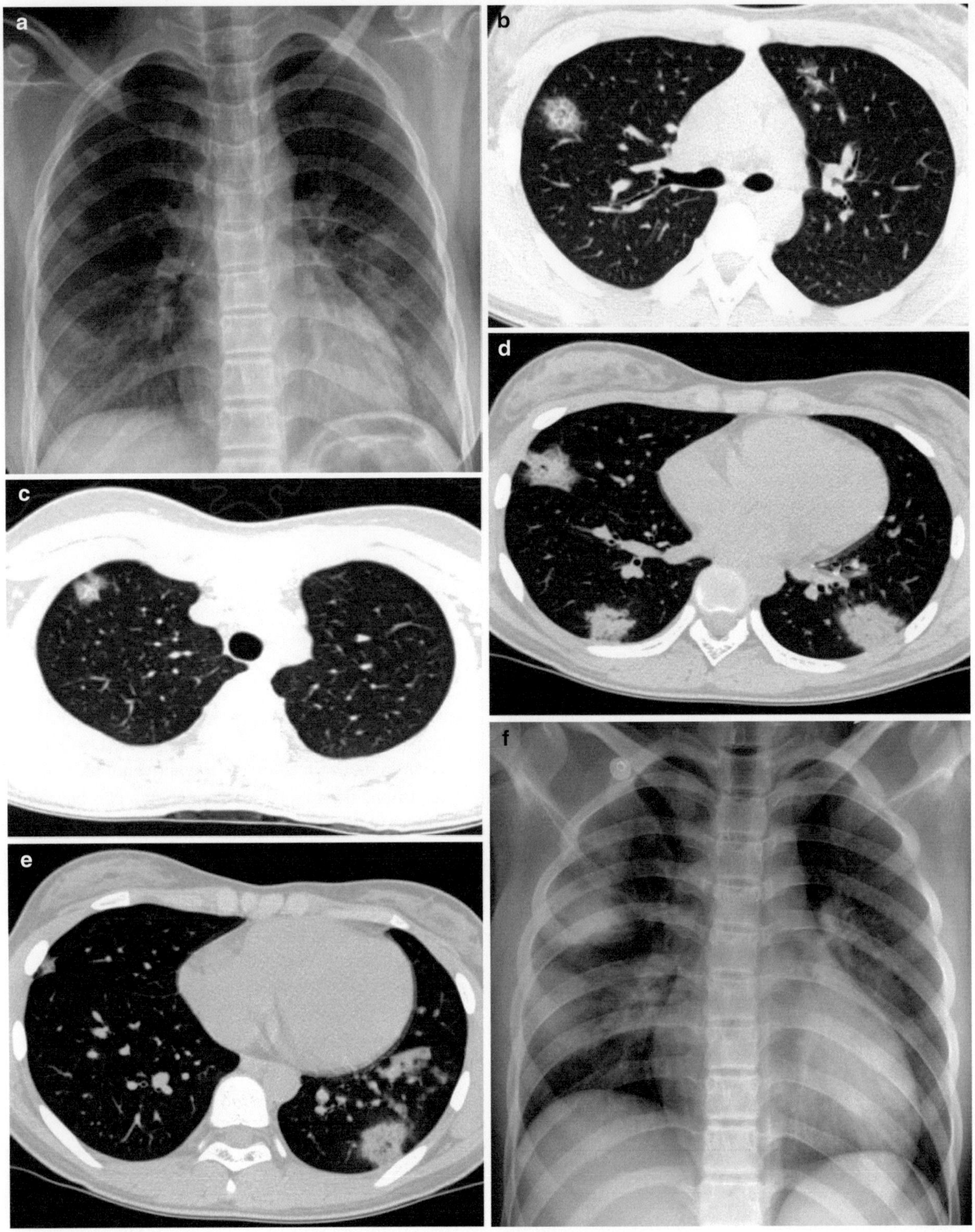

Fig. 11.2 (**a–n**) A female pediatric patient aged 11 years and 6 months manifesting fever for 3 days with vomiting once. The report by the Provincial Center of Disease Control showed positiveness in detection of H5N6 nucleic acid. The patient was diagnosed with pneumonia of H5N6 avian influenza in human (**a**) On day 4 post to the onset, chest X-ray showed multiple patchy opacities in the upper right lung and the lower left lung. (**b–e**) On day 5 post to the onset, chest X-ray showed multiple flaky opacities with uneven density and unsmooth border in lungs. (**f**) On day 8 post to the onset, multiple consolidations were observed in lungs in chest X-ray. (**g**) On day 12 post to the onset, reexamination with chest X-ray showed further progression of lesions, and the expansion of the consolidations. (**h–m**) On day 22 post to the onset, chest CT scans showed dots, bars and large flaky consolidations with blurred edge, uneven inner density and bronchogram sign in segments of the upper lobe, the lateral segment of the middle lobe, and the dorsal segment and lateral basal segment of the lower lobe of the right lung, as well as anterior segment of the upper lobe of the left lung and segments of the lower left lobe. (**n**) On day 26 post to the onset, chest X-ray showed obvious absorption of lesions in both lungs, and manifested fibrous streaks

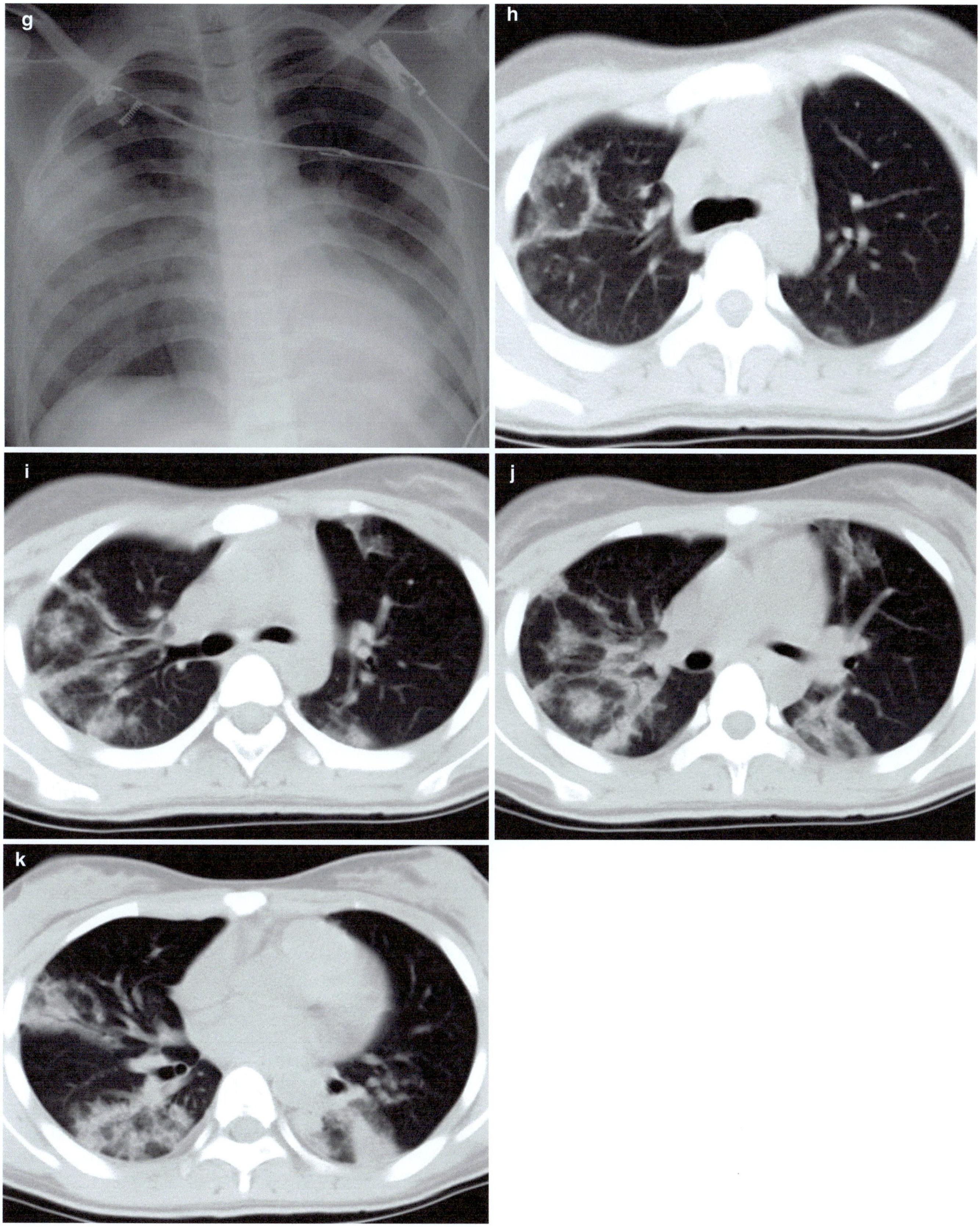

Fig. 11.2 (continued)

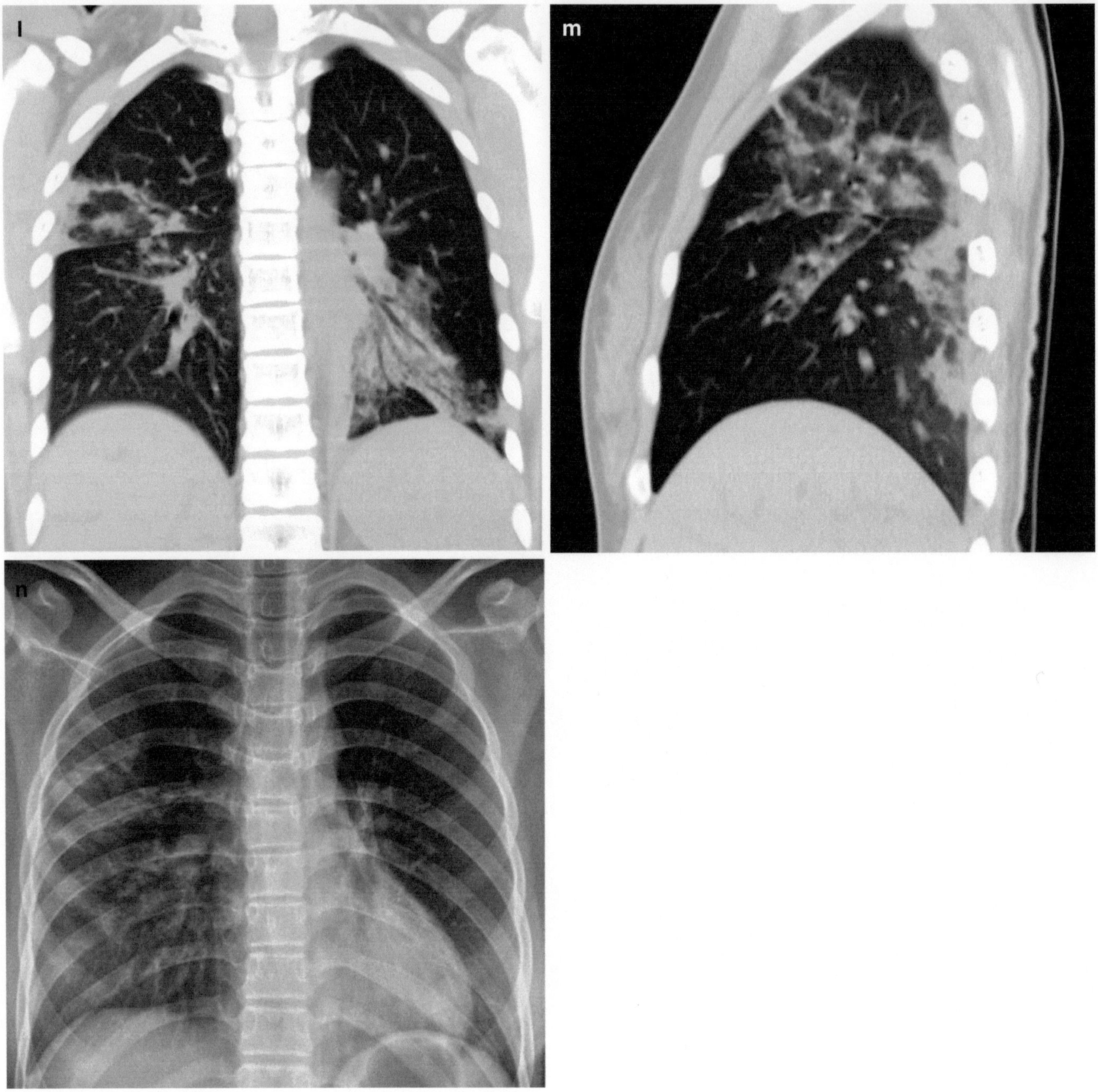

Fig. 11.2 (continued)

11.3 Diagnosis and Differential Diagnosis

I. *Diagnostic basis for H5N6 avian influenza in human*

1. Clinical symptoms. There are influenza-like symptoms such as cough and expectoration, and some patients manifest alimentary tract symptoms. Patients with severe disease may have persistent fever and rapid progression of the disease, and almost all of them have clinically obvious pneumonia, acute respiratory distress syndrome (ARDS), pulmonary bleeding, multiple organs dysfunction syndrome (MODS), shock, and Reyes Syndrome (RS). Some patients died from progressive respiratory failure, which is correlated to spreading lesion, exudation of ground glass opacities in both lungs, and occurrence of ARDS. Clinical features constituting the basis of the early diagnosis include fever, throat pain, cough, and leukopenia. Involvement of other organs includes mild-to-moderate liver damages and impairment of cardiac and renal functions in the advanced stage.

2. Epidemiology. Infectious sources are mainly birds including chickens, duck, and geese that suffer from avian influenza or carry the viruses, especially chickens. Wild birds play an important role in natural transmission of avian influenza virus. Viruses can be carried by secretion and excrement of birds, as well their feathers, organs, tissues, and eggs. More viruses are isolated from migratory waterfowls, especially wild ducks, than in other birds. The disease induced by the avian influenza virus is the severest in chicken and turkeys, and the patients have usually previous exposure to birds or visit to vegetable market. There is no report of human-to-human transmission at present, and H5N6 is a very typical avian influenza virus with an extremely low possibility of pandemics in populations.
3. Image findings. Chest CT manifests consolidations, ground glass opacities with blurred edges, and multiple exudations in lobes of both lungs; as well as central lobular nodule, mesenchymal lesions such as web-like opacities and subpleural arcs. The lesions progress and evolve rapidly, and there might be remnants of streaks, grids, thickening of lobular septum, and subpleural arc post to absorption pulmonary exudative lesions in response to active treatment is carried out.
4. Laboratory tests. There are an increase in total count of white blood cells and neutrophils, but a decrease in red blood cells and a fluctuation of lymphocytes. During the disease course, an ascending trend is observed for peripheral white blood cells and neutrophils, while the count of lymphocytes drops in the case of severe disease and rises during the recovery. Generally speaking, viral pneumonia does not induce the decrease of peripheral lymphocytes. Alanine aminotransferase and aspartate aminotransferase show gradual normalization from their significantly increased level during negative conversion of virus nucleic acid, without obvious abnormality in renal function, blood lipid, and glucose. The partial pressure of arterial blood carbon dioxide keeps increasing, and oxygen saturation changes from the low value to the normal.

II. Differential diagnosis

Imaging of H5N6 avian influenza pneumonia in human should be differentiated from that of bacterial pneumonia, mycoplasma pneumonia, and severe acute respiratory syndrome (SARS). Patchy blurred opacities are distributed in both lungs in patients infected with H5N6 avian influenza, and the disease manifests multifocal change and fast progression. Bacterial pneumonia manifests localized segmental pulmonary consolidation with pleura as the border and bronchogram inside, and there is an increase of peripheral leukocytes. Pneumonia induced by *Mycoplasma pneumoniae* has obvious seasonality and is mostly seen in children, manifesting mostly in one lung at the onset, and some lesions can involve both lungs. The imaging follow-up shows that the opacity in the lung does not change significantly within a short period of time.

The differentiation with H5N1/H7N9 avian influenza pneumonia in human [1, 4]. It depends mainly on epidemiological investigation and etiological examination. Some researchers collected the demographic characteristics, epidemiology, and clinical data of patients through the data in a standard format from China Center for Disease Control, and compared the data of 17 cases of laboratory-confirmed human infection with H5N6 avian influenza, 45 cases of human infected with H5N1 avian influenza and 782 cases of human infected with H7N9 avian influenza. It was found that human infected with H5N6 avian influenza had greater age than those infected with H5N1, and higher incidence of concurrent disease than H5N1 patients, but a younger age than those infected with H7N9. H5N6 avian influenza in human has a gender ratio similar to H5N1 and a higher proportion of female patients, while H7N9 is more commonly observed in males. All H5N6 patients have a history of exposure to live poultry, with a higher proportion of previous visits to live poultry market than H7N9 patients and H5N1 patients. It has been observed that H5N6 avian influenza in human has similar epidemiological and disease severity compared with H5N1, while milder severity and milder disease is observed in H7N9 avian influenza in human. Patients with H5N6 avian influenza are distributed geographically in Southern China and the Southwest, and the distribution of H5N1 avian influenza in human seems more extensive and more scattered. Geographic distributions of H7N9 avian are dominated by Eastern and Southern China, where there is a high density of live poultry markets.

At present, cases of H5N6 avian influenza in human are dominantly the young and the middle-aged, aged 25–58 years old, which may be related to the wide range of activities in such a population with greater risk of exposure. Now, H5N6 avian influenza in human is characterized by severe diseases, rapid progression, and high mortality. Its most common clinical manifestation shown by clinical data is severe pneumonia, among many other symptoms including fever and cough, and most patients die due to rapid progression of the disease. Pregnant woman with low immunity is the population highly susceptible to influenza, and viral infection causes often severe complications. Diagnosis of subtype H5N6 avian influenza is confronting great challenges, and it is hard to differentiate from other respiratory diseases based on clinical symptoms. Molecular biological diagnostic approaches are required eventually through determining the size of genetic fragments with PCR for viruses isolated. Oseltamivir is one of the main antiviral drugs for treating highly pathogenic avian influenza in human. Outcomes of the treatment for cases such as H7N9 imply that oseltamivir launched within 48 h post to the onset may reduce the mortality. Therefore, oseltamivir should be given as soon as possible to clinically suspected cases, before the pathogen is identified. Only oral preparation is available for oseltamivir, which is not suitable for patients with severe diseases. Injection of neuraminidase inhibitor palamivir, however, is a convenient option for severe patients. Noninvasive mechanical ventilation and glucocorticoids are also effective treatments for highly pathogenic influenza in human. Because of continuous mutation of virus, Traditional Chinese Medicine and herbs are of specific advantages in controlling highly pathogenic avian influenza in human, and this disease can be controlled, using Traditional Chinese Medicine integrated with Western Medicine.

11.4 Report of the First Case in the World

11.4.1 Case 1

1. *General information of the patient*

   The patient was a 50-year-old male was admitted on April 21st, 2014, with the chief complaint of "fever and cough for 8 days and dyspnea with bloody sputum for 1 day". Eight days before admission (i.e., April 13th, 2014), he began to have chills and fever, complicated with general aching and runny nose. He took oral drugs including Sanjiu Ganmao Granules prescribed by the local clinic, and the disease did not ameliorate. On April 18th, his symptoms deteriorated, including cough, chill, fever, general aching, and headache, complicated with obvious anorexia and fatigue. He was treated with compound Aminophenazone and Barbital Injection and dexamethasone at the clinic, but there was still no amelioration. He had abdominal discomfort on April 19th, 2014, and was treated with mezlocillin, levofloxacin, omeprazole at the local primary hospital, but his symptoms didn't ameliorate obviously and he manifested gradually dyspnea, polypnea post to activities, and a little bloody expectoration. On April 20th, 2014, his chest X-ray at the primary hospital showed the large flaky consolidation in the left lung, and nodular and patchy consolidations in the upper right lung. He was diagnosed as suspected highly pathogenic avian influenza after consultation of municipal experts, and treated with oseltamivir (150 mg bid) and methylprednisolone (40 mg bid). On April 21st, the report of virus nucleic acid by local disease control center showed positiveness in H5N6 viral nucleic acid and then he was transferred to the designated hospital for treatment.
2. The patient was a hawker in the local live poultry market and engaged in live poultry trading for years. After the market was closed, he used to raise the unsold birds temporarily in his own courtyard. There were deaths of a goose, 2 ducks, and 5 chickens between April 13th and 17th. One hundred forty four specimens were obtained from his surrounding environment and underwent RT-PCR detection. Three specimens showed positiveness in influenza A and all specimens showed negativeness in influenza H5. Virus H5N6 was detected in dead domestic poultries, suggesting the source of viral infection might be the infected poultries. The patient had 47 close contacts, including 12 medical practitioners, 7 family members, 2 patients in the same ward, and 26 other persons, who did not manifest any influenza-like symptoms during isolation observation up to 2 weeks, and negativeness in influenza virus was shown by RT-PCR for throat swab specimens from 46 close contacts.
3. Physical examination at admission: Temperature 37.3 °C, pulse 96 beats/min, respiration 30/min, and blood pressure 106/74 mmHg. Face of acute illness, poor spirit, left lung percussion dullness, with a small amount scattered moderate-fine moist rales. Clear percussion of the right lung percussion and clear breath sound, without dry or wet rales. There was no other special positive sign. The patients had been engaged in trading and cultivation of domestic birds for a long time, and there were deaths of his birds. He had eaten some of them.

   Results of virus nucleic acids detection from the Provincial Disease Control Center on April 22nd, 2014, showed positiveness in H5N6 avian influenza virus. On April 22nd, the patient had dyspnea and restlessness, and the oxygen saturation decreased to about 70%. There was no improvement, though the oxygen concentration of continuous noninvasive ventilation was adjusted to 100%. The patient was given immediately endotracheal intubation for invasive mechanical ventilation, and the hypoxia was slightly ameliorated. Blood gas analysis showed a pH of 7.48, partial pressure of oxygen of 54.0 mmHg, partial pressure of carbon dioxide of 34.0 mmHg, and standard bicarbonate of 26.40 mmol/L. The condition of the patient kept worsening, and his blood pressure began to decrease gradually at night. The airway secretion was light red watery sputum, and the arterial oxygen saturation was maintained only at about 80%. His disease worsened further and the dysfunction in ventilation and air exchange were difficult to correct. Cardiopulmonary arrest occurred eventually on April 23rd, 2014, and the patient died post to unresponsiveness to the rescue. Pathological analysis post to autopsy showed that the causes of death were

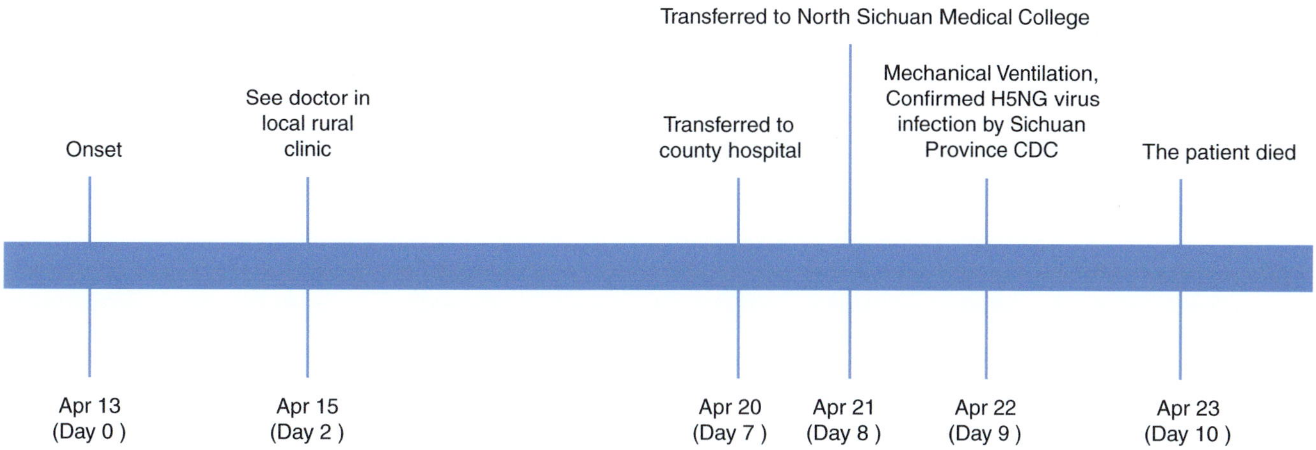

Fig. 11.3 Course of medication

severe pulmonary infection, pulmonary injuries, and extensive consolidation, which resulted in serious dysfunction of lung ventilation and ventilation function causing severe ARDS. It was confirmed further to be positiveness in H5N6 avian influenza virus by the Chinese Disease Control Center on May 6th, 2014. The onset and treatment for the patient are illustrated by the chart (Figs. 11.3 and 11.4).

4. *Laboratory examinations*

   On the day of admission to the designated hospital, blood routine showed WBC of 1.48×10^9/L, neutrophil ratio of 82.4%, and lymphocyte ratio of 12.8%. Arterial blood gas analysis showed oxygen partial pressure of 55.0 mmhg, carbon dioxide partial pressure of 34.0 mmHg, oxygen saturation of 91.0%; ESR CRP of 252.00 mg/L, procalcitonin PCT of 3.600 ng/mL. Blood biochemistry showed aspartate aminotransferase of 84.4 U/L and creatinine of 70.8 μmol/L. Reexamination of arterial blood gas at 19:20 on April 21st, 2014, showed the oxygen partial pressure of 50.0 mmHg, carbon dioxide partial pressure of 34.0 mmHg, and oxygen saturation of 88.0%. Noninvasive ventilator was used to support respiration with enhancement of respiratory tract management. Viral cultivation and genetic sequencing were used to detect the pathogen concerning etiological test, and in the advanced stage, RNA extraction and PCR typing were used for genome sequencing, primary analysis, and deep sequencing, which showed positiveness in H5N6 viral nucleic acids.

5. Image manifestations

   Chest X-ray on day 7 post to the onset showed the large flaky consolidation in the left lung with a dense opacity and unclear structures in the left hilum. An exteriorly widened and interiorly thinned opacity was noticed in the middle right lung with a clear border. There was a ground glass opacity in the lower right lung, with blurred right costophrenic angle (Fig. 11.5a). CT scans on day 8 post to the onset showed a large flaky consolidation in the left lung with bronchogram inside, and consolidations in the middle and lower right lung with subpleural ground glass opacities. In the upper right lung, there were small nodules and fibrous streaks (Fig. 11.5b–g).

6. Discussion

   The patient was a middle-aged male with history of exposure to live poultry, characterized clinically in fever and cough for 8 days complicated with dyspnea and bloody expectoration [6]. Because of unresponsiveness to treatment based on a diagnosis of common cold, he was transferred to a superior hospital for further examination and suspected of viral pneumonia, and image findings also support the presence of severe pneumonia in the lungs. Probable highly pathogenic avian influenza in human was considered, based on consultation by experts. He received antivirus medication and methylprednisolone, but his disease was not controlled effectively. Subsequent chest CT scans showed flaky consolidations in both lungs, suggesting that the disease aggravated rapidly in the patient post to viral infection and pulmonary disease spread fast with severe injuries in lungs infected, which caused severe dysfunction of pulmonary ventilation and air exchange, thereby resulting in severe ARDS. The patient died post to unresponsiveness to rescue. It was diagnosed later to be H5N6 avian influenza in human by the Chinese CDC Laboratory. This was the first case in the world with rapid progression, manifesting more extensive lesions in lungs compared with pneumonia induced by H7N9 avian influenza, and showing dominantly pulmonary consolidations. Besides, influenza-like symptoms such as fever and cough observed clinically in this case that were similar fundamentally to those of H7N9 avian influenza pneumonia, the symptom of bloody expectoration also appeared in the patient, which seemed

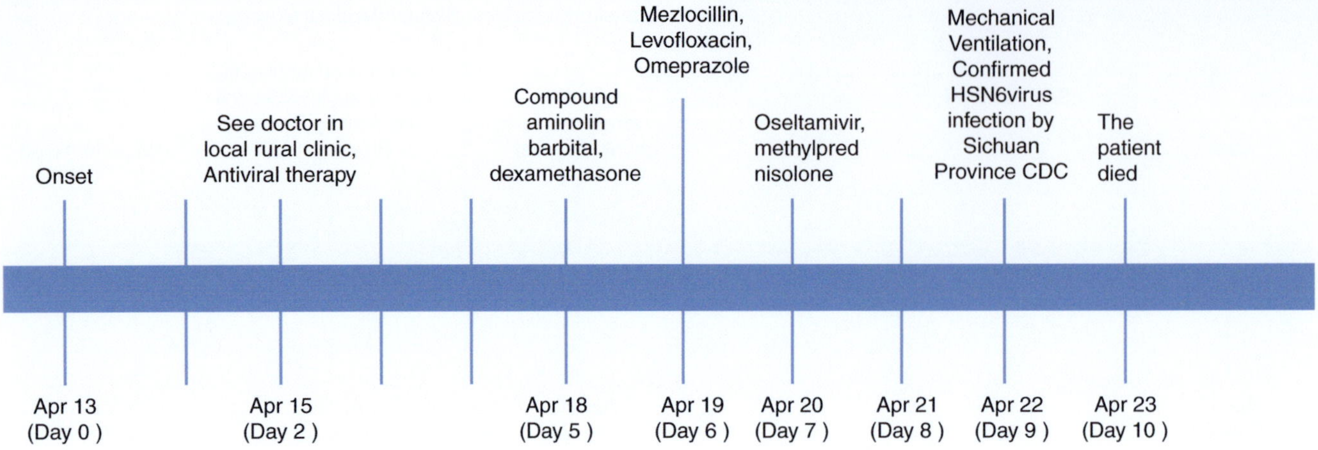

Fig. 11.4 Treatment course of the patient

rare in cases of avian influenzas in human other than H5N6 avian influenza. No human-to-human transmission for this disease has been reported clinically.

11.4.2 Case 2 (Introduction of the First Cured Case in the World)

I. Abstract of the disease history

A 59-year-old male was admitted with the chief complaint of "fever for 14 days with polypnea for 9 days." He had fever for 14 days with the temperature varying between 39 and 40 °C before admission, complicated with chill and, without cough or expectoration or bloody sputum. He had no chest tightness or chest pain. No significant improvement was found post to the treatment of self-administered Compound Pseudoephedrine Hydrochloride Tablets. His symptoms aggravated on day 10 post to the onset, and he sought medical advice at a local hospital. The disease was considered to be bacterial infection and he received anti-infection treatment with details unknown, showing poor responsiveness. Then he was hospitalized in a local primary hospital and chest radiographs showed multiple lung infection in both lungs. WBC 6.6 × 10^9/L, N 91.6%, Lym 5%, PCT1.21 ng/mL. Laboratory tests showed WBC 6.6 × 10^9/L, N:91.6%, Lym 5%, and PCT 1.21 ng/mL. Ceftazidime and moxifloxacin hydrochloride tablets were given for anti-infection, with noninvasive ventilator-assisted ventilation. On day 12 post to the onset, the polypnea aggravated and SPO_2 was 50–70% and he received tracheal intubation for assisted ventilation, when throat swab was found positive in subtype H5 avian influenza virus, with feces fungi (4+) and sputum fungi (1+). The diagnosis was considered to be "highly pathogenic avian influenza with severe pneumonia." The patient received treatments with imipenem, oseltamivir, methylprednisolone sodium succinate, but he responded poorly.

Previous history: He was diagnosed with colon cancer 1 year before this admission, when he underwent resection of sigmoid colon cancer at another hospital, followed by 4 cycles of postoperative chemotherapy. No recurrence of tumor was found during reexamination in another hospital 2 months before the admission. He had pulmonary tuberculosis unconfirmed 30 years before, which had been cured.

Physical examination: T36.6 °C, SPO_2 95%, in tracheal intubation assisted ventilation. Weakened vocal tactile fremitus. Percussive dullness, with weakened pulmonary sound in both lungs in auscultation and moist crackles in both lower lungs.

Epidemiological investigation showed that the patient had been to vegetable market to buy live birds prior to the onset, and there was the site for poultry slaughtering.

II. Image findings

The first chest X-ray (Fig. 11.6a) on day 6 post to the onset: multiple patchy blurred opacities in the upper right lung and both lower lungs, dominantly in the lower left lung, with partial consolidation in the posterior basal segment of the lower left lung. The second chest X-ray on day 8 post to the onset showed multiple bilateral pulmonary patchy blurred opacities and consolidations dominated by lesions in both lower lungs, which increased obviously compared to previous image. Chest X-ray examined on day 9, 10, and 13, respectively showed exudatives in both lungs, and gradual increase of pulmonary lobes involved by lesions infused into an enlarged area, and developing gradually into the complete lungs manifesting consolidations in the middle and lower pulmonary fields and blurred patchy opacities in both upper lungs. The first CT scans (Fig. 11.6b–d) on

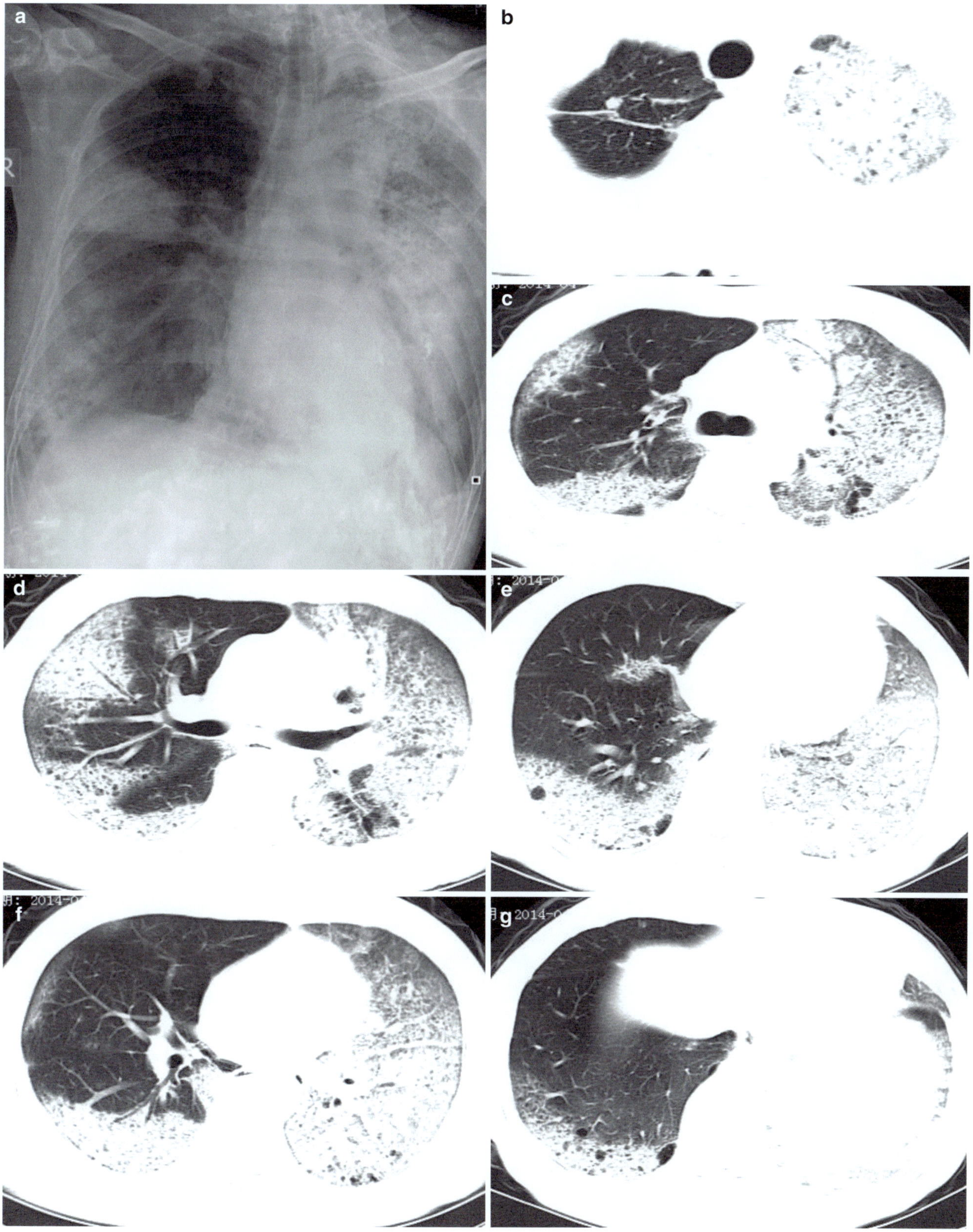

Fig. 11.5 (**a–g**) A 50-year-old man, with H5N6 avian influenza in human. (**a**) On April 20th, 2014, (day 7 post to the onset). Chest X-ray showed a large flaky consolidation in the left lung, with consolidations and ground glass opacities in the middle and lower right lung. (**b–g**) On April 20th, 2014 (day 8 post to the onset), plain CT scans of the chest show the large flaky consolidation and mesenchymal high-density opacity with bronchogram inside in the left lung. A flaky consolidation is observed in the right lung with bronchogram inside. There were nodules and streaks in the upper right lung and the right subpleural ground glass opacities

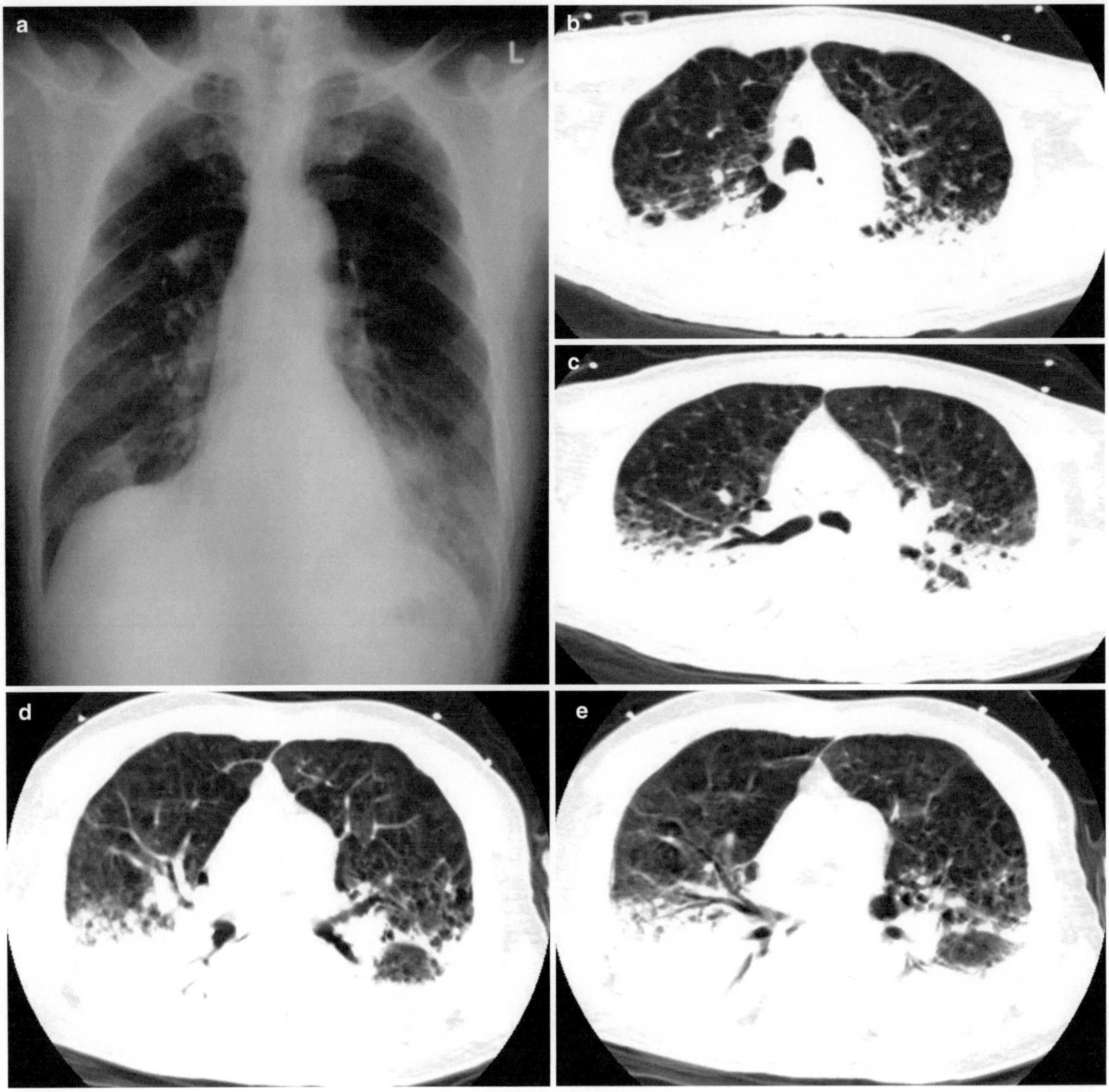

Fig. 11.6 (**a–m**) A 59-year-old male diagnosed as H5N6 avian influenza in human. (**a**) Partial ground glass opacities in bilateral lower pulmonary fields shown by chest X-ray on day 6 post to the onset, with more obvious manifestation in the lower left pulmonary fields. (**b–e**) On day 14 post to the onset, chest X-ray showed large flaky consolidations in both lungs with bronchogram inside, which was dominated by lesions in the lower lobes. (**f–i**) Chest CT scans on day 23 post to the onset showed the absorption of majority of flaky consolidations shown by the previous image, and fibrous streaks and partial ground glass opacities in both lungs. (**j–m**) Chest CT scans on day 50 post to the onset showed roughly absorption of lesions in both lungs, leaving only nodules in the upper right lung and fibrous streaks in both lungs

day 14 post to the onset showed multiple blurred opacities and dominantly consolidations in both lungs, and lesions were distributed mainly in dorsal lower fields of both lungs. A tuberculoma with calcification was observed in the posterior segment of the upper right lung. A small amount of bilateral pleural effusion was observed, with slightly more volume on the left and compression of partial pulmonary tissues of posterior basal segment of both lower lungs. Reexamination of CT scans (Fig. 11.6e–i) on day 23 post to the onset showed multiple lesions in both lungs, which decreased significantly compared with the previous image, reduced bilateral pleural effusion, and amelioration of partial compressive atelectasis in both dorsal lungs.

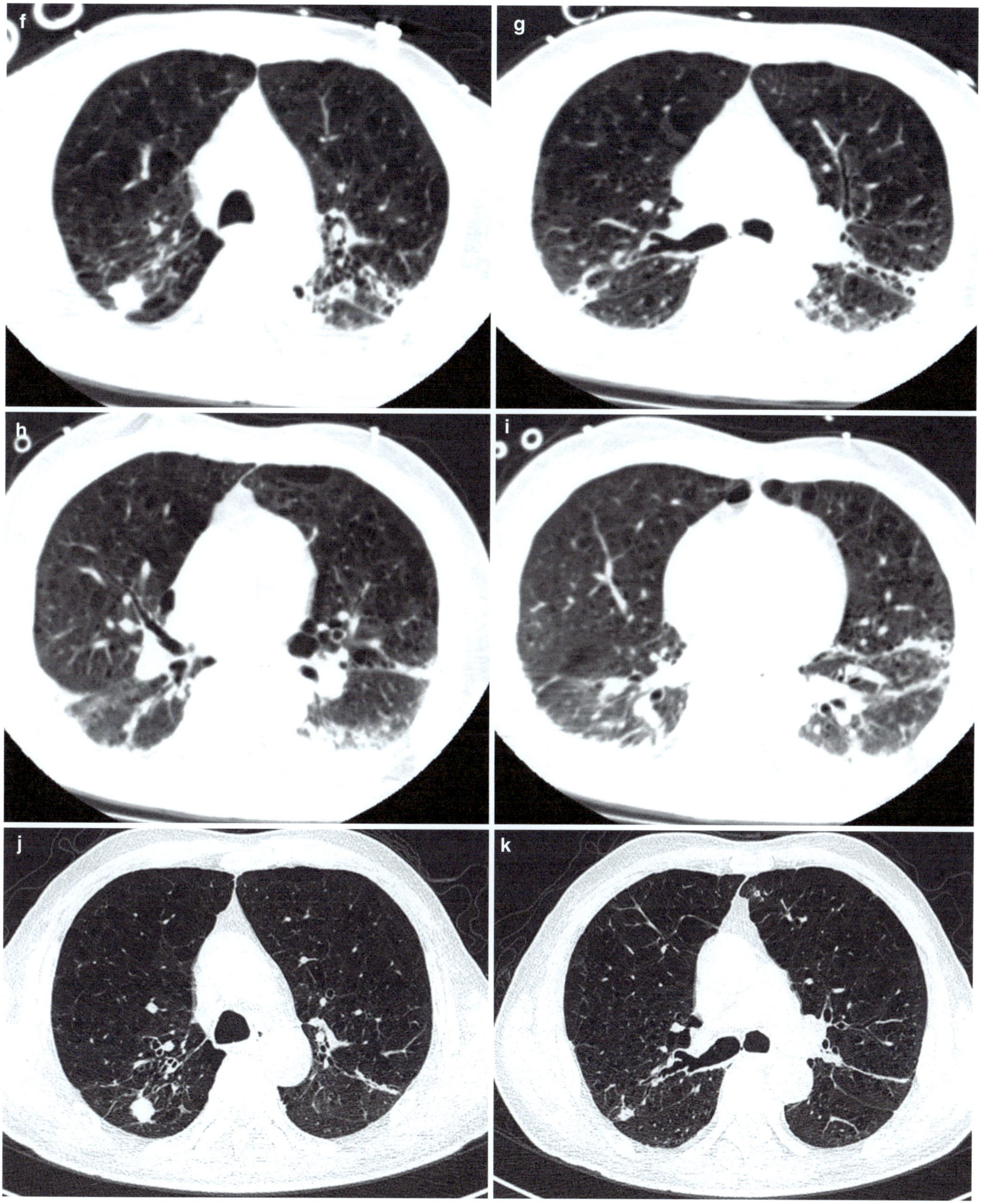

Fig. 11.6 (continued)

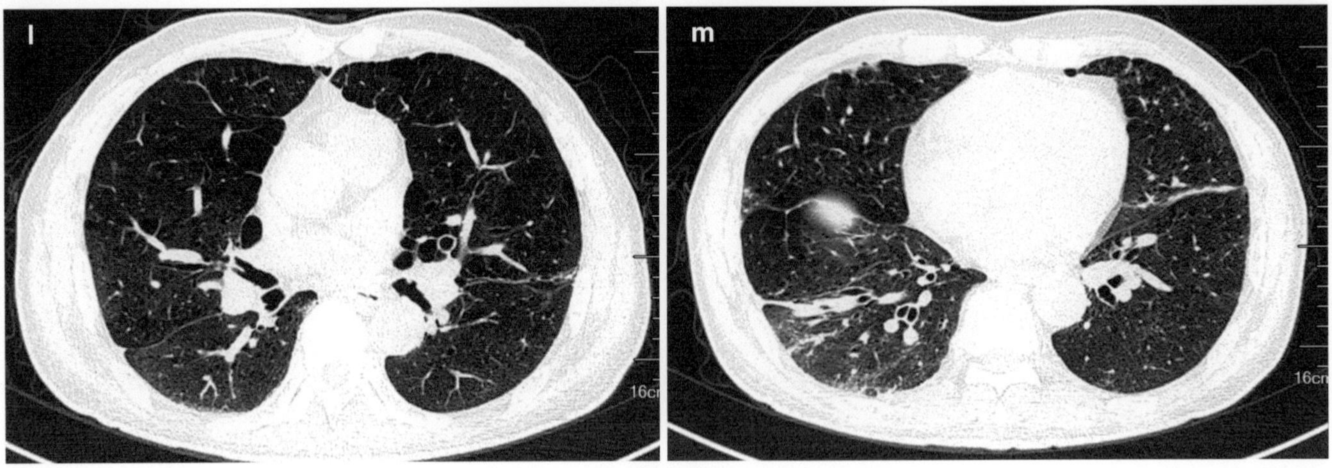

Fig. 11.6 (continued)

Reexamination of CT scans (Fig. 11.6j–m) on day 50 post to the onset showed absorption of most of the lesions with scattered streaks in both lungs.

III. *Discussion*

Avian influenza virus belongs to Orthomyxoviridae and influenza A virus. Avian influenza virus particles are polymorphous, with a spherical diameter of 80–120 nm and envelope. The nucleocapsid inside virus particles is in spiral symmetry with a diameter of about 10 nm. The infectious source is speculated to be birds carrying H5N6 avian influenza viruses or their secretion or excrement. It spreads mainly through the respiratory tract, and there is no definite evidence for human-to-human direct transmission [7, 8]. There is no definite evidence for human's susceptibility to H5N6 avian influenza virus, and the high-risk populations include mainly practitioners in breeding, sales, slaughtering and processing of birds, and those exposed to birds within 1 week prior to the onset.

Image findings, in this case, showed pneumonia induced by H5N6 avian influenza in human with pulmonary exudatives at the onset, manifesting patchy blurred opacities and consolidations which are mostly multiple and scattered, distributed mainly in the middle and lower pulmonary fields and involving both lungs. Lesions progressed rapidly and are fused and enlarged with increased area of consolidation involving multiple lobes and segments of both lungs. The signs above seemed consistent with basic profiles of pneumonia induced by avian influenza as reported by literatures. Small amount of pleural effusion occurred on day 14 as shown by CT scans, which seldom appears in patients with pneumonia induced by avian influenza. At this timepoint, *Acinetobacter baumannii* was detected clinically in sputum culture for this patient with avian influenza, which was considered to be the pleural effusion caused by the complicated bacterial infection. Thereafter anti-inflammatory treatment was strengthened clinically, and lesions were controlled gradually until the patient was cured and discharged.

This patient had a history of exposure to birds and their secretion and excrement within 1 week prior to the onset. Chest X-ray showed multiple exudative lesions in both lungs distributed randomly and involving multiple pulmonary lobes, with tendency of infusion, enlargement, and pulmonary consolidation within hours or 48 h, and an increase of area for more than 50%. The probable diagnosis of H5N6 avian influenza in human was suggested, based on clinical symptoms, signs, and laboratory tests, while the confirmed diagnosis requires also support from etiological tests.

This disease should be differentiated from bacterial pneumonia, mycoplasma pneumonia, and SARS, concerning image findings. Patients with H5N6 avian influenza show pulmonary patchy blurred opacities distributed in both lungs appearing multiple-focal lesions and a fast progression. In comparison, bacterial pneumonia manifests localized segmental pulmonary consolidation, accompanied commonly with increase of leukocytes in peripheral blood. Mycoplasma pneumonia has the obvious seasonality and occurs mostly in children with its onset commonly in unilateral lung and sometimes involving both lungs. Its pulmonary opacities do not change obviously within a short period of time, as shown by image follow up. Its differentiation from the other infectious viral pneumonia is based mainly on epidemiological investigation and etiological tests.

References

1. Lu P. Epidemiologic and imaging features of avian influenza in human: the globally first case occurring in China. Electron J Emerg Infect Dis. 2017;2(2):124–6.
2. Lu J, Zhang D, Wang G, et al. Research progress on highly pathogenic avian influenza H5N1 virus. Int J Virol. 2007;14:65–8.

3. De Jong MD, Bach VC, Phan TQ, et al. Fatal avian influenza A (H5N1) in a child presenting with diarrhea followed by coma. N Engl J Med. 2005;352:686–91.
4. Shi R, Shi C, Ma Q, et al. Value of clinical radiology in diagnosis and treatment for H7N9 avian influenza in human. Electron J Emerg Infect Dis. 2016;1(1):50–2.
5. Fouchier RA, Schneeberger PM, Rozendaal FW, et al. Avian influenza A virus (H7N7) associated with human conjunctivitis and a fatal case of acute respiratory distress syndrome. Proc Natl Acad Sci U S A. 2004;101:1356–1361.7.
6. Ling S, Yang C, Li Z. An analysis on clinical rescue of the globally first pregnant women infected with H5N6 avian influenza. Crit Care Med China. 2016;28(11):988–93.
7. Yang ZF, Mok CK, Peiris JS, et al. Human infection with a novel avian influenza A (H5N6) virus. N Engl J Med. 2015;373(5):487–9.
8. Joob B, Viroj W, et al. H5N6 influenza virus infection, the newest influenza. Asia Pac J Trop Biomed. 2015;6:434–7.

H10N8 Avian Influenza in Human

12

Yu-lin He, Fei Shi, Chuan-jun Xu, Bu-dong Chen, Ying-ying Deng, and Pu-xuan Lu

12.1 Overview

H10N8 is one of the subtypes of avian influenza virus (AIV), and its nomenclature is based on the protein hemagglutinin HA subtype 10 and neuraminidase NA subtype 8 in the surface of the virus. Given the structural characteristics that there is only one arginine and no other basic amino acids near the cleavage site of the H10N8 protein hemagglutinin (HA) precursor, the ability of H10N8 to infect poultry is relatively low. However, the pathogenicity of the virus after infecting humans is significantly enhanced, and even leads to death of infected patients, suggesting that its pathogenic ability may change greatly after crossing the species barrier [1]. According to the report from Chinese Center for Disease Control and Prevention, three cases infected with H10N8 avian influenza virus pneumonia have been reported globally as of July 2018. At present, the route of human-to-human transmission of H10N8 is not clear, but the reported cases all had a history of exposure to poultry. Especially when they were suffering from the diseases which could weaken body's resistance or immunity, the morbidity of post-infection disease was increased and the prognosis is poorer. Since the first case was reported in Nanchang, Jiangxi Province, China in December 2013, two more cases infected with H10N8 have been reported subsequently in Nanchang, Jiangxi Province. Two out of the three cases died and one case was improved and discharged. In the two deaths, one patient had a history of concurrent hypertension and prostatic hyperplasia, while the other had a history of concurrent hypertension and coronary heart disease, as well as thymoma resection before 2 years.

Subtype H10N8 is quite different from the previously reported viruses. It has been adapted to mammals, and its hemagglutinin of H10 has a high affinity to humans [2]. Compared to the critically ill patients with severe and unexplained pneumonia at the diagnosis, some patients with mild and hidden infection are more likely to be ignored. Therefore, it is not clear whether there are patients with mild and hidden H10N8 infection in the population [3–5]. Human infection with H10N8 shows an interval of 4–5 days from exposure to poultry markets contaminated with H10N8 to the onset of illness. The disease is progressing more rapidly, more severe, and has a higher mortality than human infection with H7N9 avian influenza. However, the source, infectivity, pathogenicity, and transmission route of H10N8 are still unclear, and no evidence of human-to-human transmission has been found [6].

12.2 Image Findings

12.2.1 Chest X-Ray

During the incubation period, the chest X-ray has no abnormal changes and shows a negative result. In the early stage of the disease, the increased and thickened lung texture with disorder arrangement can be observed. Part of them are grid-like changes (Fig. 12.1a), which may be accompanied with

Y.-l. He (✉)
Department of Radiology, The First Affiliated Hospital of Nanchang University, Nanchang, Jiangxi, China

F. Shi
Emergency Department, Institute of Shenzhen Respiratory Diseases, Shenzhen People's Hospital, The Second Clinical Medical College of Jinan University, The First Affiliated Hospital of Southern University of Science and Technology, Shenzhen, Guangdong, China

C.-j. Xu
Department of Radiology, The Second Hospital of Nanjing, Nanjing University of Chinese Medicine, Nanjing, China

B.-d. Chen
Department of Radiology, Beijing Ditan Hospital, Capital Medical University, Beijing, China

Y.-y. Deng
Department of Radiology, Yantian District People's Hospital, Shenzhen, Guangdong, China

P.-x. Lu
Department of Medical Imaging, Shenzhen Center for Chronic Disease Control, Shenzhen, Guangdong, China

C. Qiu et al. (eds.), *Avian Influenza in Human*, https://doi.org/10.1007/978-981-16-1429-3_12

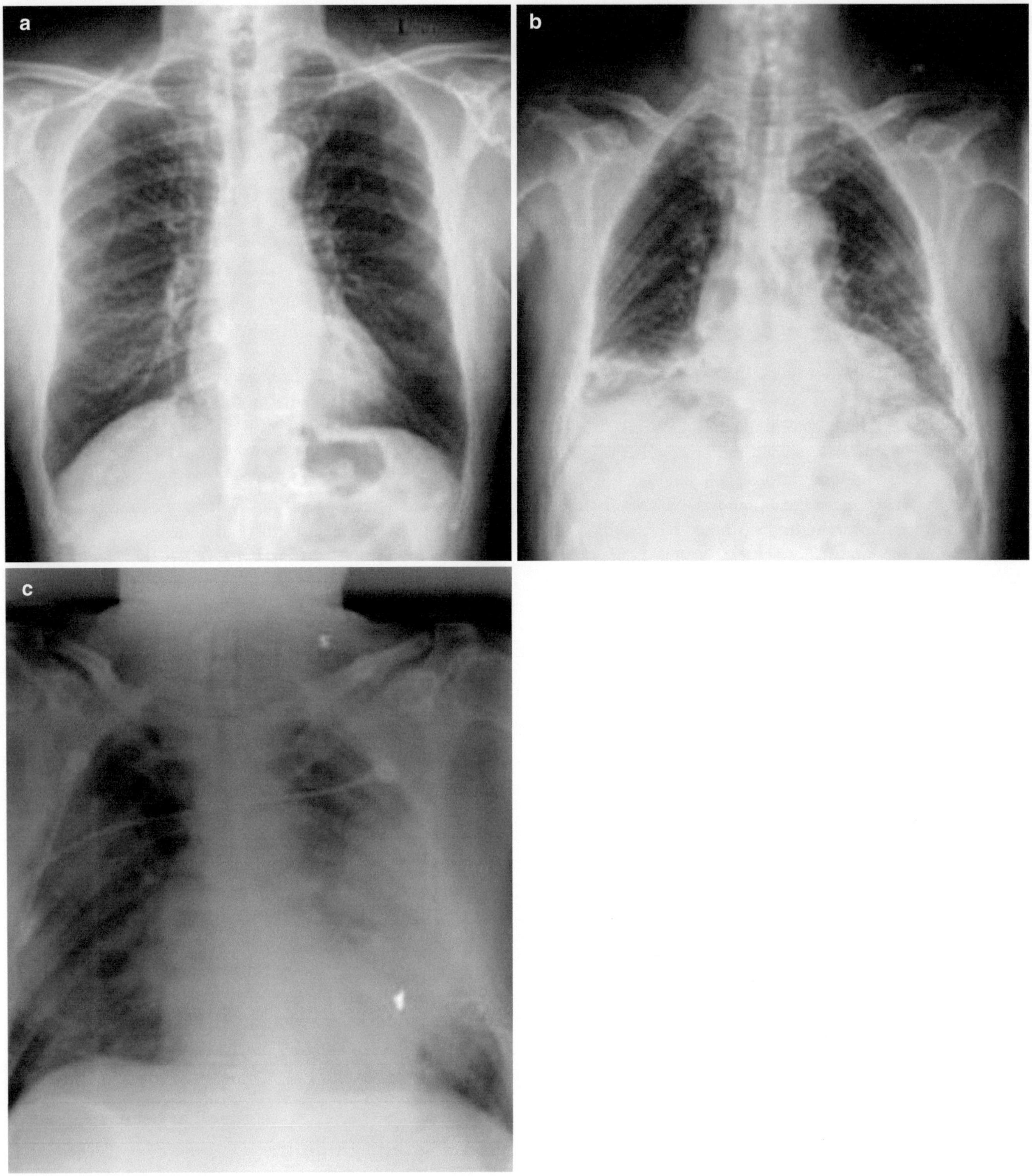

Fig. 12.1 (**a**–**c**) The patient was a 75-year-old man. He had a fever for 2 days with fatigue and anorexia. He had a history of exposure to live poultry in a week prior to the onset of the symptoms. He was infected with H10N8 avian influenza. (**a**) Jan 26th, 2014. At the time of admission, the chest X-ray showed only thickening of markings in both lungs, especially in the lower right lung. (**b**) February 3rd, 2014. The chest X-ray showed a lamellar shadow in the lower right lung field and a small lamellar shadow in the middle field of the left lung, indicating the progress of the disease. (**c**) February 5th, 2014. The chest X-ray showed large lamellar shadows in both lungs, suggesting that the lesions were progressing significantly

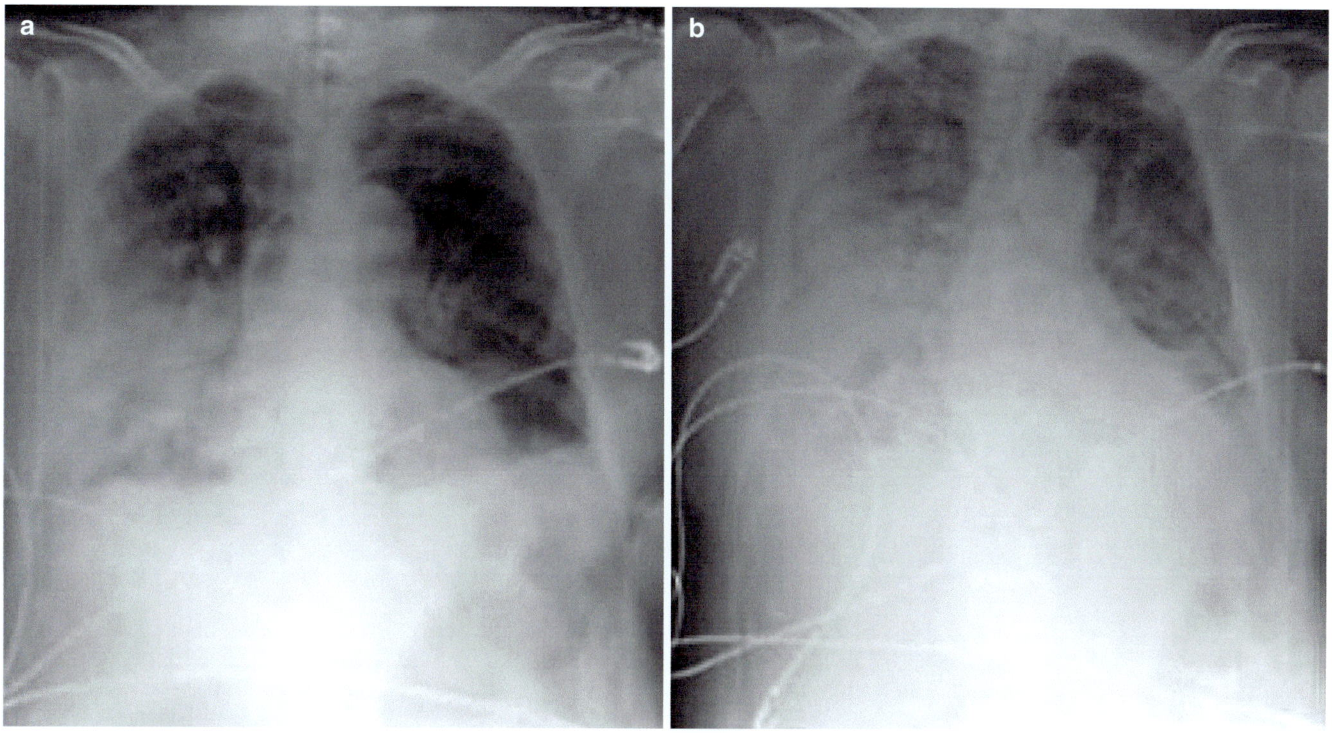

Fig. 12.2 (**a**–**b**) The female patient was 73 years old. She was admitted to hospital with chief complaint of cough, sputum, and chest tightness for 3 days and fever for 1 day. She had been to the live poultry market with a brief stay 1 week before the onset. The patient was infected with H10N8 avian influenza pneumonia. (**a**) December 3rd, 2013. The chest X-ray showed a large lamellar consolidation in the middle and lower fields of the right lung, and lamellar shadows in the left lower lung. Both hila were enlarged and thickened, the boundary was blurred, and the left costophrenic angle became blunt. (**b**) December 4th, 2013. The shadows of both lungs were further enlarged, and the costoprenic angle became blunt on both sides. Furthermore, bilateral pleural effusion increased

small patchy opacities in the lung field, indicating mesenchymal change is the main lesion in the early stage. As the disease progresses, the symptoms become severer, and there are large lamellar shadows in the lung field with blurred boundaries (Fig. 12.1b, c). Dynamic reexamination of chest X-ray show that the lesion progresses rapidly, the patchy shadow area expands significantly, the density increases greatly, and new lesions form a "white lung" appearance, indicating that the disease has entered the stage of severe pneumonia (Fig. 12.2a, b). The lesions may involve hila of lung, leading to enlargement and thickening of both hila with blurry boundary. They can also involve the pleural cavity and cause pleural effusion. The patient can progress to ARDS, manifesting dyspnea and decreased blood oxygen saturation. Most of the lesions can be absorbed if the patient has received significantly effective treatment. Patients with incomplete absorption may have fibrosis in various degrees, manifesting strip in imaging (Fig. 12.3a–d).

12.2.2 CT Image

The higher density resolution of CT helps to display earlier lesions. In the early stage, it mainly manifests consolidations and ground glass opacities with unclear boundaries. If the patient is not diagnosed and treated in time, the disease can progress quickly from one segment/lobe to multiple segments/lobes, or from the unilateral to the bilateral (Fig. 12.4a–d). Hilar involvement can lead to enlargement of both hila with increased density, which is caused by lymphadenopathy due to lymphadenitis. Interstitial involvement may cause lobular septa and thickening of the lobular core to form a grid-like change. Pleura involvement may cause free pleural effusion and interlobular effusion (Fig. 12.4e–j). These signs are particularly clear in HRCT. If the condition improves, the dynamic reexamination of CT shows absorption of the consolidation and ground glass opacity. The density decreases, the area is reduced, and the absorption of pleural effusion

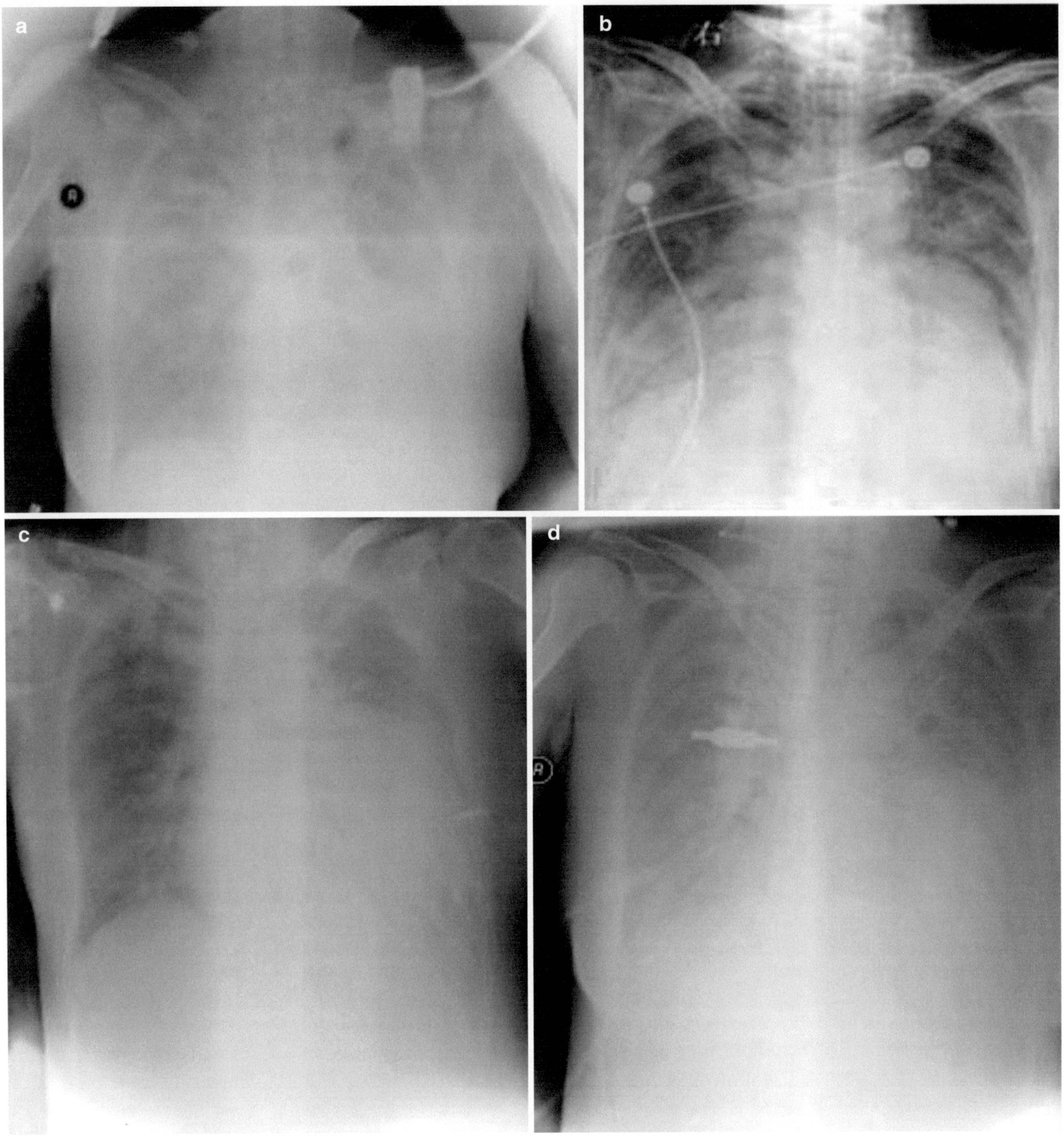

Fig. 12.3 (**a**–**d**) A 55-year-old female was admitted to the hospital with a chief complaint of cough and sputum for 12 days, a high fever for 6 days, and dyspnea for 5 days. She had a history of exposure to bazaars. The patient was infected with H10N8 avian influenza pneumonia. (**a**) January 21st, 2014. Chest X-ray showed multiple patches in both lungs, most notably in the lower left lung. (**b**) January 24th, 2014. Chest X-ray showed progression and aggravation of lesion in the right lung. (**c**) January 28th, 2014. Chest X-ray radiograph showed gradual aggravation of two pulmonary lesions and formation of "white lung". (**d**) February 7th, 2014. The shadows of the two lungs shown by chest X-ray were generally absorbed, and pulmonary transparency was restored to normal

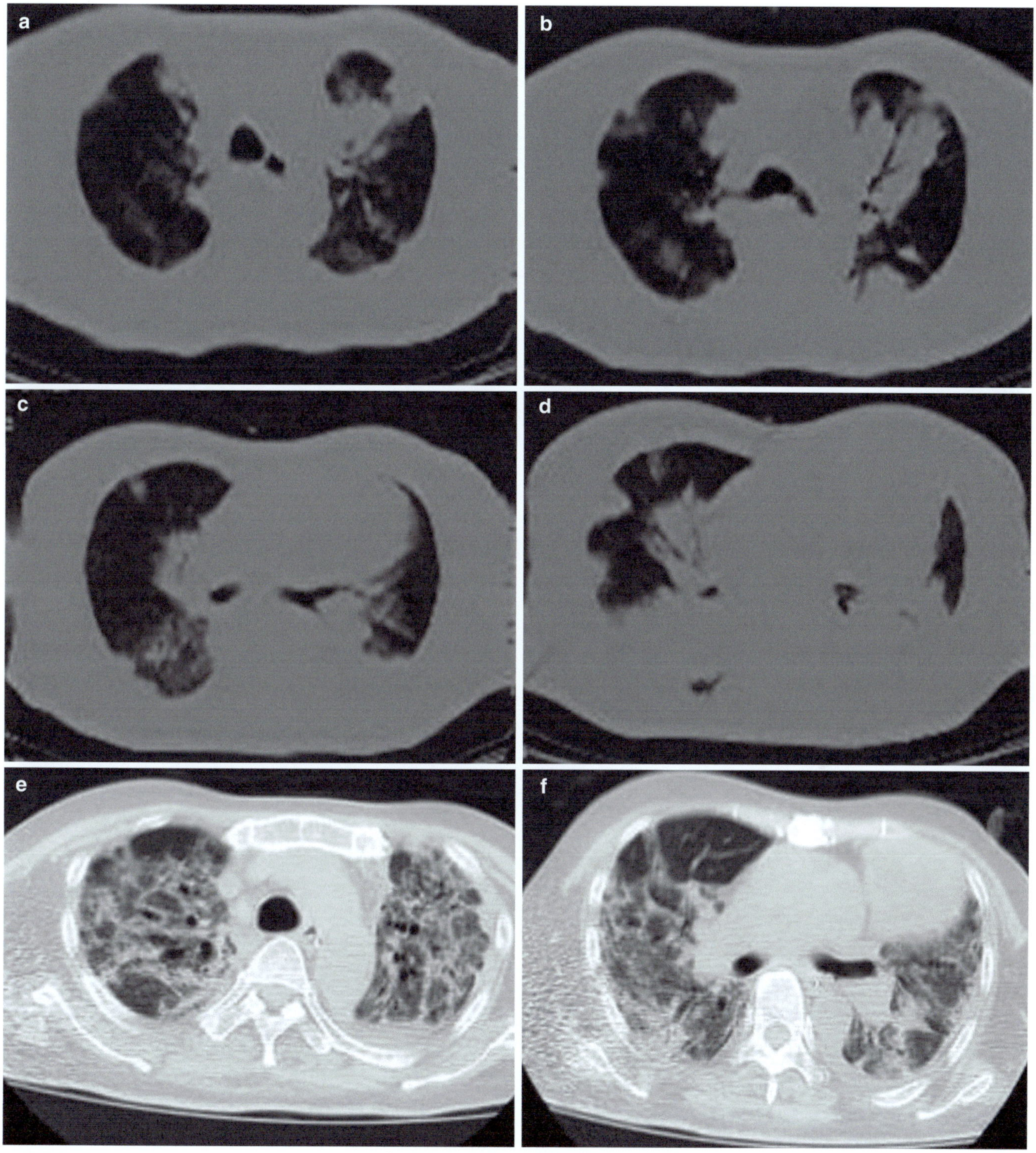

Fig. 12.4 (**a–p**) The patient was a 55-year-old woman. She was admitted to hospital with the complaint of fever and cough, with exposure to live poultry before the onset. The patient was infected with H10N8 avian influenza pneumonia. (**a–d**) January 15th 2014. Chest CT showed multiple patchy consolidations in both lungs, with severer manifestations in the left lung, complicated with inflated bronchial signs. The two lungs were scattered with patchy shadows mostly located under the pleura. (**e–j**) February 11th 2014. Reexamination of chest CT after treatment showed most of the consolidations of the two lungs were absorbed. Both lungs showed dilated bronchi and fibrous cords. There was effusion in the left pleural cavity, and space-occupying lesions in the lower left lung. (**k–p**) November 11th 2016. Chest CT (in the transverse and coronal positions) reexamined 2 years and 9 months after the onset of the disease showed remnant extensive fiber cord and small amount of ground glass opacities in both lungs

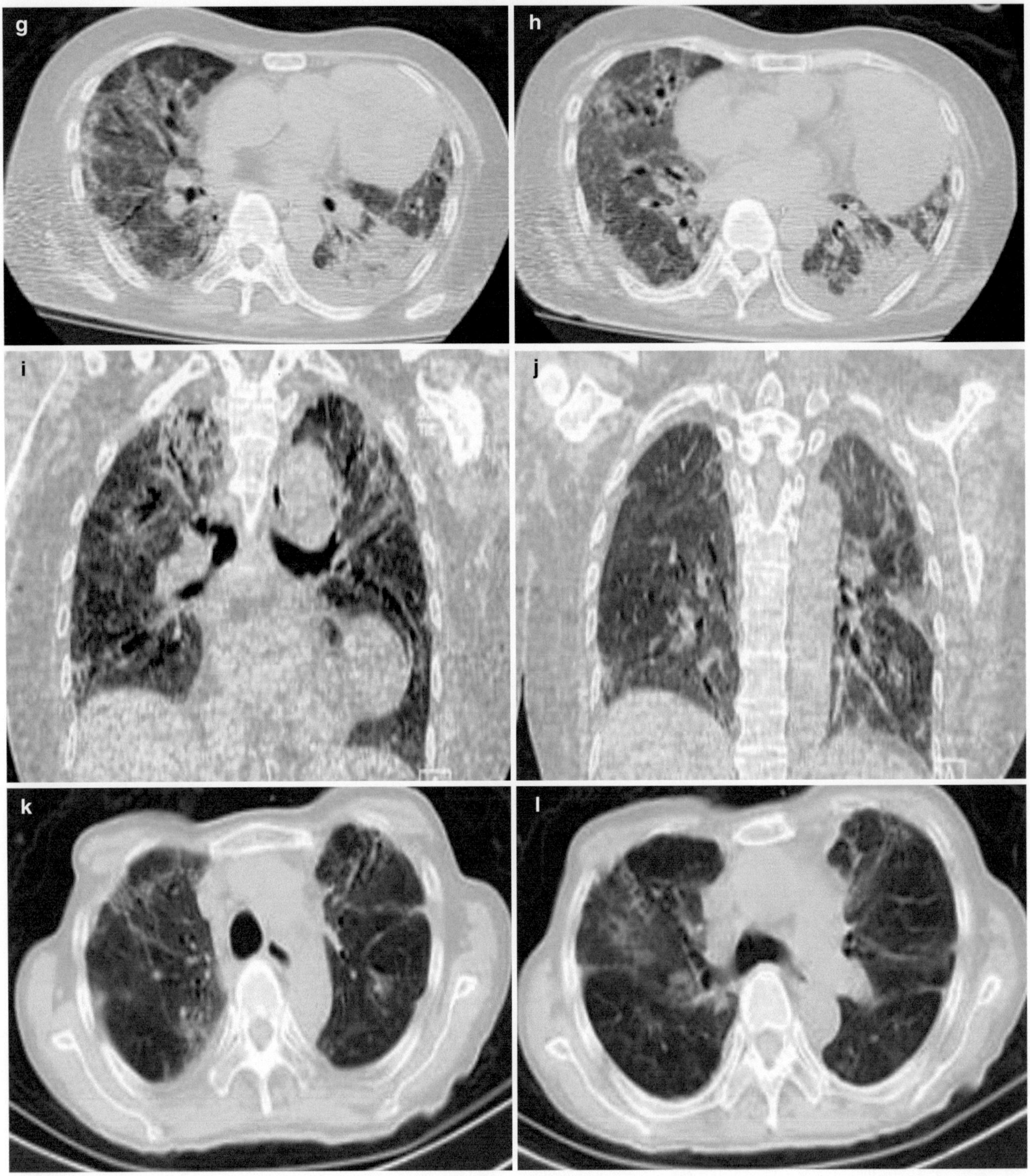

Fig. 12.4 (continued)

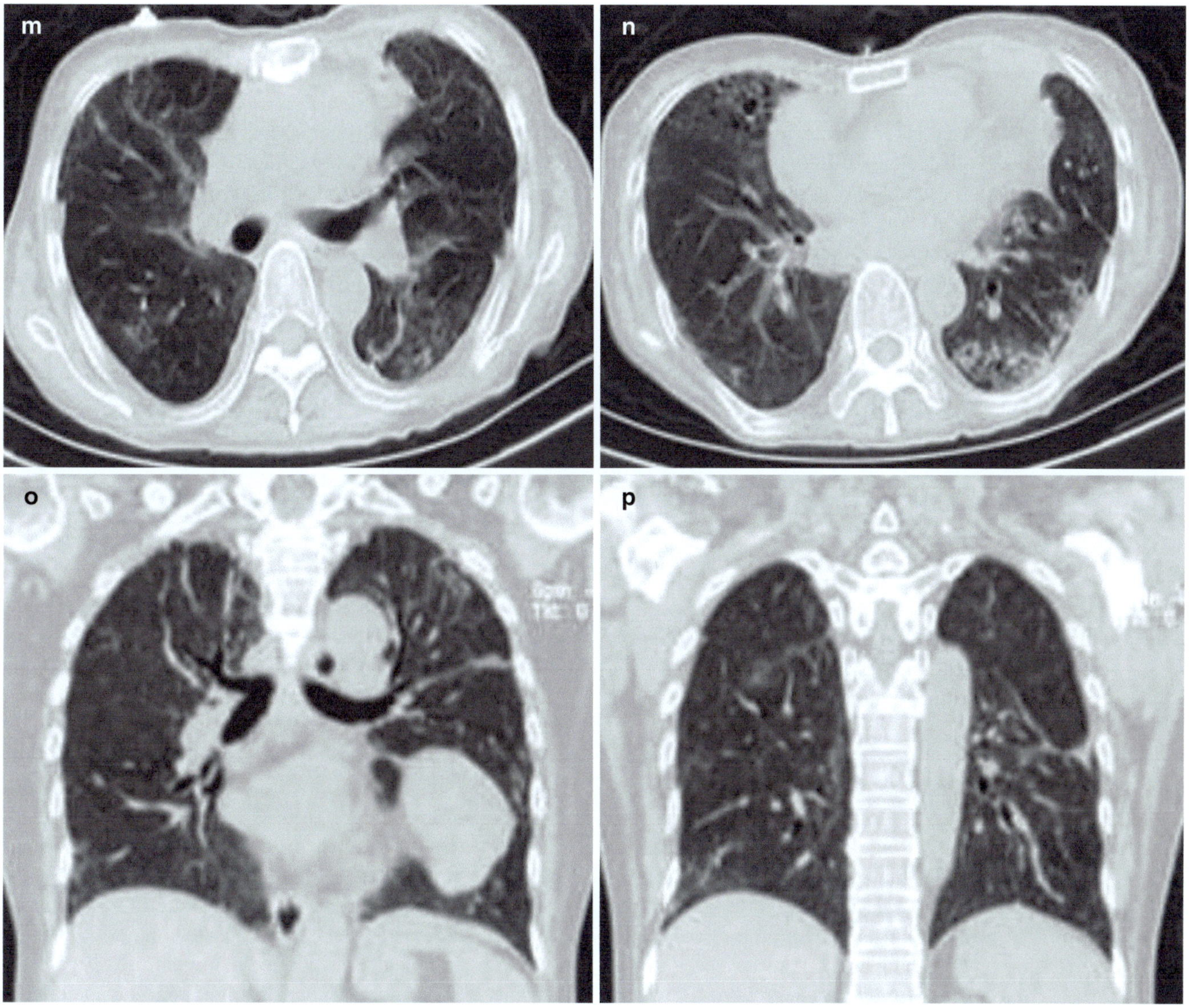

Fig. 12.4 (continued)

disappears. However, in the late stage of the disease, the two lungs manifest often the band-shaped shadow formed by fibrosis post to the absorption of lung consolidation, and even secondary traction bronchiectasis (Fig. 12.4k–p).

12.3 Imaging Diagnosis and Differential Diagnosis

I. *Imaging diagnosis*

- The imaging findings of human infection with H10N8 avian influenza virus pneumonia lack typical features. In plain film of the chest, markings of both lungs were thickened and arranged disorderly with grid-like shadows and lamellar consolidations in pulmonary fields. The hila were enlarged, thickened, and blurred. Patchy consolidations in the lungs with air bronchial signs and ground glass opacity suggest the diagnosis of viral pneumonia. If these findings are combined with the patient's epidemiological investigation, human avian influenza viral pneumonia can be highly suspected. The diagnosis still depends upon the patient's deep sputum collected for test of viral nucleic acid [7]. In view of the positive correlation between imaging changes and inflammatory indicators such as viral load, neutrophil number, and C-reactive protein, dynamic imaging review can be used clinically to evaluate the severity and responses in patients in clinical practice.

II. *Differential diagnosis*
1. Human infection with H10N8 avian influenza pneumonia has more overlapping manifestations with other subtypes of avian influenza virus pneumonia in imaging, especially H7N9 avian influenza pneumonia. H10N8 is difficult to differentiate from H7N9 based on imaging examination alone. Only the combination of the patient's age, epidemiological characteristics, and other relevant clinical data can help to distinguish the two subtypes. For example, human infections with H9N2 tend to infect children with poor resistance [8], while human infections with H5N1 tend to infect males.
2. *Differentiation from pneumonia induced by H1N1 of influenza A virus*: A H1N1 virus pneumonia is more common in young people, pregnant women, and people with underlying diseases, and most of them have cold-like symptoms. The typical imaging manifestations are multiple subpleural patchy consolidations and ground glass opacities in both lungs, showing "patches"-like changes. However, human infection with H10N8 manifests mainly lamellar consolidation and ground glass opacities, with the distribution of lesions at both hila and along the bronchial vascular bundle.
3. *Differentiation from common influenza virus pneumonia*: The latter demonstrates mostly thickening of the interlobular septum to form a subpleural grid-like shadow in the early stage. Localized ground glass shadows appear after the progression of the disease, with obvious subpleural distribution and multiple occurrences, which is different from the former characterized by obvious lung consolidations.
4. *Differentiation from pulmonary tuberculosis*: The latter is a chronic infectious disease spread via respiratory droplets. The disease progresses slowly and is calculated in months. Flocculent exudation, clustered small nodules, and caseous necrosis are more common on the image. The disease is characterized by multiple lesions, polymorphology, multiple calcifications, formation of eccentric cavity pointing toward the hila in some of the patients, and sprouting sign if it is dissolved and spreads along trachea. It is easy to distinguish from the former.
5. *Differentiation from pulmonary fungal infection (pulmonary aspergillus disease)*: The clinical onset of the latter is quite dangerous. Most patients have underlying diseases that cause a decrease in resistance, and the images are mostly characterized by nodules, plaques, and consolidations, which may be accompanied by "halo signs" without obvious aerial bronchogram. Cavitation and air crescent sign may appear when the condition ameliorates. Residual filaments or nodules are often seen in the cavity, thereby forming "hole-silk sign," which is easy to distinguish from the former characterized by multiple consolidations and ground glass opacities.
6. *Differentiation from mycoplasma pneumonia*: The latter can affect children and adults, but it is more common in children. Mild clinical symptoms in contrast to severe image findings are its typical feature. Image findings include many interstitial changes such as early bronchial vascular bundles and lobular septal thickening. The bronchial wall is markedly thickened. The progression of the disease can form large patches of high-density shadows, sprouting sign, and peripheral ground glass opacities, thereby forming "tree fog sign." There is no complete aerial bronchogram in the consolidation, and the bronchus is often narrowed and filled with shadows with slightly increased density.

12.4 The First Reported Human Infection with H10N8 Avian Influenza Pneumonia in the World

I. *Brief introduction to the case*

A 73-year-old woman was admitted to the hospital on November 30, 2013, with a chief complaint of cough, expectoration, and chest tightness for 3 days and fever for 1 day. Three days before admission, she had cough with white sputum, chest tightness, and shortness of breath post to exertion, and then developed fever with a body temperature of 38.6 °C complicated with chills, but without other accompanying symptoms such as abdominal pain, diarrhea, headache, and muscle soreness. Physical examination on admission: body temperature 39.1 °C, no cyanosis of perilabial mucosa, slight pharyngeal congestion, and no swelling of bilateral tonsils. The sound of respiration in both lungs was coarse. Fine moist rales could be heard in the right lung, without wheezing, or pleural friction sounds in both lungs.

Laboratory examination: Blood routine examination: C-reactive protein >200.00 mg/L, white blood cell 10.34×10^9/L, lymphocyte percentage 7.0%, neutrophil percentage 76.4%. Results of arterial blood gas analysis: PH value 7.48, arterial oxygen partial pressure 57 mmHg, arterial carbon dioxide partial pressure 32 mmHg. Biochemical examination: normal results were observed for creatine kinase, lactate dehydrogenase, aspartate aminotransferase, and alanine aminotransferase.

Image findings: Plain chest CT scans (2013-12-01) showed large solidification in the lower right lung with aerial bronchogram, the uneven-density patchy shadow with unclear edges in the left lower lung. A little thickening of interlobular septa in both lower lungs was found, with inter-lobar effusion at the right oblique fissure. Pulmonary infection was considered (Fig. 12.5a–h). The

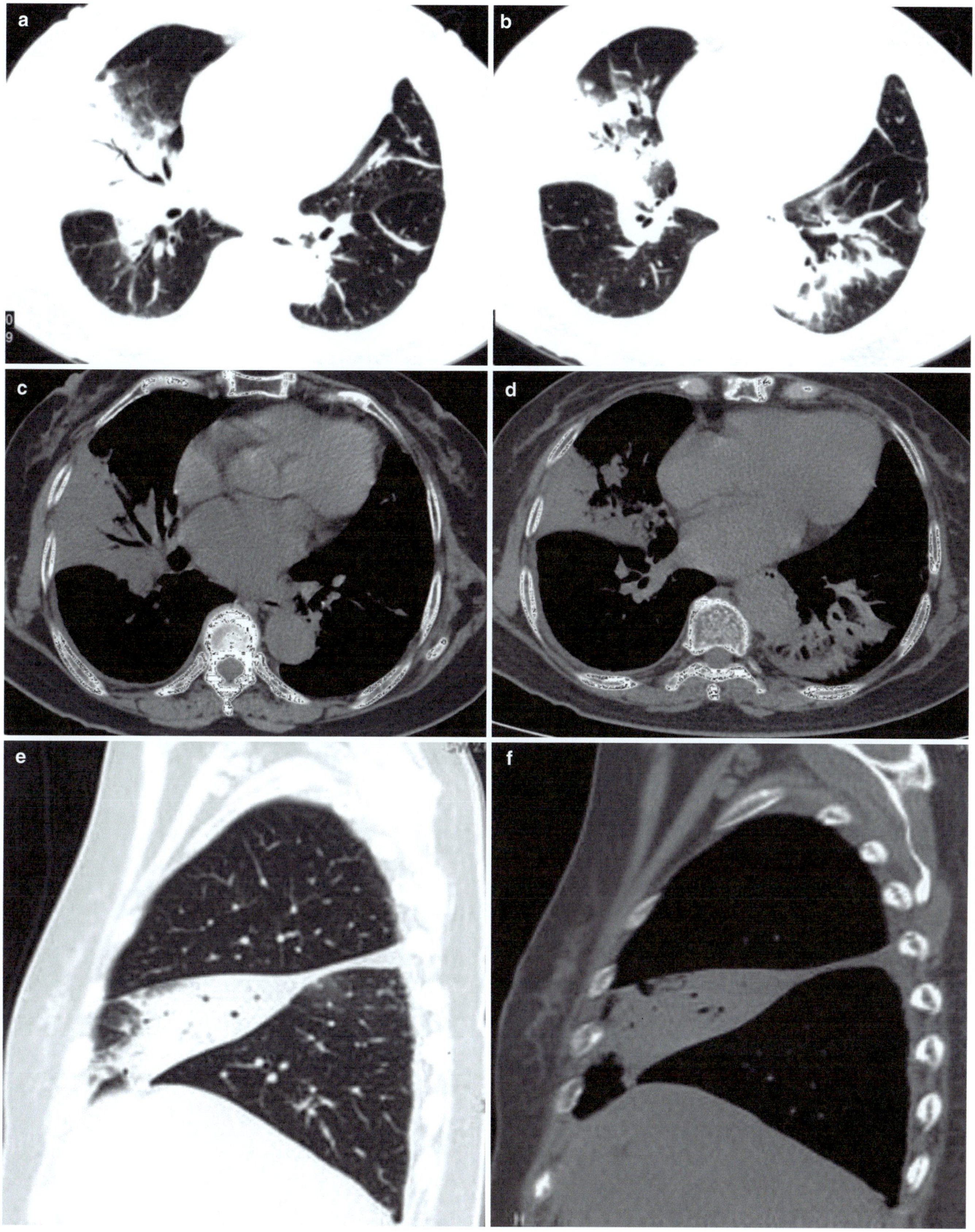

Fig. 12.5 (**a**–**h**) 2013-12-01 Plain chest CT scan on February 1st, 2013, showed a large consolidation shadow in the middle and lower lobe of the right lung with air bronchogram, and a patchy shadow with heterogeneously raised density in the lower left lung

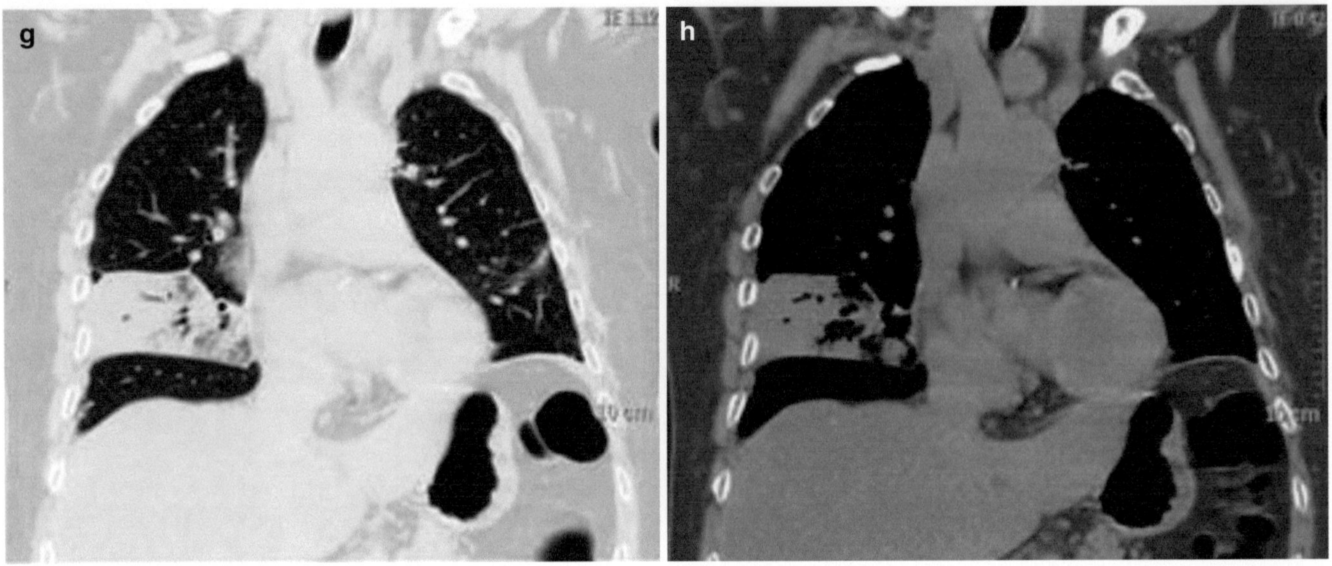

Fig. 12.5 (continued)

patient had a past history of thymoma excision in 2012 because of "myasthenia gravis and thymoma." Since the operation, she had been on the treatment of brompistigmine tablets 60 mg tid po. However, the patient still complained of chest tightness and shortness of breath post to exertion, though she was occasionally competent with out-of-bed activities.

The main diagnoses on admission: (1) severe pneumonia; (2) type I respiratory failure; (3) myasthenia gravis; (4) post to thymoma resection.

After admission, cefotaxime sodium and levofloxacin were given for anti-infection treatment, but the patient did not respond well. On December 2, 2013, the patient was transferred to the intensive care unit due to respiratory failure.

Blood routine examination on December 2, 2013, showed that C-reactive protein >200.00 mg/L, white blood cell 12.09 × 10^9/L, lymphocyte percentage 2.4%, neutrophil percentage 94.3%. Blood gas: PH 7.26, arterial partial pressure of oxygen 68 mmHg, arterial partial pressure of carbon dioxide 48 mmHg, showing the deterioration compared with the condition at admission. Immediately after the transference to the intensive care unit on December 2, the patient was given meropenem and vancomycin against infection, and provided with pressurized oxygen inhalation connected to the ventilator for auxiliary respiration. At night, her blood oxygen saturation kept dropping, and the tracheal intubation was given to connect to the ventilator for auxiliary respiration. A large amount of pink watery sputum and non-foaming sputum were sucked out of the tracheal intubation. No obvious rales were heard in both lungs. On December 3, the patient developed septic shock.

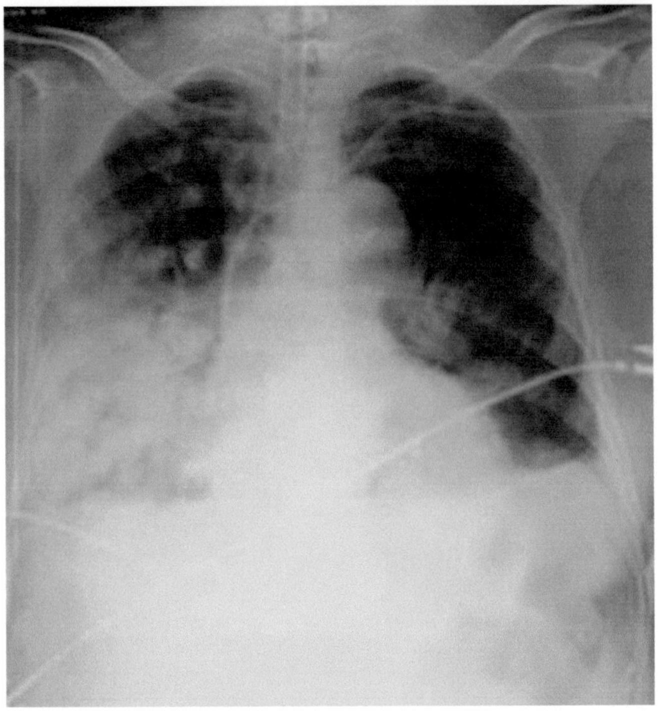

Fig. 12.6 The bedside chest X-ray on December 3rd showed large consolidations in the middle and lower fields of the right lung, with blurred boundaries. A small lamellar shadow was observed in the lower left lung. Both hila increased in size with raised density, and the left costophrenic angle became dull

Bedside chest X-ray on December 3, 2013, showed large consolidations in the middle and lower fields of the right lung, with blurred boundaries. There was a patchy shadow in the lower left lung. Bilateral hilar enlargement with increased density was observed, with blunting of the left costal diaphragmatic angle (Fig. 12.6). Compared with chest CT on admission, new lesions were found in the left lung with partial interstitial changes (hilar enlargement and concentration). It indicated rapid progression of the disease. After repeated inquiries about the patient's medical history, it was revealed that the patient's housekeeper had flu symptoms recently, and the patient herself had a history of poultry contact. Judging from the rapid progression of pulmonary lesions of the patient in combination with the patient's epidemiological history, the possibility of "avian influenza and other viral infections" could not be ruled out. Bedside isolation was provided and tamiflu antiviral therapy was given. On December 3, the blood routine examination showed that the percentage of lymphocytes and neutrophils were 4.2% and 93.4%, respectively. The results of arterial blood gas analysis showed that PH was 7.30, arterial blood oxygen partial pressure was 39 mmHg, and arterial carbon dioxide partial pressure was 43 mmHg. In addition, oliguria occurred.

On December 4, 2013, blood routine examination showed white blood cell 7.00 × 10^9/L, lymphocyte percentage 3.1%, neutrophil percentage 93.5%. Blood gas: PH 7.12, arterial partial pressure of oxygen 45 mmHg, arterial partial pressure of carbon dioxide 66 mmHg. Urea nitrogen 12.20 mmol/L, creatinine 189.0 μmol/L, and anuria appeared.

On December 4, 2013, bedside chest X-ray (Fig. 12.7) showed that the shadow of both lungs was enlarged further, and bilateral costal diaphragmatic angle became dull (pleural effusion) compared with the image on December 3. Blood oxygen saturation kept decreasing, and the condition continued to deteriorate. Deep sputum viral nucleic acid detection was performed for the patient.

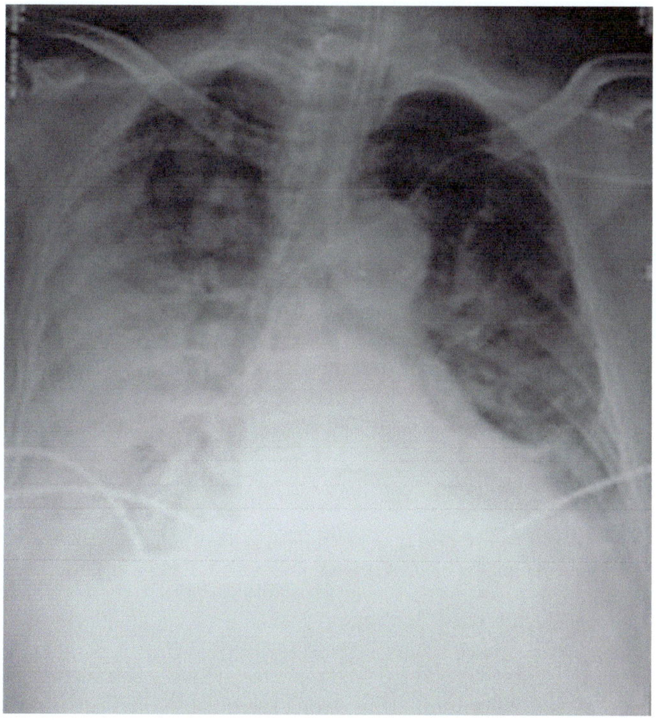

Fig. 12.7 The chest radiograph at the bedside on December 4th, 2013, showed that the shadows of both lungs were further enlarged with bilateral pleural effusions, in comparison with findings shown by chest X-ray on December 3rd

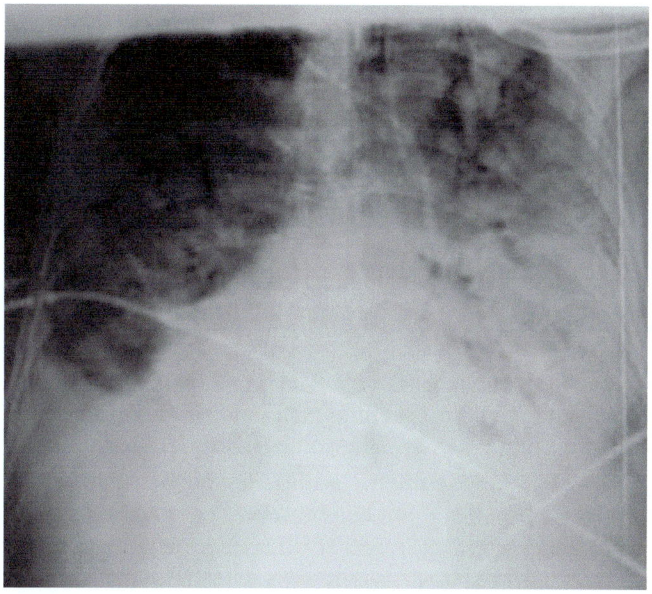

Fig. 12.8 Bedside chest X-ray on December 5th, 2013, showed that shadows of both lungs were further enlarged, and the pleural effusion significantly increased compared with image findings on December 4th

On December 5, 2010, bedside chest X-ray (Fig. 12.8) showed that the shadows of both lungs were enlarged further compared with that on December 4th, and the amount of pleural effusion significantly increased. The patient had liver damage, renal failure, and coagulation failure, indicating multiple organ failure. The patient died on December 6. Chinese Center for Disease Control and Prevention reported on December 10 that the patient was a case of H10N8 avian influenza in human.

II. *Discussion*

In 2012, Jiao et al. [9] reported the discovery of H10N8 avian influenza virus in ducks. On January 30th, 2013, the Third Affiliated Hospital of Nanchang University admitted a patient who was confirmed by the Chinese Center for Disease Control and Prevention to be infected with the subtype H10N8 of avian influenza. The patient was the world's first case of viral pneumonia induced by N10N8 avian influenza infection. Avian influenza viruses belong to the genus Influenza A of the orthomyxoviridae family. H10N8 avian influenza virus is a virus produced by the recombination of multiple gene fragments [9], and the complete genome series analysis of this type of avian influenza virus strain has been completed at present [10]. The H10N8 avian influenza virus was first discovered and isolated from waters or poultry

[9, 10], and the H10N8 avian influenza virus found in this case was a human infection of this type.

Except for subtypes H5 and H7, all Avian Influenza A including 18 subtypes of HA and 11 subtypes of NA (e.g., subtypes H7N2, H7N3, H9N2, or H10N7 [1–14]) are considered to be low pathogenic avian influenza viruses. The lower respiratory tract diseases caused by these avian influenza viruses are characterized by mild (conjunctivitis or uncomplicated influenza-like illness), moderate symptoms of infection. However, it is worth noting that low pathogenic viruses are precursors of highly pathogenic ones [15, 16], and there is a high risk of pathogenicity. Therefore, although highly pathogenic avian influenza viruses are limited to the subtypes H5 and H7, other subtypes with potential threat to public health [9] should not be ignored when attention is paid to subtypes H5, H7, and H9. This case of human infection with H10N8 avian influenza virus is a good warning.

The patient's condition develops and evolves very fast. The evolution process and characteristics of chest images are as follows: (1) Lobar consolidation and segmental exudation: on the first day of admission, the patient's chest CT showed a large area of consolidation in the middle and lower right lung with air bronchogram, a patchy exudation was seen in the lower left lung with unclear boundary. In addition, there was a little thickening of the lobular septa of both lower lungs and interlobar effusion in the right lung. The patient showing a disease with exudate extending up to 3 pulmonary lobes was categorized into the type of severe pneumonia. (2) Diffuse exudative consolidation of both lungs: bedside chest X-ray within 48 h post to admission showed large fusion of the right lung lesions, and exudative lesions larger than the previous images were also seen in the lower left lung, occupying an increased area and involving more lobes in comparison with the image on admission, which suggested the disease entered the clinically critical stage. (3) Image features of the patient were consistent with the clinical manifestations. Bedside chest X-rays performed for 3 consecutive days post to treatment in the intensive care unit (ICU) showed that lung lobes involved increased in number and area of lesions expanded and fused rapidly within a short period of time.

The patient's condition developed and evolved rapidly, featuring typical manifestations of acute respiratory distress within a short period, with continuous drop of blood oxygen saturation followed by instantly respiratory failure. Despite the ventilator-assisted breathing, no amelioration was achieved for hypoxemia in the patient. The patient's image findings and the evolution of clinical symptoms suggested that they were consistent with the diagnosis of viral pneumonia [16]. According to the characteristics of the current epidemiological diseases, the possibility of human avian influenza was considered. The treatment was based on the "Regimens for Diagnosis and Treatment for Human Infection with H7N9 Avian Influenza," [17] and diagnostic and therapeutic measures were adopted, which were timely, standardized, and scientific. However, image changes of human infection with H10N8 avian influenza pneumonia were compared with those of human infection with H7N9 avian influenza, and the two were difficult to distinguish in terms of image changes [17]. In addition, based on the characteristics of image changes alone, this case also needed to be differentiated from bacterial pneumonia and pulmonary fungal infection characterized by large lamellar exudates as the main manifestations. In this case, a few interstitial changes were observed in both lungs, which were helpful to indicate viral pneumonia. However, the diagnosis of human avian influenza ultimately depends upon pathogenic examination as the "gold standard," especially the confirmation of the subtype [18].

Human infection with avian influenza virus A usually occurs after contact with poultry, which should draw widest attention [19]. In this case, the source of infection of the H10N8 avian influenza virus was not clear. Wild birds, domestic poultry, and aquatic environment may all play an important role in the spread of this type of avian influenza virus [19]. At present, there is no definite evidence of interhuman transmission. The family members who were in close contact with this patient and the medical staff who treated him had negative pathogenic examinations.

In summary, the chest image of patients infected with H10N8 avian influenza pneumonia mainly shows progressive consolidation and exudation of both lungs with interstitial changes, which may be complicated with pleural and interlobular effusion. Fibrotic changes may occur during the absorption period. Dynamic observation for image changes can comprehensively and objectively reflect the course of the disease and assess its severity.

References

1. Chen H, Yuan H, Gao R, et al. Clinical and epidemiological characteristics of a fatal case of avian influenza A H10N8 virus infection: a descriptive study. Lancet. 2014;383(9918):714–21.
2. Vachieri SG, Xiong X, Collins PJ, et al. Receptor binding by H10 influenza viruses. Nature. 2014;511(7510):475–7.
3. Li Q, Zhou L, Zhou M, et al. Preliminary report: epidemiology of the avian influenza A (H7N9) outbreak in China. N Engl J Med. 2013;370(6):1668–77.
4. Chen EF, Chai CL, Sun JM, et al. Epidemiological characteristics and control strategies of human infection with avian influenza A (H7N9) virus in Zhejiang province. Chin J Public Health. 2013;29(5):625–7.

5. Cowling BJ, Jin L, Lau EH, et al. Comparative epidemiology of human infections with avian influenza A H7N9 and H5N1 viruses in China: a population-based study of laboratory-confirmed cases. Lancet. 2013;382(9887):129–37.
6. Chen Y, Liang W, Yang S, et al. Human infections with the emerging avian influenza A H7N9 virus from wet market poultry: clinical analysis and characterisation of viral genome. Lancet. 2013;381(9881):1916–25.
7. El Zowalaty ME, Bustin SA, Husseiny MI, et al. Avian influenza: virology, diagnosis and surveillance. Future Microbiol. 2013;8(9):1209–27.
8. Wenzhong H, Qianqian Z, Puxuan L, et al. Clinical imaging descriptive study of the first case of human infection with avian influenza H9N2 virus in the world. Electron J Emerg Infect Dis. 2016;1(1):18–22.
9. Jiao P, Cao L, Yuan R, et al. Complete genome sequence of an H10N8 avian influenza virus isolated from a live bird market in southern China. J Virol. 2012;86(14):7716.
10. Zhang H, Xu B, Chen Q, et al. Characterization of an H10N8 influenza virus isolated from Dongting lake wetland. Virol J. 2011;8(8):42–51.
11. Aamir UB, Naeem K, Ahmed Z, et al. Zoonotic potential of highly pathogenic avian H7N3 influenzaviruses from Pakistan. Virology. 2009;390(2):212–20.
12. Blair PJ, Putnam SD, Krueger WS, et al. Evidence for avian H9N2 influenza virus infections among rural villagers in Cambodia. J Infect Public Health. 2013;6(2):69–79.
13. Ostrowsky B, Huang A, Terry W, et al. Low pathogenic avian influenza A (H7N2) virus infection in immunocompromised adult, New York, USA, 2003. Emerg Infect Dis. 2012;18(7):1128–31.
14. Arzey GG, Kirkland PD, Arzey KE, et al. Influenza virus a (H10N7) in chickens and poultry abattoir workers, Australia. Emerg Infect Dis. 2012;18(5):814–6.
15. Agusto FB, Gumel AB. Qualitative dynamics of lowly- and highly-pathogenic avian influenza strains. Math Biosci. 2013;243(2):147–62.
16. He J, Li J, Lu P, et al. Radiological description about the globally first case of human infected avian influenza virus (H10N8) induced pneumonia. Radiol Infect Dis. 2016;3(1):44–7.
17. Alexander DJ. An overview of the epidemiology of avian influenza. Vaccine. 2007;25(30):5637–44.
18. National Health and Family Planning Commission of the People's Republic of China. Diagnosis and treatment of human infection with H7N9 Avian Influenza (2nd edition, 2013). Chin J Crit Care Med. 2013;6(3):34–7.
19. Gao R, Cao B, Hu Y, et al. Human infection with a novel avian-origin influenza A (H7N9) virus. N Engl J Med. 2013;368(20):1888–97.

13 H9N2 Avian Influenza in Human

Qian-qian Zhang, Kai Zhou, Wen-zhong Hou, Ru-ming Xie, Yu-lin He, and Pu-xuan Lu

13.1 Introduction

Subtype H9N2 of avian influenza virus (AIV) was first detected by Homme PJ et al. in the respiratory tract of turkeys in Wisconsin, USA in 1966 [1]. Since the 1990s, this virus has been spreading more and more widely, and has become endemo epidemic in many countries in Asia, the Middle East, and North Africa [2]. In China, H9N2 has been prevalent in some of the provinces since 1992, and has become sporadic distribution in most regions since 1998. Hosts of H9N2 show a great diversity, including poultry (chicken, duck, pig, dog, and horse), wild birds, waterfowl, and occasionally through cross-species contamination, humans [3].

The first case of subtype H9N2 of AIV in human was reported in 1998 [4]. Since then, the virus has been distributed globally, despite its low prevalence rate. Cases of human infection have been found mainly in China (including Hong Kong) and Bangladesh with sporadic distribution. At present, 37 confirmed cases of human infection by H9N2 have been reported worldwide, with 27 cases in China (Table 13.1) including 2 deaths. The pathogenicity of H9N2 is significantly lower than that of H7N9 and H5N1 subtypes; however, it is more prone to cause human infection [27, 28]. The number of cases with detectable H9N2 in serum seems much larger than that of patients with confirmed diagnosis. This may be attributed to patients' frequent exposure to poultry [29]. It is reported that 2.3–4.6% of poultry workers are positive in H9 antibody [30]. The relatively mild symptoms caused by H9N2 are clinically difficult to distinguish from those caused by viruses H1N1 or H3N2. Most of the 27 cases infected with H9N2 avian influenza in China manifested clinical symptoms of acute respiratory tract infection, i.e., fever, cough, sore throat, and headache. The body temperature of all patients with fever was between 38.0 and 39.3 °C, and laboratory examination showed that the number of neutrophils slightly elevated. The mortality of human infection caused by H9N2 was relatively low. Two out of the 27 Chinese patients died, and both of them had underlying diseases with poor immunity. Patients infected with AVI H9N2 show good prognosis. It is a self-limited disease in patients with normal immunity, or a disease with good prognosis post to antiviral treatment in those with low immunity.

Avian influenza virus spread mainly through the oral–fecal route, animal infection, respiratory transmission, and direct contact infection. Among them, the gas transmission route results in faster and wider dissemination, thus it is the most difficult one to prevent and control. It has been confirmed by a research [31] that some natural isolates of subtype H9N2 of AIV carry concurrently point mutations of PA L627 and HA K363, which confer the capacity of aerosol transmission. Among the 27 cases of human H9N2 infection in China, 20 cases had direct or indirect history of contacting poultry. Because of the potential of H9N2 to cause pandemic influenza, prevention and control actions should be performed continuously. Though unstable to heat, H9N2 shows high resistance to low temperature. It can be inactivated at

Q.-q. Zhang
Magnetic Resonance Room, Zhoukou Central Hospital, Zhoukou, Henan Province, China

K. Zhou
Shenzhen Institute of Respiratory Diseases, Shenzhen People's Hospital, The Second Clinical Medical College of Jinan University, The First Affiliated Hospital of Southern University of Science and Technology, Shenzhen, Guangdong, China

W.-z. Hou
Department of Radiology, Meizhou People's Hospital, Meizhou, Guangdong Province, China

R.-m. Xie
Department of Radiology, Beijing Ditan Hospital, Capital Medical University, Beijing, China

Y.-l. He
Department of Radiology, The First Affiliated Hospital of Nanchang University, Nanchang, Jiangxi, China

P.-x. Lu (✉)
Department of Medical Imaging, Shenzhen Center for Chronic Disease Control, Shenzhen, Guangdong, China

C. Qiu et al. (eds.), *Avian Influenza in Human*, https://doi.org/10.1007/978-981-16-1429-3_13

Table 13.1 Information of 27 human infection cases with subtype H9N2 of AVI in China

Year	Location (reference)	Age and gender	Clinical symptoms	Image findings	Poultry exposure	Remarks
1998	Shaoguan, Guangdong [5, 6]	14-year-old, male	ARI[a]	Normal	Yes	
	Shaoguan, Guangdong	43-year-old, female	ARI	Pneumonia manifestations	Yes	Death
	Shaoguan, Guangdong	9-year-old, female	ARI	None	No	
	Shaoguan, Guangdong	75-year-old, male	ARI	No abnormality in chest X-ray	Yes	
	Shantou, Guangdong	4-year-old, male	ARI	No abnormality in chest X-ray	Unknown	
	Shantou, Guangdong	1-year-old, female	ARI	No abnormality in chest X-ray	Unknown	
	Shantou, Guangdong	–	ARI	No abnormality in chest X-ray	Unknown	
	Shantou, Guangdong	–	ARI	No abnormality in chest X-ray	Unknown	
	Shantou, Guangdong	36-year-old, female	ARI	No abnormality in chest X-ray	Yes	
1999	Guangdong [5]	22-month-old, female	Fever (38 °C), cough	N.A.	No	
1999	Hong Kong [7]	13-month-old, female	Fever, vomiting	N.A.	Yes	
	Hong Kong [7]	4-year-old, female	Fever (38.9 °C), sore throat and headache	Normal chest X-ray	No	
2003	Hong Kong [8]	5-year-old, male	Mild fever, cough, mild dehydration	No abnormality in chest	No	
2007	Hong Kong [9]	9-month-old, female	Mild upper respiratory tract infection	No abnormality in chest	Yes	
2008	Shenzhen [9]	2-month-old, female	Cough, vomiting	No abnormality in chest	Yes	
2013	Shenzhen [9]	86-year-old, male	Chilliness, cough	No abnormality in chest	Yes	
	Yongzhou, Hunan [10]	7-year-old, male	Fever, runny nose	No abnormality in chest	Yes	
2015	Hefei, Anhui [11]	4-year-old, female	Fever (up to 39.5 °C), cough	No abnormality in chest	Yes	
	Chuzhou, Anhui [11, 12]	6-year-old, male	Fever (up to 38.7 °C)	No abnormality in chest	Yes	
	Chenzhou, Hunan [13]	11-month-old, female	Fever (39.2 °C)	No abnormality in chest	Yes	
	Changsha, Hunan [14]	Unknown	Fever, cough	Unknown	Unknown	
2016	Chengdu [15–17]	57-year-old, female	Cough, expectoration, dyspnea	Pneumonia manifestations	Yes	Death
	Meizhou, Guangdong [18]	6-year-old, female	Cough, fever	Pneumonia manifestations	Yes	
	Pingxiang, Jiangxi [19, 20]	4-year-old, female	Fever, sore throat, 38.9 °C	Thickening of bilateral lung markings	Yes	
	Mengzi, Yunnan [21, 22]	10-month-old, male	Fever, cough, 38.1 °C	Normal	Yes	
	Beijing [23–25]	3-year-old, male	Fever, 39 °C	Normal	Yes	
2017	Beijing [26]	32-year-old, male	Fever, malaise and headache, 39 °C	Normal	Yes	

[a]*ARI* acute respiratory tract infection

65 °C for 30 min. It is sensitive to ultraviolet radiation and can be inactivated by exposure to sunlight within several hours at room temperature on the surface of poultry feces.

13.2 Image Findings

I. Normal chest image

Among the 27 cases of human infection with subtype H9N2 AIV in China, 22 cases showed normal chest images. This is mainly due to the low pathogenicity of the subtype H9N2 AIV, which causes mild clinical signs, and the autoimmune system is sufficient to resist the virus invasion into the lungs.

II. Manifestations of bronchitis

Among the 27 cases of human infection with subtype H9N2 AIV in China, a female child aged 4 was admitted to hospital with the chief complaint of fever (temperature 38.9 °C) and pharyngeal pain. The positive laboratory tests indicated that the neutrophil percentage increased, the lymphocyte ratio decreased, and the C-reactive protein increased. The chest X-ray showed thickened lung markings. When the autoimmune system of patients cannot completely fight off the virus, a series of infections will appear in the lungs. The replication results of avian influenza virus H9N2 in human lung tissue [32] show that H9N2 is able to infect human lung tissue, and the main target cells of infection and replication are type II alveolar cells, respiratory bronchiolar epithelial cells, and bronchiolar epithelial cells. When the virus invades bronchiolar and respiratory bronchiolar epithelial cells, there are bronchiolar congestion and swelling or hyperplasia and hypertrophy of epithelial cells, showing thickening of lung markings in chest X-ray. Respiratory tract infection symptoms are found in H9N2-infected patients, including cough, fever, and sore throat. The symptoms disappear soon after receiving anti-infective treatment. The condition of the 4-year-old patient was improved and the symptoms disappeared in 2 days after receiving anti-infection and symptomatic treatment.

III. Manifestations of Pneumonia

In case of a weakened or defective immune system, the patient will show relatively severe clinical symptoms after being infected with the H9N2 subtype virus. There are 3 pneumonia cases including 2 deaths among the 27 H9N2 infection cases in China. Both deaths were adults (aged 57 and 43 years, respectively) with underlying diseases and low immunity. The image finding of the three patients with pneumonia showed the changes of viral pneumonia.

1. Signs of local exudation in pulmonary lobes and segments

   Chest X-ray and Computed Tomography (CT) showed local strip-like and patches of increased density shadow at lung with uneven density and unclear boundary. The lesions were mainly distributed in the medial and middle zones. The pathological mechanism was supposed to be that the subtype H9N2 virus invaded type II alveolar cells, and there was serous exudate in the alveolar cavity, leading to pulmonary interstitial congestion and edema, which demonstrated strip-like and patchy shadows in the lung.

2. Signs of pulmonary consolidation and pulmonary atelectasis

   Unilateral pulmonary consolidation with atelectasis. Chest X-ray and CT showed an increase in the density of the entire pulmonary lobe, containing air bronchograms inside and demonstrating uneven density. Mediastinum and main bronchus showed ipsilateral displacement, with contralateral or adjacent lobar emphysema (Figs. 13.1 and 13.2a–d).

3. Complication of pleural effusion

   Exudate was found in the pleural cavity when inflammation spread to the pleura. Chest X-ray showed the disappearance of costophrenic angles, and a shadow in increased density in unilateral lung, which was higher at the lateral and lower at the medial. The mediastinal window of CT showed a curved low-density shadow in unilateral pleural cavity, and the CT value was higher than the density of the fluid (Fig. 13.2e).

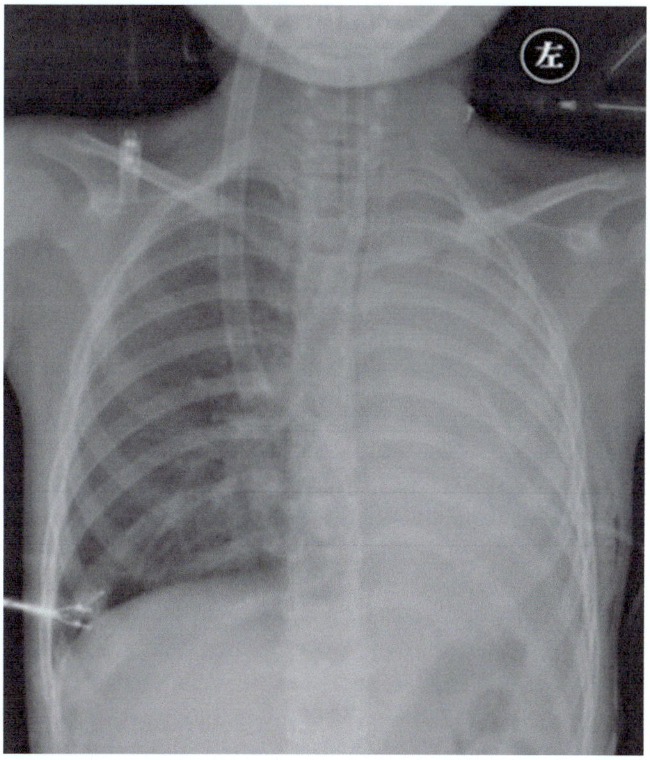

Fig. 13.1 On June 12th, 2016, day 3 post to the onset, chest X-ray showed left atelectasis, and a small amount of exudative lesions in the middle and lower fields of the right lung

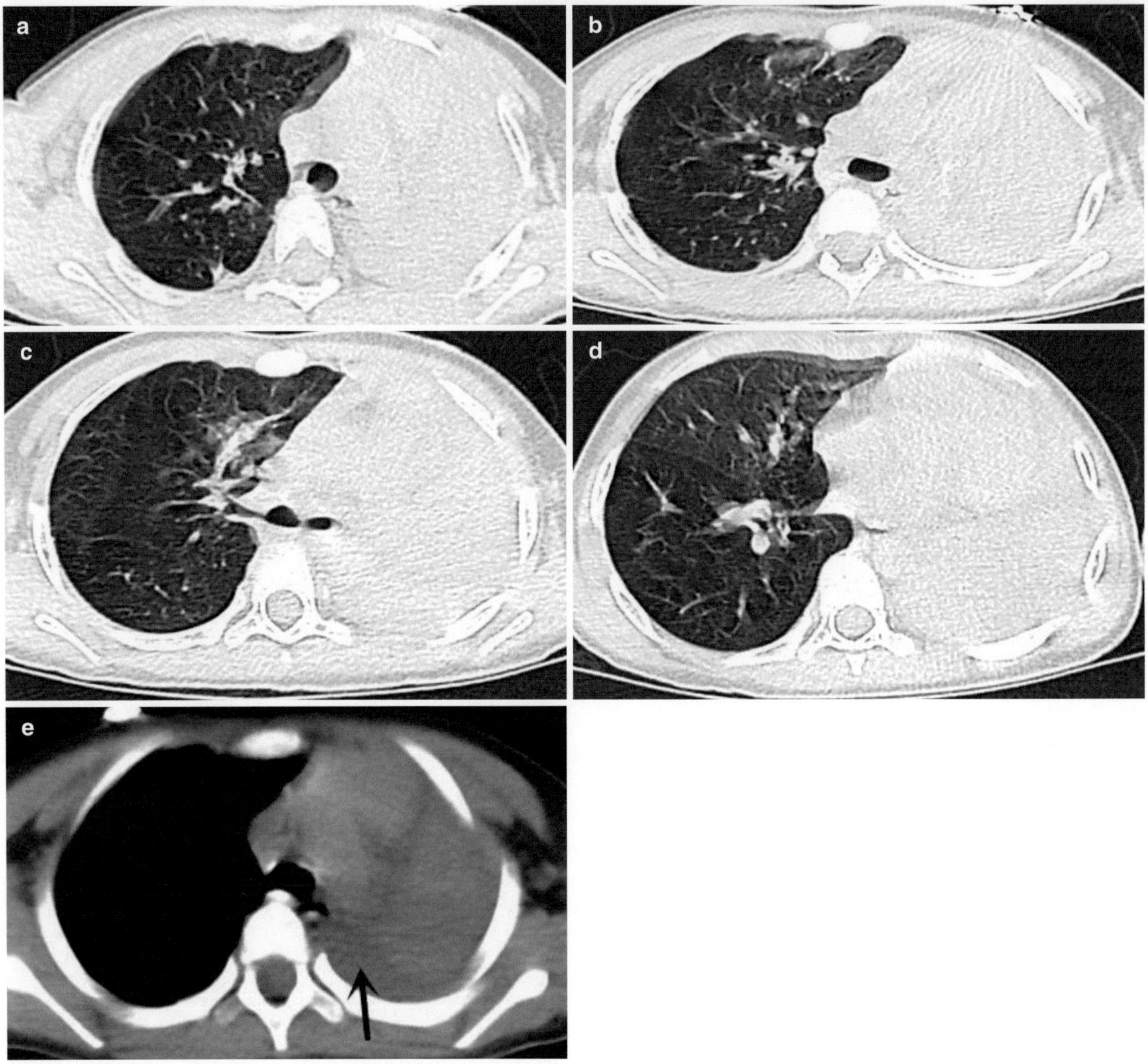

Fig. 13.2 (**a**–**e**) On June 12th, 2016, day 3 post to the onset, the right lung shown by the lung window in (**a**–**d**) demonstrated patchy ground glass opacities and strips. Left thoracic collapsed slightly with left lung atelectasis. Pleural effusion on the left side was shown by the mediastinal window of CT scans in (**e**), with the crescent low-density (black arrow)

4. Complication of fungal infection

   A patient with severe infection from Chengdu (Sichuan, China) was complicated with pulmonary fungal infection [15–17]. The patient was in a serious condition with multiple organ failure, type II respiratory failure, and hypoproteinemia. The patient was admitted twice to different hospitals for diagnosis and treatment, and secondary fungal infections appeared, including infection with *Cryptococcus*, *Candida albicans*, and *Mucorales* infection. This might be caused by the use of antibiotics, glucocorticoids, and low resistance of the patient. H9N2 combined with fungal infection demonstrated mainly extensive exudative lesions of both lungs, characterized by severe pneumonia with extensive exudative lesions of both lungs and uneven density as shown by chest X-ray and CT scans.

5. Dynamic change of image findings

   The dynamic change of pneumonia caused by subtype H9N2 avian influenza virus was not so rapid. The prognosis would be better in case of a diagnosis and active treatment performed timely. The dynamic

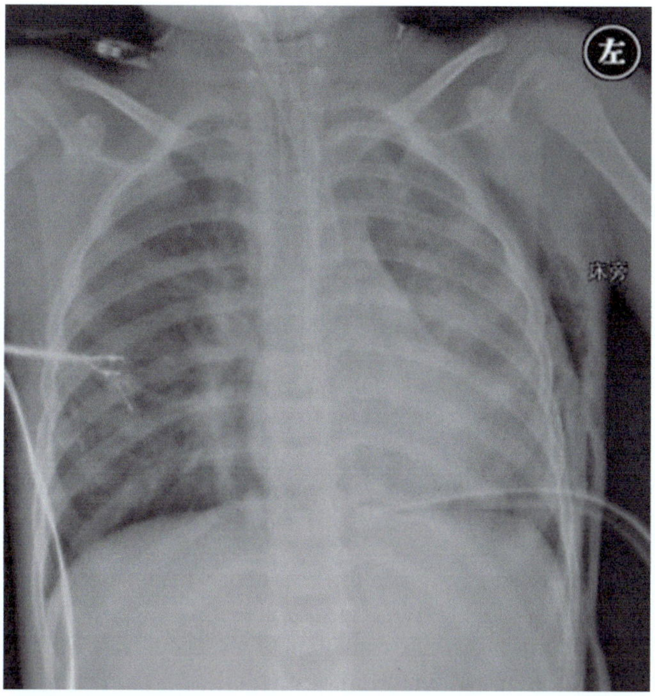

Fig. 13.3 On June 13th, 2016, day 4 post to the onset, the previous left atelectasis had been obviously re-expanded as shown by reexamination of chest X-ray, the left lung showed exudative lesions, the right lung lesions had increased. The lesions showed unclear borders, and the bilateral lesions are mainly located in the medial and middle zones

changes are characterized by the lesions growing out of nothing, the shadow with increased density changing from speckles to patches with unclear border, lesions in both lungs distributed mainly in the medial and the middle zones and persisting for 7–9 days followed by their gradual absorption, and a trapezoidal tendency including an early stage, a progressive stage, and an absorption stage with a certain degree of migration. The lesion could not be fully absorbed in the recovery stage, and the fibrotic shadow with clear boundary was observed in the lesion area (Fig. 13.3).

13.3 Differential Diagnosis

It is relatively rare for human infection with subtype H9N2 AIV. It has no specific image findings in the H9N2-infected patient with lung infection, thus it is difficult to distinguish it from bacterial and other viral pneumonias according to image findings. The confirmation of diagnosis needs clinical laboratory examination. However, it has significant differences compared with the consolidation pneumonia.

1. Differentiation from Influenza A H1N1 Virus Pneumonia

   The most common image findings of influenza A H1N1 virus pneumonia are ground glass opacity and consolidations in the upper lung. It is easy to distinguish from subtype H9N2 AIV pneumonia when H1N1 virus pneumonia demonstrates the ground glass opacity. Ground glass opacity of H1N1 virus pneumonia is characterized by the distribution mainly along the bronchus and in subpleural area as well as the wide spread, in contrast to relatively limited distribution in most of ground glass opacities caused by subtype H9N2 avian influenza virus. However, it is difficult to distinguish these two types of pneumonia when the main findings are pulmonary consolidations. Aerial bronchogram with or without staged atelectasis can be observed in the consolidation commonly seen in bilateral lower pulmonary fields in patients with influenza A H1N1 virus pneumonia, which shows also lesions demonstrating focal, multiple, or diffuse distributions. In comparison, pneumonia caused by H9N2 subtype avian influenza virus in human is characterized by the absence of obvious aerial bronchogram in the consolidation, and possible complication of atelectasis dominated by a distinguishable distribution in the medial-middle pulmonary zones. Despite clinical manifestations categorizable as self-limiting respiratory infections for both, influenza A H1N1 infection manifests mostly severe influenza symptoms, and less commonly mild respiratory symptoms. They can be differentiated roughly based on clinical symptoms combined with image findings, though the confirmation is dependent on the virological examination by the laboratory [33].

2. Differentiation from subtype H7N9 AIV pneumonia in human

   H7N9 and H5N1 dominate pneumonias induced by avian influenza viruses in human. Both are highly pathogenic and H7N9 is the most common one, which has been listed by the Chinese CDC as one of the infectious diseases requiring yearly statistics. H7N9 infection results in severe clinical manifestations and severe lung infection. Its dynamic change includes the early onset, the progression stage, and the recovery stage. The dynamic changes showed by images reveal that the scope of lesions and the degree of consolidation caused by pneumonia triggered by H7N9 or H5N1 are much wider and more severe than those by H9N2. The image findings of pneumonia caused by H7N9 show dominantly solitary lamellar, multiple lamellar, or larger lamellar consolidations at the early stage, followed by a variation of the lesion progressing from one to multiple pulmonary fields within 3–7 days, with the severest state reached on day 8–14. The lesions may coexist in a variety of forms, and lung consolidation may contain aerial bronchogram in most cases. The most common complication in pneumonia caused by H5N1 and H7N9 infections is pulmonary fibrosis, while the lesions can almost be fully absorbed after the recovery stage for H9N2 pneumonia. Although it has a cord-like fibrosis, it is less severe than H5N1 and H7N9 pneumonia [34, 35].

3. Differentiation from bacterial pneumonia

   Bacterial pneumonia manifests the consolidations in lobes, segments or subsegments, and the lesions are relativity limited. This is similar to the manifestations of subtype H9N2 AIV pneumonia. However, the dynamic changes of bacterial pneumonia are limited, and it will not migrate, which is distinguishable from subtype H9N2 AIV pneumonia. Bacterial pneumonia can also be complicated with atelectasis and pleural effusion, and in severe cases, it may induce abscess complicated with cavitation. Most cases of bacterial pleural effusion are purulent, which is different from the bloody pleural effusion caused by H9N2.

13.4 The First Case Report Worldwide

In August 1998, it was first confirmed that avian influenza (H9N2) virus could infect humans, but there is no abnormality in the lungs and no image data available. So far, there have been three reports of human infection with H9N2 subtype avian influenza pneumonia, but no relevant clinical imaging data are available due to the death of two adult patients. The detailed clinical imaging findings of a child with pneumonia caused by infection with subtype H9N2 avian influenza virus are reported as follows.

1. Clinical history and epidemiological history

   The patient was a 6-year-old female who lived near the poultry wholesale market and had occasionally entered the market to play prior to the onset of the disease. She had a contact history with poultry, while the type of poultry was not clear. Her family members had no contact history with poultry. On June 10th, 2016, the child had paroxysmal nonirritating cough without apparent inducement, accompanied by laryngeal noise sputum. There was no hoarseness, barking cough, nasal congestion, runny nose, dizziness, or headache. At the onset, she had no obvious wheezing, shortness of breath, or symptoms of cyanosis. The child had low fever at the early stage without chills. She was given oral medication (with details unknown) for treatment at a local health center, but the effect was not good and she got fever repeatedly. On the night of June 11th, 2016, she had a high fever up to 39.7 °C complicated with chills but no convulsions, while coughing more frequently than before, having shortness of breath accompanied by obvious wheezing. She also vomited once with a large amount, but without coffee-like or bile-like substances. She was admitted to the hospital on the morning of June 12th, 2016.

2. Clinical symptoms and signs

   The physical examination: body temperature 38.4 °C; pulse 180 beats/min; breathing rate 48/min; blood pressure 110/68 mmHg; body weight 16 kg. Consciousness; normal spirit and reaction; tachypnea; nares flaring; no facial cyanosis; moderate three-concave sign; pharyngeal congestion, and degree-II swelling of bilateral tonsils with hyperemia but no purulent spots; the trachea displaced to the right, the fullness of the left thorax, without deformation of the right thorax; clear sound on percussion for the right lung, and dullness for the left; weakened breathing movement on the left with weakened speech tremor; thickened breath sounds for the right lung with a moderate amount of fine moist rales and wheezing sounds; and significantly weakened breath sounds for the left lung.

3. Laboratory examination

   The white blood cell and neutrophil count increased, with elevated erythrocyte sedimentation rate. Pleural effusion: turbidity, coagulum, with the red blood cell count of 106,000 (10^6/L), white blood cell count of 276 (10^6/L), and positiveness in Rivalta. On June 15th, 2006, the throat swab test was positive for H9N2 performed by Meizhou CDC, which was confirmed based on reexamination by Guangdong Provincial CDC on June 18th.

4. Imaging examination and dynamic demonstration

   The patient received a chest X-ray on day 3 post to the onset. Results showed that the left chest slightly collapsed with atelectasis of the left lung, and patches were observed in the right lung (Fig. 13.1). Chest CT scans performed on the same day found atelectasis on the left lung, the left pleural cavity had a small amount of effusion, and the right lung showed patchy ground glass opacities and strip consolidations (Fig. 13.2a–e). The chest X-ray was reexamined after 24 h, showing the recruitment of the left lung and patches in both lungs (Figs. 13.3, 13.4 and 13.5). Later, chest CT reexamination was performed on day 22 and 55 post to the onset, showing lesions in both lungs were obviously absorbed and there were fibrotic strips, which suggested changes of pulmonary fibrosis (Figs. 13.6a–e and 13.7a–c).

5. Treatment and prognosis

   The patient received treatments after the admission on June 12th, 2016, including airway patency maintenance, anti-infection, expectorating and cough relieving, spasm-relief spraying, and support of internal environment stability. Rescue was performed twice for the patient due to low blood oxygen saturation (75% and 80%, respectively) on June 12th and 13th, respectively. Thoracentesis was performed with closed drainage, and tracheal intubation ventilator was used to assist breathing during rescue. Poultry contact history was reported during ward round

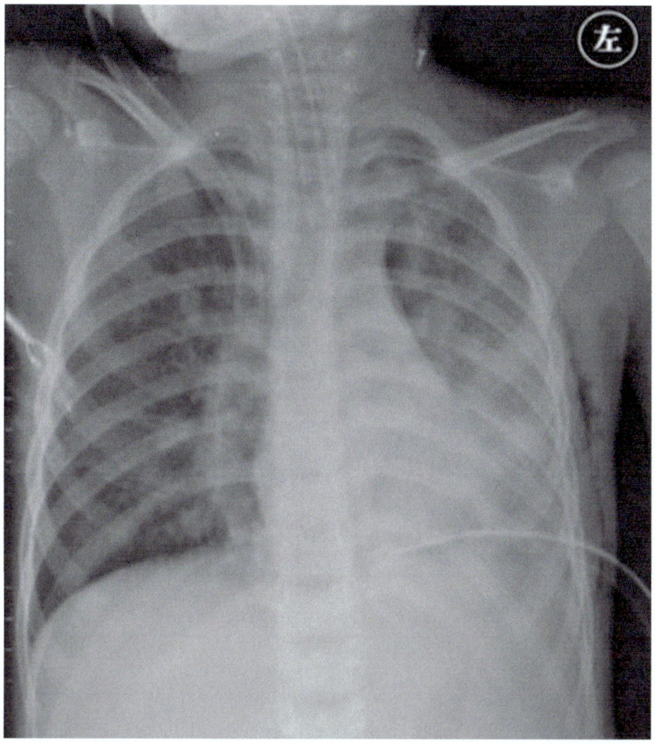

Fig. 13.4 On June 14th, 2016, day 5 post to the onset, reexamination of chest X-ray showed that the upper field lesions of the two lungs became smaller than before, and the border became clear. The border of some lesions in the middle and lower fields became clearer than before, and the lesion in the lower left lung was blurred

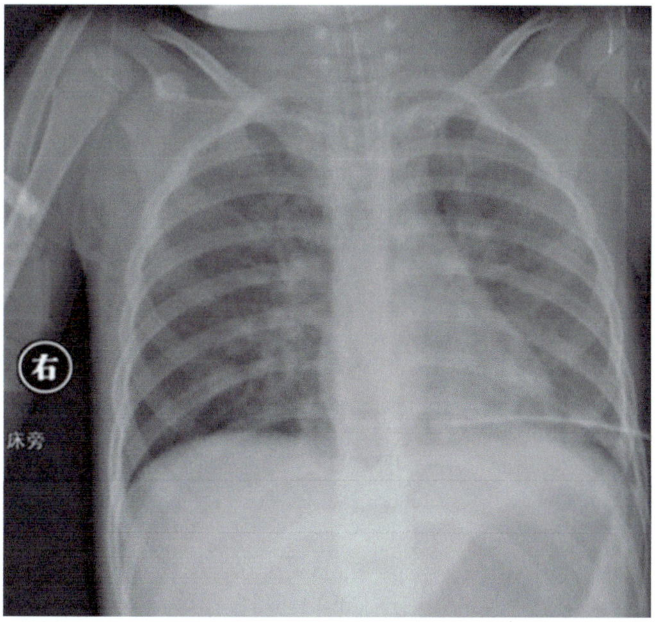

Fig. 13.5 On June 18th, 2016, day 9 post to the onset, the reexamination of chest X-ray showed obvious absorption of lesions of lateral zones of both lungs, decreased number of lesions in the middle zone than before, and clearer border of medial lesions, as compared with previous image findings

on the morning of June 13th. Subsequently, oseltamivir antiviral therapy was added to the treatment. The fever of the child had been gradually controlled as of June 15th. The ventilator parameters were gradually reduced, and the blood oxygen saturation increased beyond 96%. The child was isolated since the H9N2 result was positive as shown by the throat swab influenza virus test. The symptoms of the child improved as a result of antiviral treatment and auxiliary ventilator therapy. The isolation was ended till double influenza virus tests were negative on June 23rd and 24th, respectively. This patient was transferred to the pediatrics of general ward on June 25th and discharged on July 3rd after recovery.

6. Discussion

The causality for AVI infection, in this case, might be the poor immunity of the young child with a history of poultry exposure. The initial symptoms included paroxysmal nonirritating cough with phlegm in the throat and low fever at the onset, which was unresponsive to medication for common cold. Symptoms worsened on the next day, manifesting high fever with chills, frequent cough, and obvious wheezing. The patient's body temperature fluctuated between 38.5 and 40.5 °C on day 1 post to admission. Chest CT showed that left atelectasis is combined with left pleural effusion. The left main bronchus, as well as lobar and segmental bronchus, seemed unclear, and a small amount of exudative lesions was observed in the lower right lobe. Previous study reported that edema, congestion, and hemorrhage could be found in lungs of H9N2-infected mice [36]. Hemorrhagic fluid was also drained from the thoracentesis of this patient. The child had phlegm in his throat on day 2 post hospitalization. After a moderate amount of yellow viscous sputum was sucked out by respiratory tract clearing, chest X-ray reexamination showed left lung atelectasis had been significantly improved, and no foreign matters could be found based on CTVR. These suggested that the left atelectasis may be due to sputum obstruction. Therefore, sputum excretion care should be given time to patients with H9N2 virus infection. An antiviral drug, oseltamivir, was added on day 2 post to the admission, and the body temperature of patient fluctuated between 37.0 and 39.5 °C on day 3 post to the admission. On day 4, the patient's fever was gradually controlled, the exudative lesion was absorbed, and the patient's symptoms improved significantly, indicating that the antiviral drug oseltamivir had a certain efficacy on H9N2 infection. Negative conversion was noted for serum virus test on H9N2 for the child on June 23rd and 24th, 2016. The child's illness lasted 14 days from the onset of the disease to the negative conversion in serum virology, and the fever fluctuation lasted 15 days (Fig. 13.8). The laboratory tests showed that white blood

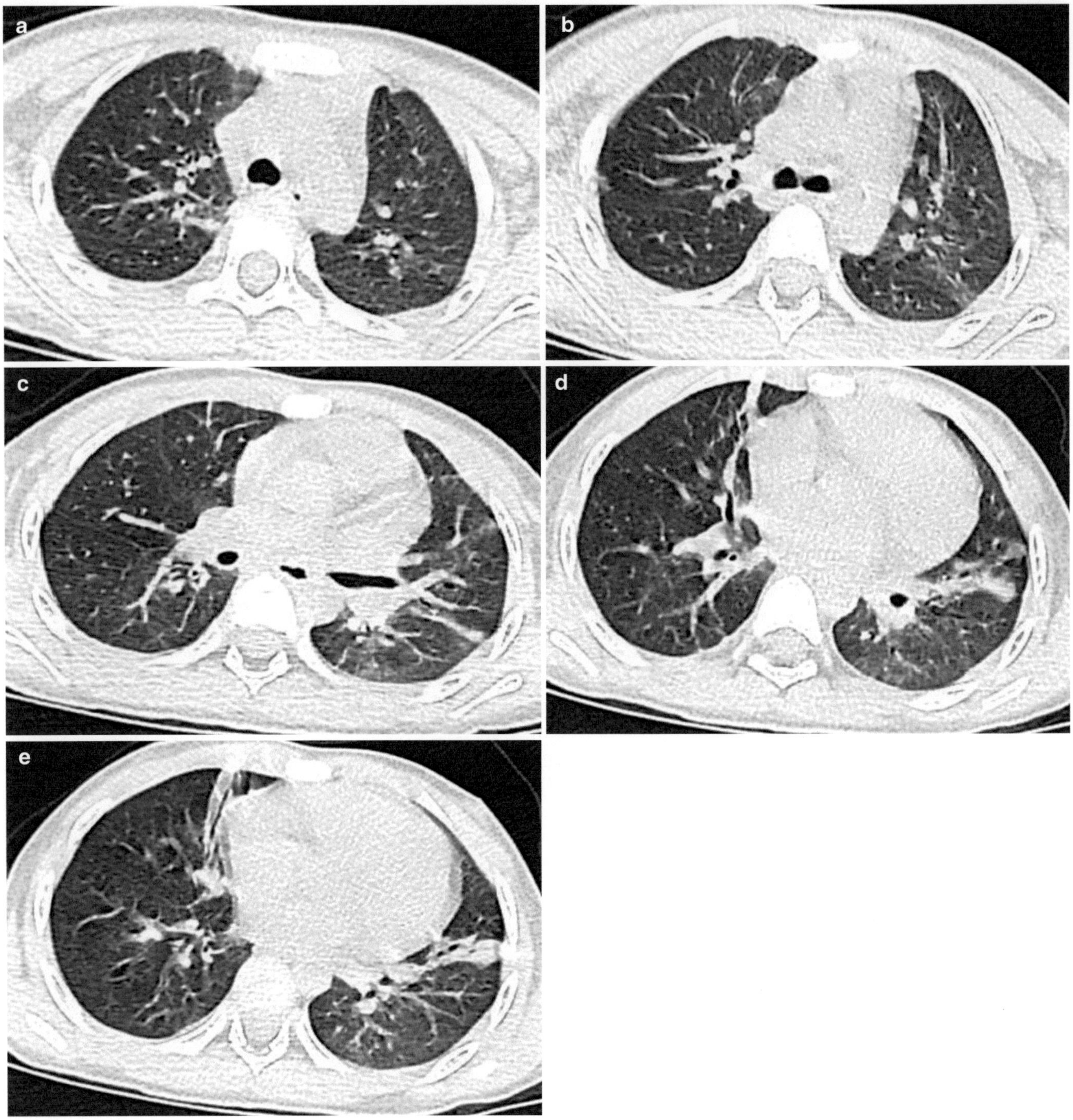

Fig. 13.6 (**a–e**) On July 2nd, 2016, day 22 post to the onset, CT scans showed strips with increased density and patchy ground glass opacities in both lungs, with bronchiectasis in the right lung

cell count increased (dominantly the increase of neutrophil granulocytes), lymphocytes decreased, and erythrocyte sedimentation rate increased post to admission, without any other abnormality in laboratory test on blood. These suggest that there was a significant correlation between negative conversion in virology and improvement of clinical symptoms, which was similar to outcomes of clinical symptoms and laboratory tests for infections by the other subtypes of avian influenza viruses.

Chest image findings demonstrated a dynamic process. The lesions appeared out of nothing, with an extension from small to large for diseases dominantly distributed in the medical and middle zones from June 12th to 13th. Pulmonary lesions were partially absorbed

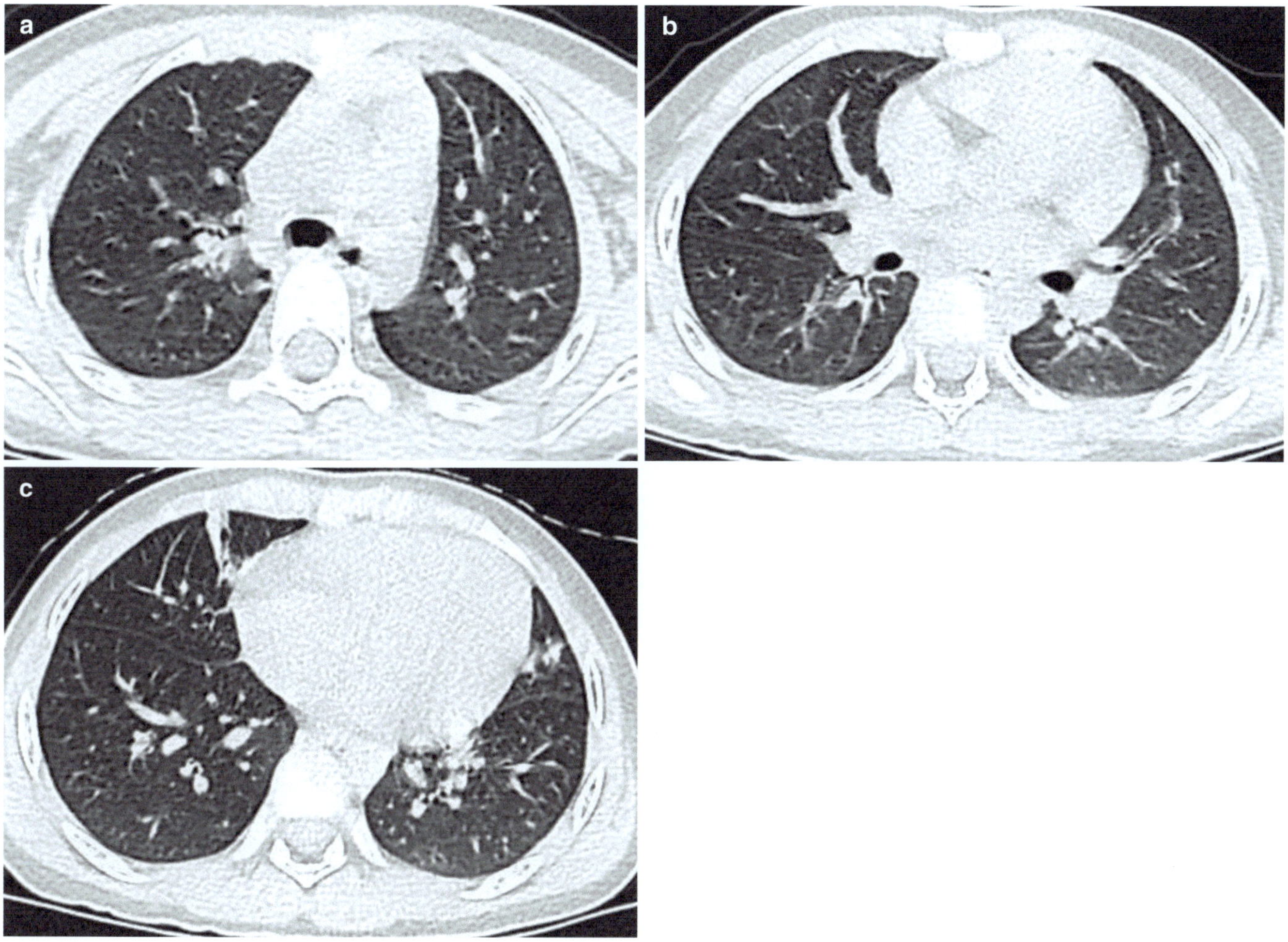

Fig. 13.7 (**a–c**) On August 5th, 2016, day 55 post to the onset, the fibrotic strips were shown in the medial segment of the middle right lobe and the anterior medial basal segment of the lower left lobe were shown by CT reexamination, and the remaining lung lesions were generally absorbed

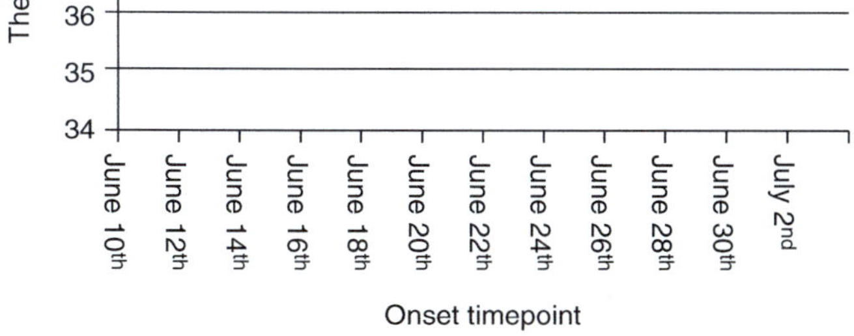

Fig. 13.8 Fluctuation of body temperature [22]

while a few new lesions appeared on June 14th. The reexamination of the chest X-ray showed that the lesion area shrank gradually and was absorbed day by day. Chest CT showed a small amount of strips and exudation in the medial segment of the middle right lobe and the anterior medial basal segment of the lower left lobe and the inferior lingular segment of the upper left lobe on July 2nd. CT reexamination in 1 month post to the discharge showed only a small amount of fiber strips in the medial segment of the middle right lobe without any other abnormality in the lungs. This was partially similar to the changes of pulmonary fibrosis in the late absorption stage in human infection with H7N9 avian influenza, characterized by fibrous cords, grids, subpleural and/or bilateral pulmonary small patchy shadows, and small ground glass opacities observed in both lungs [35, 37, 38]. The progress in lung images of human H9N2 avian influenza infection, in this case, was basically the same as the dynamic changes of chest images of other subtypes of avian influenza virus pneumonia, i.e., the initial stage of onset during day 1–3, the peak period during day 4–13, and the absorption during day 14 and later. However, it was not as severe and rapid as human infection with H7N9 and H5N1 avian influenza [35–39].

H9N2 subtype AIV post to infection in human shows the virulence inferior to that of subtypes H7N9 or H5N1, thus its clinical manifestations are mostly flu-like symptoms with rare changes of pulmonary inflammation. The imaging findings are dominated by exudative patchy ground glass opacities, and pulmonary interstitial fibrosis can be detected even during the recovery period. Therefore, clinicians should consider the possibility of human avian influenza virus infection for children with a history of poultry contact and complicated with fever and lung infections. The prognosis is generally good if antiviral treatment and reasonable care are provided as soon as the etiology is clarified.

References

1. Homme PJ, Easterday BC. Avian influenza virus infections. I. Characteristics of influenza A-Turkey-Wisconsin-1966 virus. Avian Dis. 1970;14(1):66–74.
2. Khan SU, Anderson BD, Heil GL, et al. A systematic review and meta-analysis of the seroprevalence of influenza A (H9N2) infection among humans. J Infect Dis. 2015;212(4):562–9.
3. Su W, Wang C, Luo J, et al. Testing the effect of internal genes derived from a wild-bird-origin H9N2 influenza A virus on the pathogenicity of an A/H7N9 virus. Cell Rep. 2015;13(6):1283.
4. Guo Y, Li J, Cheng X. Discovery of men infected by avian influenza A (H9N2) virus. Zhonghua Shi Yan He Lin Chuang Bing Du Xue Za Zhi. 1999;13(2):105–8.
5. Peng G, Ni H, Liu S, et al. Etiological surveillance for influenza in populations in Guangdong Province in 1999–2000. Chin J Epidemiol. 2002;23(2):154.
6. Zou Y, Li Y, Ye J, et al. Monitoring report for human infection with avian influenza H9N2 found in Shaoguan City. Chin J Epidemiol. 2000;4:303.
7. Peiris M, Yuen KY, Leung CW, et al. Human infection with influenza H9N2. Lancet. 1999;354(9182):916–7.
8. Butt KM, Smith GJD, Chen H, et al. Human infection with an avian H9N2 influenza A virus in Hong Kong in 2003. J Clin Microbiol. 2005;43(11):5760–7.
9. https://www.chp.gov.hk/sc/index.html
10. Huang Y, Li X, Zhang H, et al. Human infection with an avian influenza A (H9N2) virus in the middle region of China. J Med Virol. 2015;87(10):1641–8.
11. He J, Liu L, Hou S, et al. Genetic characteristics of 2 strains of virus H9N2 infecting human in Anhui Province. Chin J Epidemiol. 2016;37(5):708–13.
12. Zhang Y, He J. Laboratory diagnosis and viral sequence analysis for the first case of human infection with avian influenza H9N2 in Chuzhou City. Chin Healthcare Nutr. 2016;18:63–4.
13. Huang Y, Chen B, Zhang H, et al. Characteristic analysis on one case of avian influenza subtype H9N2 infecting an infant. Chin J Exp Clin Virol. 2017;31(5):419–23.
14. Huang Z, Ou X, Yuan J, et al. Characteristic analysis on HA genetic sequence in the first case of human infection with avian influenza virus H9N2 in Changsha City. Chin J Zoonoses. 2016;32(11):997–1000.
15. Yang L, Du X, Zhang X. Investigation and analysis on the first case of human infection of avian influenza H9N2 in Chengdu City. Chin J Zoonoses. 2017;33(3):245–9.
16. Wang Y, Lu L, Feng C, et al. Transference path in clinical treatment for the first case of human infection of severe avian influenza H9N2 in Sichuan Province in 2016. World Latest Med Inf. 2016;16(88):152–3.
17. Wang Y, Li J, Wang L, et al. Analysis on treatment and rescue of the first case of human infection with severe avian influenza H9N2 in Sichuan Province in 2016. Chin J Respir Crit Care Med. 2016;15(4):415–7.
18. Hou W, Zhang Q, Luo C, et al. A descriptive study on clinical imaging in the first case of viral pneumonia induced by avian influenza virus subtype H9N2 infecting human in the world. Electron J Emerg Infect Dis. 2016;1(1):18–22.
19. Yue G, Wu X, Yi A, et al. Investigation and analysis on the first case of a child infected with avian influenza subtype H9N2 in Jiangxi Province. Mod Prev Med. 2017;44(5):785–789, 792.
20. You S, Feng X, Liu X, et al. An epidemiological investigation on the first case of human infection of avian influenza H9N2 in Jiangxi Province. Mod Prev Med. 2017;44(5):782–4.
21. Huang Y, Jing Z, Tong J, et al. An investigational and disposal report on 1 case of human infection with avian influenza H9N2 in 2016 in Mengzi City of Yunnan Province. J Med Pest Control. 2017;33(10):1085–7.
22. Luo C, Zhao X, Ning D, et al. Discovery and response to the first case of human infection of avian influenza H9N2 in Yunnan Province. Chin J Zoonoses. 2017;33(3):214–44.
23. Zhu R, Sun Y, Wang F, et al. A case of human infection of avian influenza virus H9N2 found in children in Beijing. Chin J Pediatr. 2017;55(1):69.
24. Ma J, Wen W, Huang L, et al. An epidemiological survey on the first case of human infection of avian influenza H9N2 in Beijing. Int J Virol. 2017;24(2):81–4.
25. Pan Y, Cui S, Sun Y, et al. Human infection with H9N2 avian influenza in northern China. Clin Microbiol Infect. 2018;24(3):321–3.
26. Li L, Yang P, Pan Y, et al. Epidemiological investigation and analysis on one case of human infection with avian influenza H9N2 in Beijing City. Int J Virol. 2017;24(5):342–6.
27. Liu Y, Lu E, Wang Y, et al. Analysis of characteristics of avian influenza infection in poultry workers in Guangzhou. Chin J Epidemiol. 2009;30(11):1111–3.
28. Wu ZQ, Zhang Y, Zhao N, et al. Comparative epidemiology of human fatal infections with novel, high (H5N6 and H5N1) and low (H7N9 and H9N2) pathogenicity avian influenza A viruses. Int J Environ Res Public Health. 2017;14(3):E263.
29. Sun Y, Liu J. H9N2 influenza virus in China: a cause of concern. Protein Cell. 2015;6(1):18–25.
30. Huang R, Wang AR, Liu ZH, et al. Seroprevalence of avian influenza H9N2 among poultry workers in Shandong Province, China. Eur J Clin Microbiol Infect Dis. 2013;32(10):1347–51.
31. Zhong L, Wang X, Li Q, et al. Molecular mechanism of the airborne transmissibility of H9N2 avian influenza A viruses in chickens. J Virol. 2014;88(17):9568–78.
32. Zhang Z, Fan X, Chen X, et al. Replication of avian influenza virus H9N2 in human pulmonary tissue. J Virol. 2013;29(2):206–9.
33. Li H, Lu P, Shi Y, editors. Imaging of influenza, vol. 1. Beijing: Science Press; 2016. p. 93.
34. Lu P, Zhou B, editors. Clinical imaging diagnosis of emerging infectious diseases, vol. 7. Beijing: Peoples' Medical Publishing House; 2013. p. 87.

35. Lu P, Zeng Z, Zheng P, et al. Imaging manifestation and dynamic variation characteristics of severe pneumonia induced by avian influenza virus H7N9 infecting human. Radiol Pract. 2014;29(7):740–4.
36. Zhang C. An investigation on subtype H9N2 of avian influenza virus infecting minks. Beijing: China Agriculture University; 2016.
37. Li J, Zeng Z, Lu P, et al. Imaging follow up and investigation on pneumonia induced by avian influenza virus H7N9 infecting human. Radiol Pract. 2016;31(3):228–31.
38. Zeng Z, Lu P, Zhou B, et al. Imaging of severe pneumonia induced by avian influenza. J Tuberc Lung Health. 2014;3(1):25–8.
39. Lu P, Zhu W, Ye R, et al. CT manifestations and dynamic changes in severe viral pneumonia induced by avian influenza subtype H5N1 infecting adults. Chin J CT MRI. 2007;5(1):31–4.

14 H7N4 Avian Influenza in Human

Yi-bo Lu, Wei Huang, Sheng-xiu Lv, Qiu-ting Zheng, Pu-xuan Lu, and Jin-ping Wu

14.1 Overview

Avian influenza virus belongs to influenza A virus in the family Orthomyxoviridae. According to the different hemagglutinin proteins, the virus can be divided into different subtypes, of which the outbreak of subtype H7 in birds has attracted much attention because of its high pathogenicity. H7N4 [A (H7N4) virus] belongs to one of the newly discovered subtypes. The H7N4 influenza virus can infect not only poultry but also humans. H7N4 avian influenza in human is an acute respiratory infectious disease caused by a novel variant H7N4 avian influenza virus. The main clinical manifestations include influenza-like symptoms such as fever, cough, and runny nose. It progresses rapidly and may develop into viral pneumonia complicated possibly with respiratory failure. Any delay in detection or treatment may lead to death [1–4].

Avian influenza is often seasonal, common in winter and spring, and tends to be endemic locally or on a large scale. H7N4 avian influenza virus was first detected in two commercial chicken farms near Tamworth town, Australia, in November 1997 [5]. As of July 2018, only 1 clinical case of human infection with influenza A (H7N4) virus was reported in the Third People's Hospital of Changzhou, Jiangsu Province, China, and was clinically cured. To date, there is no evidence of efficient human-to-human transmission of avian influenza A (H7N4) virus.

Y.-b. Lu
Department of Radiology, Third People's Hospital of Changzhou City, Changzhou, Jiangsu, China

W. Huang
Bacteriology & Antibacterial Resistance Surveillance Laboratory, Shenzhen Institute of Respiratory Diseases, Shenzhen People's Hospital, The Second Clinical Medical College of Jinan University, The First Affiliated Hospital of Southern University of Science and Technology, Shenzhen, Guangdong, China

S.-x. Lv
Department of Radiology, The Fourth People's hospital of Nanning, Nanning, Guangxi, China

Q.-t. Zheng
Department of Medical Imaging, Chongqing Public Health Medical Center, Chongqing, China

P.-x. Lu
Department of Medical Imaging, Shenzhen Center for Chronic Disease Control, Shenzhen, Guangdong, China

J.-p. Wu (✉)
Department of Radiology, Third People's Hospital of Changzhou, Changzhou, Jiangsu, China

14.2 Diagnosis and Differential Diagnosis

I. Image findings

X-ray image findings show scattered, ill-demarcated patchy and small patchy shadows in both lungs. With the development of the disease, the lesions can further fuse with each other, showing a lobar distribution and a small amount of pleural effusion.

Image findings in CT scans show multiple patchy ground glass opacities (GGOs), mixed GGOs, consolidations, and lobar pulmonary consolidations in both lungs. It can be distributed in pulmonary lobules, subsegments, segments, and lobes. The lesions are mainly in the lower lobes of both lungs. The lesions in the middle and upper lung fields of both lungs appear later than those in the lower lung fields. The early image findings of the lesions in the lungs show small lamellar GGOs. With the progression of the disease, they then develop into GGOs mixed with patchy consolidations. Pulmonary lesions have a wide distribution range, rapid progression, and slow absorption. Air bronchogram is observed in the segmental consolidation, without bronchiectasis or stenosis. Pleural effusion will progress with intrapulmonary lesions and demonstrate an increase in the amount of effusion. Improvement and absorption of both pulmonary lesions are evidenced in a decrease in the amount of pleural effusion, thereby indicating a close correlation between pleural effusion and the condition of diseases in both lungs. No significant lymphadenectasis is observed for mediastinal, hilar, or axillary lymph nodes [6].

C. Qiu et al. (eds.), *Avian Influenza in Human*, https://doi.org/10.1007/978-981-16-1429-3_14

II. Essentials for diagnosis

A history of exposure to live poultry in the high incidence season of influenza. The image findings show multiple lamellar lesions in both lungs, which progress rapidly and are refractory to antibiotic treatment. The diagnosis of viral pneumonia can be established by excluding pneumonia caused by other pathogens. The definite diagnosis needs to be confirmed by laboratory nucleic acid testing (NAT) for avian influenza virus.

III. Differential diagnosis

1. Differentiation from viral pneumonia of human infection with H9N2/H7N9 avian influenza

In the early stage of viral pneumonia of human infection with H9N2/H7N9 avian influenza, inflammation mainly involves a single lobe or segment, followed by rapid development of inflammation in multiple lobes and segments, demonstrating GGOs and consolidations. Severe disease progression and delayed treatment will easily lead to residual pulmonary fibrosis in the lung during the period when outcome is observed. If the diagnosis and treatment of human infection with H7N4 avian influenza pneumonia are timely, the prognosis will be good, and only a small amount of fibrous stripes would remain on imaging without pulmonary interstitial fibrosis. However, pneumonia of human infection with avian influenza H7N4 virus has basically the same pulmonary imaging characteristics as pneumonia of H9N2/H7N9 avian influenza virus, and clear differentiation depends on virus isolation and NAT [7–11].

2. Differentiation from SARS

Chest X-ray findings of SARS: Small or large lamellar GGOs are observed at the early stage of lesion, which is focal and can be unilateral or bilateral. The lesions are mostly single, and sometimes multiple. In the progressive stage, the disease is aggravated, and the small lamellar shadow in the early stage becomes large lamellar, multiple, or diffuse. The lesions progress from the unilateral to the bilateral, from one to multiple lung fields. The lesions are in the shape of lobes or segments, or are quasi-circular in varying sizes. Lesions are often multiple and variable, and lesions of various forms may coexist. Generally, the recovery period is in week 2–3 post to the onset of disease, during which the lesion shrinks and the density gradually decreases or the lesion disappears. Pulmonary interstitial hyperplasia may occur concurrently during absorption of intrapulmonary lesions, and some may develop into pulmonary interstitial fibrosis. The pulmonary lesions of adult SARS change rapidly, and the old and new lesions can alternate or reoccur.

CT findings of SARS: GGOs and interstitial thickening are the main image findings of SARS, and CT examination can reveal signs that cannot be found by X-ray, including small patchy light-density GGOs, thickened interlobular septa and intralobular interstitial thickening in fainter GGOs, subpleural fine lines and reticular structures, and crazy paving appearance. Only large vascular branches and obviously thickened interlobular septa can be seen in the medial side of higher density GGOs. In a few cases, lesion consolidation is observed, with signs of air bronchogram and bronchiolectasis. Human infection with H7N4 avian influenza pneumonia is similar to it, but interstitial changes are not as obvious as those of SARS, and pulmonary interstitial fibrosis may not occur in patients treated on time.

3. Differentiation from lobar pneumonia

It is common in young adults, and the main pathogen is *Streptococcus pneumoniae* causing acute pulmonary inflammation with acute clinical onset and specific features including common complications of high fever, cough, and rusty sputum.

Chest X-ray findings: The X-ray signs appear later than clinical symptoms. Because the alveolar exudates are not numerous and the alveoli are still inflated during the early pathological stage of lobar pneumonia (congestion, on day 1–2 post to onset), the whole chest X-ray usually shows no positive findings, or shows only increased lung markings in the lesion area, slightly lower transparency of the lung field or blurred opacities with slightly higher density. When the lesion progresses to the consolidation stage (including the red hepatization and gray hepatization; on day 2–6 post to onset), the alveoli are filled with exudates, and the whole chest X-ray shows a homogeneous-density shadow distributed in the lobes, and the lesions are limited by interlobar fissures. The air bronchogram appears as a result of the consolidation of the pulmonary tissue against the air-containing bronchi. In the dissipation stage (1 week after onset), the exudate in the alveoli begins to be dissolved and absorbed, and the alveoli are inflated. The whole chest X-ray shows that the density of the consolidation area in the affected lobe gradually decreases, and the lesions dissipate, which demonstrate mostly scattered patchy shadows in different sizes and heterogeneous density, with fibrous stripes after absorption, which can gradually return to normal.

CT image findings: The main CT signs correspond to the pathological changes, air bronchogram is observed in the lobar or segmental consolidations, the volume of consolidated lobe is equal to that in the normal condition, and the edge of the lesion area seems straight and limited by the interlobar fissure. The lesions in the dissipation stage show scattered patchy shadows differing in size and density, and only stripe shadows or complete dissipation of the lesions can be observed after further absorption of the lesions.

The imaging findings for human infection with H7N4 avian influenza pneumonia are similar to those of lobar pneumonia. However, the latter generally involves unilateral lung, commonly the right lung with rare cases of multiple lobar involvement, while the former often involves multiple lobes, with a wider range and rapid progression.

4. Differentiation from *Mycoplasma pneumoniae*

   Chest X-ray findings: It shows increased lung markings, and diffuse nodular/reticular shadows distributed in segment or both lungs. Rapid changes in pulmonary images are one of its characteristics, and it is common that one lesion dissipates and new infiltrative changes appear elsewhere, with segmental atelectasis occurring when exudates obstruct bronchioles. Pulmonary lesions often dissipate in 2–3 weeks, or are postponed occasionally to 4–6 weeks.

   CT imaging findings: The image findings are diverse, demonstrating mainly interstitial pneumonitis, bronchitis, and even lobar pneumonia. Because mycoplasma pneumonia involves the pulmonary interstitium, CT shows lobular GGOs, which may show large consolidations. A small amount of pleural effusions occur in about 1/5 of cases. Hilar lymphadenectasis can be seen in children. Most patients with mycoplasma pneumonia have mild symptoms, including only low fever and cough, and sometimes a small amount of white viscous sputum. Few positive signs in the lungs with obvious image findings are an important feature. *Mycoplasma pneumoniae* usually involves unilateral lung and rarely multiple lobes on imaging, while H7N4 avian influenza pneumonia often involves multiple lobes. Moreover, laboratory examination of *Mycoplasma pneumoniae* shows positiveness in mycoplasma antibody, and the ratio of cold agglutinin test increases (up to 1:64) in week 2–3 post to onset. Based on these imaging characteristics, therefore, it can be differentiated from human infection with H7N4 avian influenza, considering also serum agglutinin test and serum specific antibody assay.

5. Differentiation from *Klebsiella pneumoniae*

   Klebsiella exists in the intestine and oropharynx of healthy individuals and is a conditioned pathogen. It induces infections mostly in hospitals and can also be transmitted by close contact between patients. Patients with low immunity, or exposure to immunosuppressants, hormones, or broad-spectrum antibiotics are susceptible to infection. *Klebsiella* enters the lungs through the respiratory tract, causing exudation and confluent consolidation in the lobes and segments, and the lesions are mainly distributed in the subpleural area, resulting in interlobar fissure descending due to the viscous and heavy exudate of the lesions. The capsule of *Klebsiella* leads to necrosis and liquefaction of the tissue, thus single or multiple cavitations may appear in the lungs. In comparison, human infection with H7N4 avian influenza pneumonia often involves multiple lobes, with a broader range and rapid progression. Like other avian influenza pneumonia, it generally does not lead to necrosis of pulmonary tissues such as multiple cavitation [12, 13].

14.3 First Human Infection Reported Worldwide

1. Case data

   The patient, a 68-year-old woman, was a poultry farmer from Liyang, Changzhou City, Jiangsu Province with a history of slaughtering live poultry 3 days before the onset. On December 25, 2017, the patient developed chills and fever, complicated by a little cough without hemoptysis. She had fatigue, muscle soreness, and other symptoms, which were not taken seriously. On December 30th, the patient had syncope, fecal and urinary incontinence, and disturbance of consciousness, and later she woke up spontaneously.

   On January 1st, 2018, the patient was admitted to the Third People's Hospital of Changzhou, Jiangsu Province.

   Physical examination upon admission: Body temperature 36.5 °C, pulse 60 bpm, respiratory rate 22/min, oxygen saturation 96% (oxygen inhalation at 5 L/min). The patient had clear consciousness, listlessness, shortness of breath, and no cyanosis. Breathing sounds were coarse in both lungs, and scattered crackles could be heard in both lower lungs. The heart rate was regular without pathological murmur. No abdominal abnormality. Physiological reflexes were present and pathological reflexes were not elicited. Laboratory tests: on admission (January 1st, 2018), peripheral WBC 12.36 × 10^9/L, neutrophil percentage 78.6%, elevation of C-reactive protein (range: 23.3–39.3 mg/L). Bacterial culture and identification showed *Klebsiella pneumoniae* on January 8th, 2018, and normal bacterial growth on January 9th, 2018.

2. Confirmed diagnosis and epidemiological investigation

   On day 3 post to the admission (January 3rd, 2018), the Third People's Hospital of Changzhou City sampled the throat swab and sent it to the CDC of Changzhou City, based on the patient's epidemiological history. After PCR NAT, it was determined that the patient was positive in subtype H7 of avian influenza virus. Since the existing subtypes of avian influenza virus were all negative, the sample was urgently sent to the CDC of Jiangsu Province for review. On January 4, 2018, the sample was tested by the CDC of Jiangsu Province, and suspected to be avian influenza H7N4 subtype by gene sequencing. The sample was finally confirmed to be subtype H7N4 of avian influenza based on gene sequencing in China CDC, and was disclosed on February 13, 2018.

   The CDC of Changzhou City, Jiangsu Province sampled and traced the suspected exposure sites of the case, and found that among the poultries tamed by the patient, 6 chickens and 12 ducks were positive in avian influenza H7N4 virus. However, there were no deaths. Twenty-eight (28) persons who had been in close contact with the patient were medically observed for 1 month, and there were no abnormal findings.

3. Treatment

   The patient was admitted to the hospital on January 1, 2018. The treatment protocol was based on the Guidelines for the Diagnosis and Treatment of Human Infection with Subtype H7N9 Avian Influenza and Influenza A (H1N1): antiviral therapy with Oseltamivir Phosphate Capsules (Kewei) 75 mg (q12h), anti-infective therapy with Moxifloxacin Hydrochloride and Sodium Chloride Injection 0.40 g (qd); and Methylprednisolone 40 mg (q12h). After active and effective treatment, the clinical symptoms and signs disappeared, and three throat swab NATs were negative in H7N4 [3]. On January 22, 2018, the patient was cured and discharged.

4. Dynamic changes in images
   (a) On day 5 post to the onset, CT revealed a lamellar heterogeneous hyperdense shadow in the lower right lung (see Fig. 14.1a–d). CT scans on day 9 post to onset showed large lamellar GGOs and pulmonary consolidations in both lower lobes, and the extent of the lesion expanded, suggesting that the disease entered the progressive stage (see Fig. 14.2a–e). On days 11 and 15 post to onset, CT examination revealed that some lesions in both lungs began to be slightly absorbed (see Fig. 14.3a–e). CT scans on day 21 post to the onset showed that the extent of consolidation in the lesion area of both lower lobes shrank, the density of patchy consolidation in the middle and upper lobes of the right lung became fainter, and no new GGO appeared in the lungs (see Fig. 14.4a–d). On reexamination around the 50th day of onset, most of the lesions of the patient were absorbed, with residual fibrous lesions in both lower lungs (see Fig. 14.5a, b).
   (b) Pulmonary CT findings of the patient were mainly pulmonary parenchymal lesions, lamellar GGOs mixed with consolidations in the lower lobes of both lungs, and air bronchogram was seen in the pulmonary consolidations. Patchy GGOs were observed in the middle and upper lung fields of both lungs. The manifestations varied according to the temporal sequence and severity of pulmonary involvement. The lower lobes of both lungs were involved earlier and the lesions progressed rapidly, showing mixed lamellar GGOs and consolidations. The middle and upper lung fields of both lungs were involved later, demonstrating the first scattered patchy GGOs, followed by patchy pulmonary consolidations, and CT findings reflected the development of pulmonary lesions.
   (c) During the development of the lesions, the interstitial changes in the lungs were not significant, and no significant dilatation or stenosis was seen in the images of bronchi.
   (d) The pleural effusion shown is correlated with the development of pulmonary lesions, demonstrating lesions in the lower right lobe and a small amount of pleural effusion on the right side. The lesions in both lungs progressed rapidly, with a small amount of bilateral pleural effusion. The amount of bilateral pleural effusion was reduced along with the stabilization of pulmonary disease and the start of absorption.
   (e) Mediastinal, hilar lymph nodes, and axillary lymph nodes did not show significant enlargement [6] (Fig. 14.1a–d).

5. Discussion

   This case had a definite history of exposure to live poultry during winter, the avian influenza season, and was admitted with a diagnosis of severe pneumonia. The patient's samples underwent escalated screening by three-level CDCs in Changzhou, Jiangsu and China respectively, and was confirmed to be subtype H7N4 of influenza avian in human. This was the first case in the world.

   The patient had acute onset, followed by fever, cough, fatigue, and muscle soreness, among other viremia manifestations. The disease progressed rapidly into severe pneumonia and respiratory failure within a short period of time. Early laboratory tests showed leukopenia and thrombocytopenia, increased C-reactive protein, increased lactate dehydrogenase, and increased CK and AST, which were not significantly different from severe cases of H7N9 avian influenza in human. In the respect of imaging, this

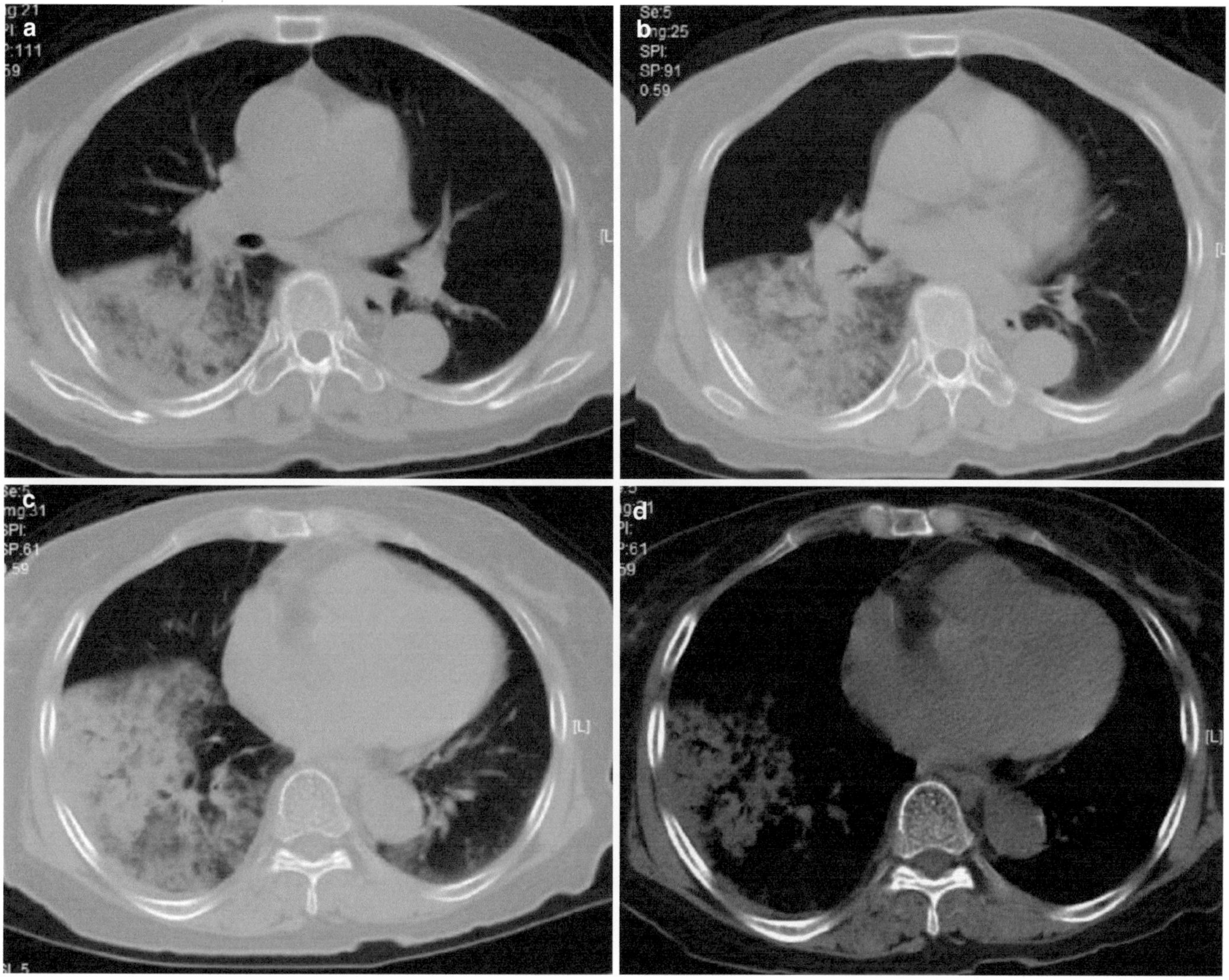

Fig. 14.1 (**a–d**) First CT on December 30, 2017 (day 5 post to onset). (**a–c**) In the lung window of chest CT, large lamellar and patchy heterogeneous high-density shadows were observed in the lower right lobe. (**d**) In the mediastinal window, a shadow of heterogeneously increased density was seen in the lower right lung, with a little pleural effusion in the right side

case showed dominantly the involvement of the lower lobes of both lungs, with postponed appearance of the lesions in the middle and upper fields of both lungs. The early manifestations were patchy GGOs, which progressed subsequently into patchy pulmonary consolidations. The lesions in both lungs progressed rapidly, with wide extent and slow absorption. Air bronchogram was observed in the segmental consolidation, with no significant dilatation or stenosis of the image of bronchi. Pleural effusion is correlated with the development of the disease in such a way that the amount of pleural effusion increased along with the progression of pulmonary lesions, and decreased along with the stabilization of pulmonary lesions. Mediastinal, hilar, and axillary lymph nodes did not show significant enlargement. After effective treatment with Oseltamivir, the thoracic lesions were gradually absorbed without pulmonary interstitial fibrosis, and only a small amount of fibrous streaks remained in both lower lungs as shown by imaging follow-up. This is significantly different from other cases of H9N2/H7N9 avian influenza viral pneumonia [14].

In this case, the diagnosis was confirmed on day 5 post to admission and effective treatment containing Oseltamivir was administrated. Although the disease developed rapidly before the diagnosis, it was quickly controlled and improved after etiological treatment [15].

The whole process of infection at early stage, disease progression, improvement, and recovery after etiological treatment, in this case, were evaluated using image findings, which showed that images played an important role in assessing occurrence, development, and outcome of the disease.

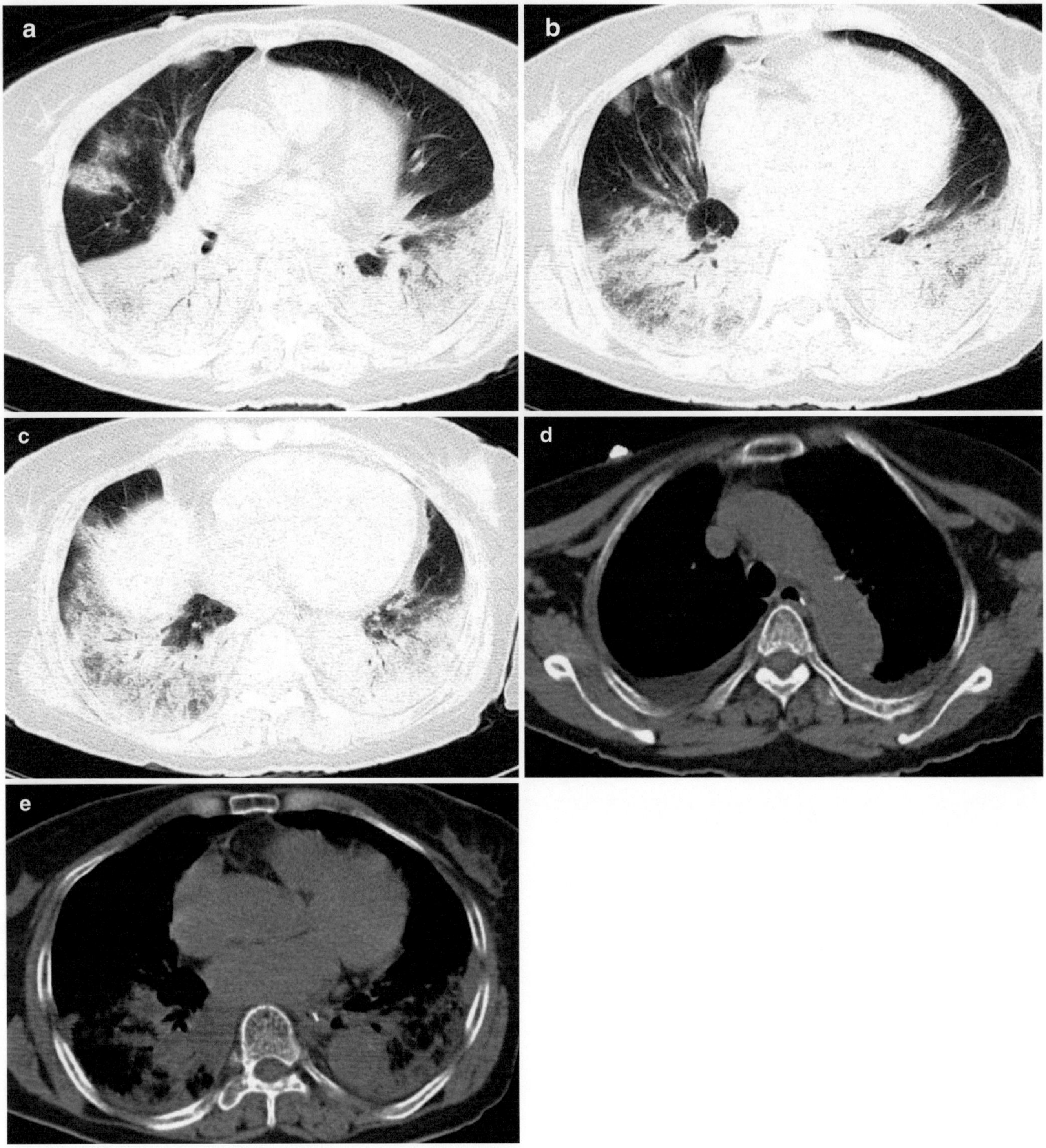

Fig. 14.2 (**a–e**) CT on day 9 post to onset (January 3, 2018). (**a–c**) Lung window of CT scans showed large lamellar GGOs and consolidations in the lower lobes of both lungs, and scattered patchy GGOs in the upper and middle right lobes and the upper left lobe; (**d**, **e**) On mediastinal window, high-density consolidations were observed in both lungs, with increased pleural effusion than before

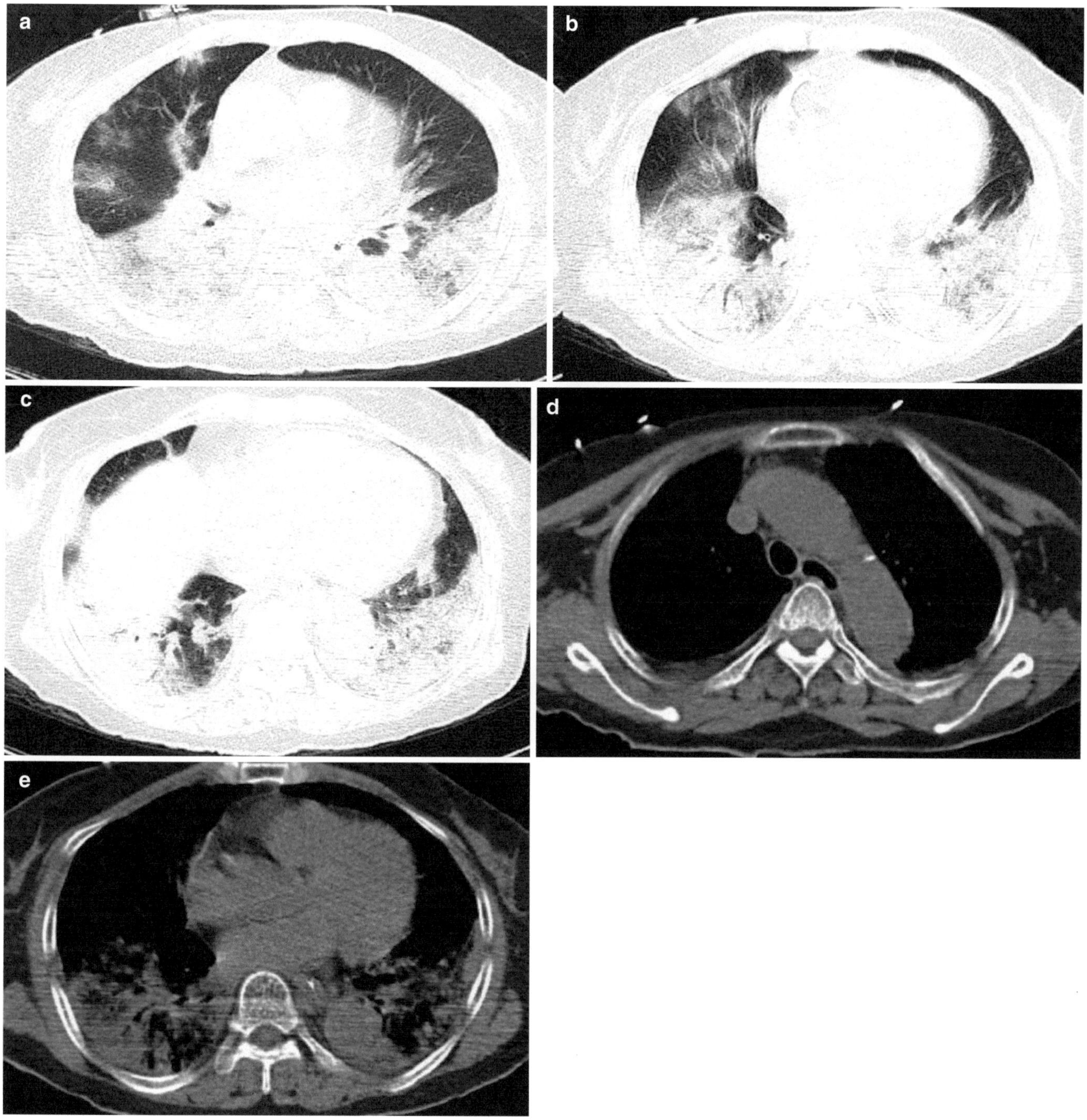

Fig. 14.3 (**a**–**e**) CT on day 11 post to onset (January 5, 2018). (**a**–**d**) In lung window, absorption of lesions in both lungs began, the extent of the lesion shrank, and the density of the lesion became lower. (**e**) In mediastinal window, there was absorption of irregular consolidation in both lower lungs and reduction of bilateral pleural effusion

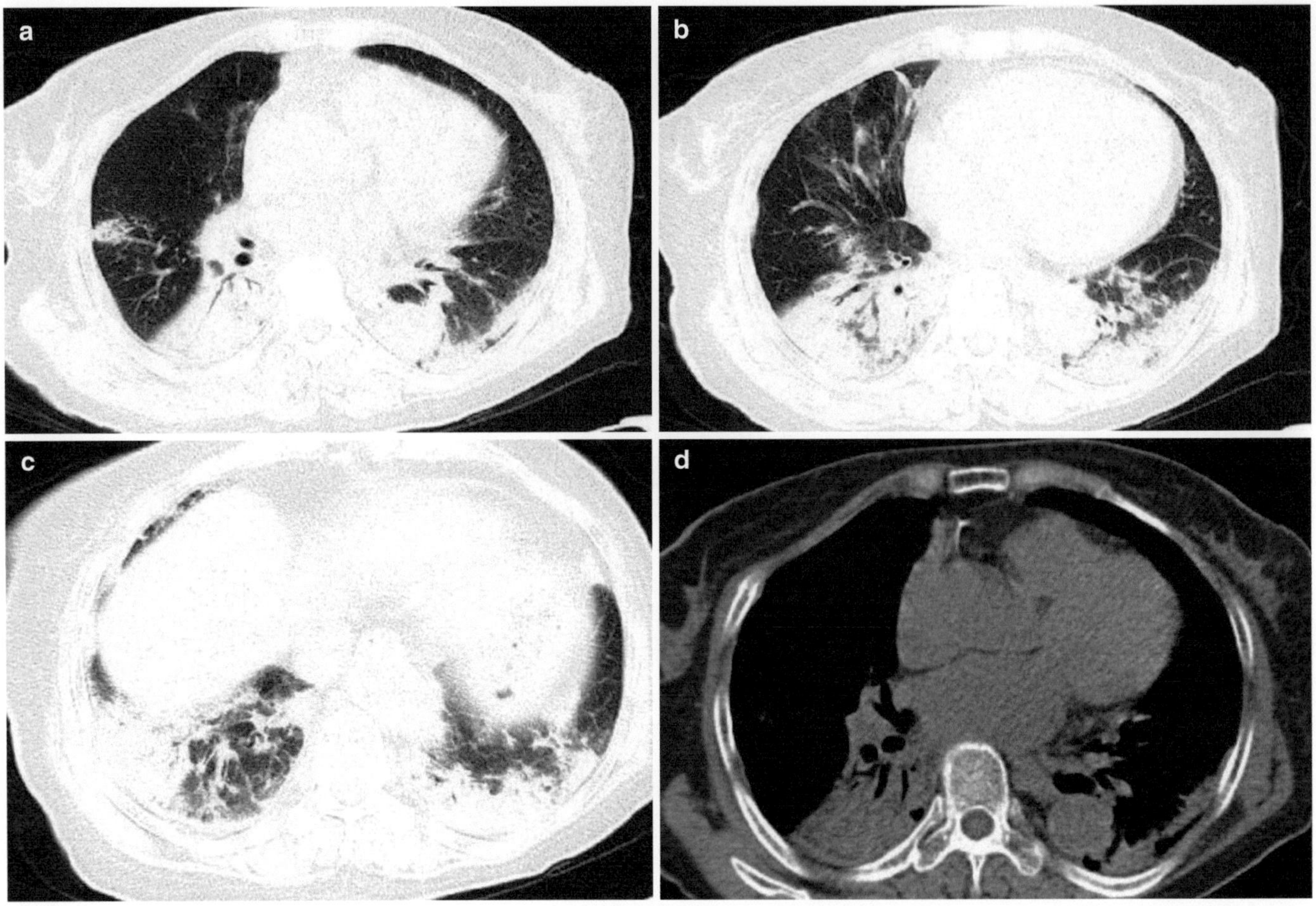

Fig. 14.4 (**a**–**d**) CT on day 21 post to onset (January 15, 2018). (**a**–**c**) In lung window, the area of lesion consolidation in the lower lobes of both lungs was reduced, the areas of patchy consolidations in the middle and upper right lobes were reduced, and most of the GGOs in both lungs were absorbed. (**d**) Pleural effusion in both sides was essentially absorbed and both pleurae were thickened

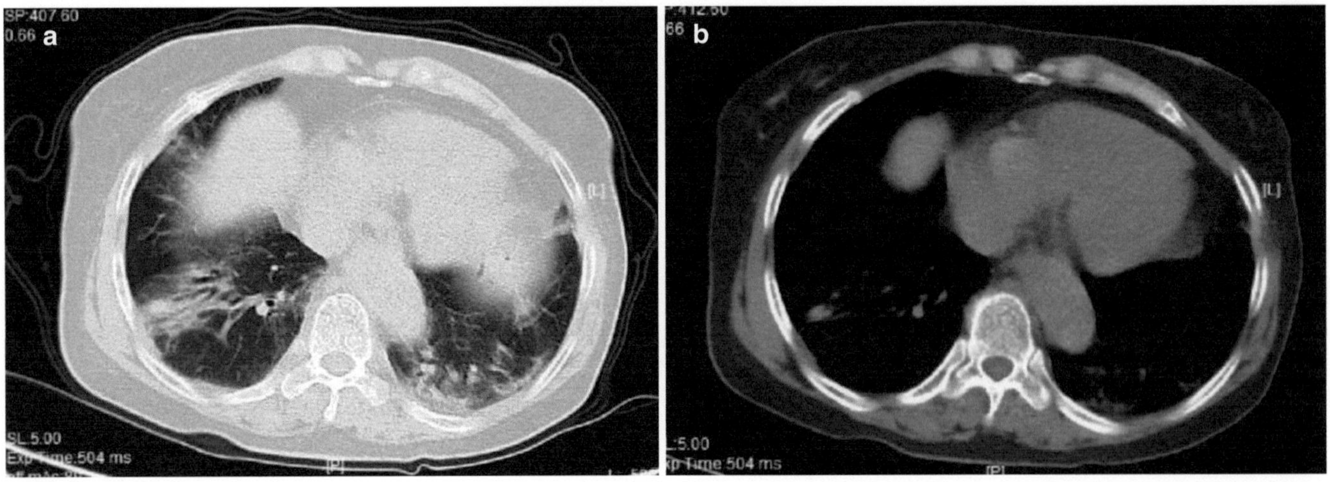

Fig. 14.5 (**a**, **b**) Medical imaging reexamination on February 10, 2018, post to discharge showed that the lesions in both lower lungs were further absorbed, with a small amount of residual fibrous stripes

References

1. Fry AM, Gubareva LV. Understanding influenza virus resistance to antiviral agents; early warning signs for wider community circulation. J Infect Dis. 2012;206(2):145–7.
2. Nagy A, Cernikova L, Křivda V, et al. Digital genotyping of avian influenza viruses of H7 subtype detected in central Europe in 2007–2011. Virus Res. 2012;31(65):126–33.
3. National Health and Family Planning Commission of the People's Republic of China. Diagnosis and treatment program of human infection with H7N9 avian influenza (version I, 2017). Chin J Clin Infect Dis. 2017;1:1–4.
4. Ministry of Health of the People's Republic of China. Diagnosis and treatment program of human infection with H7N9 avian influenza (version 2010). Int J Respir. 2011;2:81–4.
5. Li J, Zhang H, Yang L, et al. An investigation on human infection with avian influenza virus and its pathogenic mechanism. J Microbiol. 2017;37(1):94–7.
6. Jin Q, Zhang L, Yang L, et al. CT findings in the first case of viral pneumonia induced by avian influenza virus H7N4 infecting human in the world. Electron J Emerg Infect Dis. 2018;3(1):51–4.
7. Hu S, Hu C, Zhou X, et al. Characteristics of chest images in human infection with avian influenza H7N9. Chin J Radiol. 2013;47(9):775–7.
8. Gao R, Cao B, Hu Y, et al. Human infection with a novel avian-origin influenza A (H7N9) virus. N Engl J Med. 2013;368(20):1888–97.
9. Wang Q, Shi Y, Zhang Z, et al. Preliminary observation of imaging for pneumonia induced by novel recombinant avian influenza virus (H7N9) [J]. Chin J Radiol. 2013;47(6):505–8.
10. Deng Y, Huang H, Yuan J, et al. Clinical imaging diagnosis and response evaluation for pneumonia induced by avian influenza virus H7N9 infecting human. Electron J Emerg Infect Dis. 2017;2(1):46–9.
11. Hou W, Zhang Q, Luo C, et al. A descriptive investigation on clinical imaging for pneumonia induced by subtype H9N2 of avian influenza virus infecting human. Electron J Emerg Infect Dis. 2016;1(1):18–22.
12. Li C, Hu Y, Shao L, et al. Literature review and clinical analysis of 3 cases of liver abscess invasion syndrome caused by *Klebsiella pneumoniae*. J Microbes Infect. 2016;11(4):247–51.
13. Zhang C, Li X, Tai H, et al. A discussion of image findings of pneumonia induced by *Klebsiella pneumoniae*. Diagn Imaging Intervent Radiol. 2007;16(6):261–3.
14. Lu P, Deng Y. Epidemiological features and chest imaging of avian influenza in human [J]. Chin Comput Med Imaging. 2010;16(5):431–4.
15. Tong X, Wu X, Xu T, et al. An analysis on clinical rescue for the first case of human infection with avian influenza H7N4 in the world. Chin J Infect Dis. 2018;36(3):129–32.

15 Prevention of Avian Influenza in Human

Gui-lin Yang, Ling-wei Wang, Chen Qiu, Yong-yi Lu, and Yu-xin Shi

According to the Law of the People's Republic of China on the Prevention and Control of Infectious Diseases, avian influenza in human (HAI) is a category B infectious disease, but it is managed as category A infectious disease [1]. The prevention and control of avian influenza in human must be based on the basic epidemiological characteristics of avian influenza in human, while integrating the prevention and control of animal avian influenza, applying theory and methods in modern preventive medicine, viewing the three segments including source of infection, transmission routes and susceptible population, considering fully the influence of social and natural factors on avian influenza in human, and implementing comprehensive prevention and control measures [2].

G.-l. Yang (✉)
Department of Infectious Diseases, Shenzhen People's Hospital (The Second Clinical Medical College, Jinan University, The First Affiliated Hospital, Southern University of Science and Technology), Shenzhen, Guangdong, China

L.-w. Wang
Department of Respiratory and Critical Care Medicine, Shenzhen People's Hospital (The Second Clinical Medical College, Jinan University; The First Affiliated Hospital, Southern University of Science and Technology), Shenzhen Institute of Respiratory Diseases, Shenzhen, Guangdong, China

C. Qiu
Department of Respiratory Diseases, Shenzhen People's Hospital, The Second Clinical Medical College of Jinan University, The First Affiliated Hospital of Southern University of Science and Technology, Shenzhen, Guangdong, China

Y.-y. Lu
Department of Health Studies, American University, Washington, DC, USA

Y.-x. Shi
Department of Radiology, Shanghai Public Health Clinical Center, Shanghai, China

15.1 Basic Strategies for Preventive Control

Based on the experience in the control of pandemics of human and animal avian influenza in recent years, and according to the actual situation in China, the National Health Commission of China has determined the basic principles for the prevention and control of avian influenza in human, which are "governmental leadership, departmental cooperation; prevention and control according to law, scientific response; prevention prioritized, combination of prevention and control; mass prevention and control, and hierarchical responsibility" [3].

I. Governmental leadership and departmental cooperation

   Due to China's vast territory and wide range with multiple points, most of the poultry breeding conditions in rural areas are relatively backward. The prevention and control of avian influenza in human involves various aspects, and the task is very arduous. In the prevention and control of avian influenza in human, we must adopt the principle of governmental leadership and multi-departmental cooperation, keep ideological understanding in place, work measures in place, coordination and cooperation in place, political, and policy support in place to ensure the implementation of various prevention and control measures. Meanwhile, we shall strengthen leadership and maintain close cooperation to achieve the goal of keeping all regions and departments under unified leadership, with sound institutions, careful deployment, and effective measures; all regions shall be responsible for and engaged in keeping the land. Only if different departments and regions cooperate to form joint forces, can we win the warfare of preventing and controlling avian influenza in human.

II. Prevention and control according to law and scientific response

   It is necessary to strictly enforce the relevant laws and regulations of the State and conscientiously comply

C. Qiu et al. (eds.), *Avian Influenza in Human*, https://doi.org/10.1007/978-981-16-1429-3_15

with the Law of the People's Republic of China on the Prevention and Control of Infectious Diseases, The Regulations on Emergency Response to Public Health Emergencies, and the Law of the People's Republic of China on Animal Epidemic Prevention, which require that the prevention, reporting, control, and treatment of avian influenza in human, the protection of vulnerable populations and traffic quarantine should be administered in accordance with the law, and that responsibility for illegal acts should be investigated according to law. We must carry out the policy of relying on science and technology to overcome avian influenza in human and implement scientific prevention and control. We should actively develop, scientifically evaluate and popularize the application of test reagents, vaccines and drugs, strengthen clinical treatment regimens and epidemiological research, standardize prevention and control measures and operation procedures, and realize scientific and standardized prevention and control work.

III. Prioritized prevention and integration of prevention and treatment

The prevention and treatment of avian influenza in human is equally important. However, because avian influenza in human is a new infectious disease, it is not well understood, and the disease can cause serious harm to human health and social and economic development. Prevention must be emphasized. The practice of human struggle against infectious diseases also shows that prevention must be the main focus in the control of avian influenza in human.

IV. Group control, and hierarchical responsibility

The battle to prevent and control avian influenza in human needs not only the close cooperation of all regions and departments and coordinated operations, but also the motivation of general populations aiming at group control. We should conscientiously implement various policies and measures, arouse the enthusiasm of all parties and rely heavily on CPC organizations at all levels, the masses of the people, and actively carry out joint prevention and control, take prompt, decisive, and effective measures against the outbreak of the epidemic and give full play to the role of the people.

V. Epidemic surveillance, information sharing, and connectivity

The basis of prevention and control of avian influenza in human is strengthening the construction of surveillance system to ensure its sensitive and efficient operation. The key to successful prevention and control of avian influenza in human is to pay much attention to the release and exchange of relevant information, the timely reporting of information in professional organizations, and to ensure that the public can get enough official information and relevant knowledge in time. Avian influenza in human is a zoonotic disease. Health and epidemic prevention departments and animal epidemic prevention departments should strengthen cooperation. First, the two departments should establish an information exchange mechanism and exchange information on the epidemic situation in a timely manner. Second, a joint meeting mechanism should be established. The two departments should hold a meeting during prevention and control of avian influenza in human, exchanging relevant information, analyzing the situation, and studying the countermeasures. Third, coordination and cooperation mechanisms should be established and various prevention and control measures should be implemented conscientiously. The two departments have stepped up surveillance of avian influenza in human and avian influenza, respectively. In addition, it is necessary to strengthen the mechanism of sharing information with countries around the world, especially with China's neighboring countries such as Russia and Kazakhstan and to deal with new outbreaks in a timely manner. This principle must be adhered to in the near future in the prevention and control of avian influenza in human.

VI. Early detection, early reporting, early isolation, and early treatment

It is the key to take comprehensive measures to manage the source of avian influenza infection, and to make great efforts to achieve "early detection, early reporting, early isolation and early treatment," that is," four early," which is the basic requirement of prevention and control. Ensure that the "four early" measures are in place, especially during the epidemic of avian influenza in human.

15.2 Epidemic Surveillance and Early Warning

I. Surveillance of avian influenza in human

"Avian influenza in human" surveillance includes surveillance of "avian influenza in animal" outbreaks and surveillance of "avian influenza in human" outbreaks, which makes planned, systematic, and long-term observation of the occurrence, prevalence, and influencing factors of avian influenza in human and avian influenza in animals as well as timely reporting of relevant information in order to take timely preventive and control measures and evaluate their effectiveness [4, 5]. Surveillance of avian influenza in human is an important task in the prevention and control of this disease.

Surveillance has become the main content of epidemiological research and application, as well as the main method of disease prevention and control. Disease surveillance usually involves medical personnel in medical institutions. For the early detection of diseases in the population, especially the occurrence and epidemics of new infectious diseases, some scholars have put forward the theory and method of Symptom Surveillance or Syndromic Surveillance in the population. The establishment of "avian influenza in human" surveillance system has attracted almost all the theories and methods of modern epidemiological surveillance. Epidemiological investigation of cases of avian influenza in human and many local researches suggest that live poultry exposure is a key risk factor for avian influenza in human. The live poultry market may be an important source of infection. Timely and effective monitoring of epidemics of avian influenza in the live poultry market is the key factor of monitoring.

(i) Purpose of surveillance on avian influenza in human

1. Early detection and early report cases of avian influenza in human, timely and effectively take prevention and control measures to prevent the possible spread of avian influenza in human and the epidemic.
2. To understand the changes of epidemic strains of avian influenza in the local monitoring period.

(ii) Conditions for initiating monitoring

If one of the following situations occurs in the relevant areas, the emergency monitoring of avian influenza in human will be started immediately.

1. The confirmation of the occurrence of epidemic of highly pathogenic avian influenza in animals by provincial agricultural authorities
2. Occurrence of epidemic of highly pathogenic avian influenza in animals or in human in adjacent countries or regions
3. Occurrence of cases of avian influenza in human (including medical observation cases, suspected cases, clinical diagnosis cases, and confirmed cases).

(iii) Determination of monitoring scope

1. The outbreak of highly pathogenic avian influenza in animals.
2. Emergency monitoring of counties (cities, districts) with epidemic diseases in animals defined by the local agricultural authority.
3. When the animal epidemic occurs in the border township, the counties (cities, districts) adjacent to the border should carry out emergency monitoring work. The border counties (cities, districts) whose adjacent countries have the outbreak of highly pathogenic avian influenza in animals or in human should carry out emergency monitoring work.
4. Occurrence of cases of avian influenza in human.
5. Emergency surveillance is initiated in counties (cities, districts) where avian influenza in human occurs.
6. If cases of avian influenza in human are imported, the primary county (city, district) where the cases originate from should start emergency monitoring at the same time.
7. If avian influenza in human originates from laboratory pollution, the laboratory and county (city, district) where the cases are in should start emergency monitoring simultaneously.

(iv) Target subjects

Patients with fever (body temperature $\geq$ 38 °C) accompanied by influenza-like symptoms and their close contacts, in areas under surveillance.

(v) Time frame for monitoring

1. In areas where an animal epidemic occurs, emergency surveillance begins on the date of discovery of the epidemic by the agricultural authority and persists until 7 days after the ban is lifted.
2. In case of avian influenza in human without animal epidemic, emergency surveillance begins on the date of detection of the epidemic and persists until the end of the medical observation period for the last close contact with the disease.

(vi) Monitoring methodology

1. Case detection
   (1) Passive monitoring. All the cases with fever and influenza-like symptoms should be registered and reported by all levels of medical institutions.
   (2) Active surveillance.
      (a) The CDC actively tracks and investigates the reported fever-associated influenza-like cases and reports the progress to the national CDC and National Health Commission every day; (b) The CDC conducts home search, including the investigation on the presence of cases of fever and flu-like symptoms among the residents, reports the results to the national CDC and National Health Commission via Internet, and sends the patients to the hospital for treatment; (c) The CDC reports medical observation form about close contacts every day. (d) If it develops into suspected cases of avian influenza in human, it should be treated as a suspected case.
2. Epidemiological investigation, specimen collection, and detection for the cases

   The CDC should conduct a detailed epidemiological investigation of influenza-like cases within 2 h upon receipt of the report. At the same time, disease-related specimens should be collected according to relevant requirements and standards.

The specimens of upper and lower respiratory tracts should be collected for nucleic acid detection and virus isolation, and serum samples of acute and convalescent stages should be collected to detect the specific antibody of subtype A (H_XN_X).

In principle, preliminary testing is performed by the provincial disease control institution or its subordinate, while positive specimens are sent to the national CDC for review. At the same time, all localities should report the relevant epidemiological and clinical data of the cases in time, and send the relevant specimens to the higher CDC for review within 24 h according to the requirements of the National Health Commission or the national CDC.

3. Reporting and feedback

During the period of emergency monitoring, all kinds of medical and health institutions at all levels within the scope of monitoring should fill out the Emergency Monitoring Report Card for Highly Pathogenic Avian Influenza in Human and log in to China Influenza/Human Highly Pathogenic Avian Influenza Surveillance Information System to submit the report. At the same time, telephone reports to the local health administration authority and higher disease control agencies are demanded. If it is not practically feasible to carry out direct network reporting, the "Emergency Monitoring Report Card for Highly Pathogenic Avian Influenza in Human" should be reported by telephone and fax to county authority of disease prevention and control, which is responsible for the direct network reporting. Immediately after receiving the report, the disease prevention and control agency should initiate follow-up and investigation work at once, fill out the results in the Emergency Monitoring Report Card for Highly Pathogenic Avian Influenza in Human, and submit daily escalated report via email or fax to national CDC and the National Health Commission. Testing and diagnosis results from provincial or national level should be fed back timely step by step. Disease prevention and control agencies will rectify prognosis of the cases in time according to the feedback.

II. Early warning of avian influenza in human

In order to prevent and control avian influenza in human, early warning should be given and corresponding prevention and control measures should be taken to prevent the spread of avian influenza in human and its possible epidemic.

1. Pneumonia with unknown etiology [6, 7].

   Pneumonia with unknown etiological diagnosis is considered, if all of the four criteria are met: (1) fever (≥38 °C); (2) Image findings of pneumonia or acute respiratory distress syndrome (ARDS); (3) decreased or normal leukocyte count, decreased differential lymphocyte counts in early onset; (4) No obvious response to standard antibiotic treatment for 3–5 days.

2. Case of avian influenza in human requiring early warning

   A case of pneumonia with unknown etiology which meets one of the following conditions can be classified as an early warning case of avian influenza in human.

   (1) Pneumonia with unknown etiology in persons exposed to poultry (persons raising, selling, slaughtering, and/or processing poultry, veterinarians, and persons who kill and/or dispose sick or dead birds and/or disinfect epidemic sites, etc.).
   (2) Pneumonia with unknown etiology in persons who may be exposed to avian influenza viruses or potential infectious materials.
   (3) Death due to pneumonia with unknown etiology with SARS excluded.

3. Investigation of early warning cases

   After the early warning cases are found, the CDC should immediately carry out epidemiological investigations and collect specimens for examination.

4. Isolation and management of early warning cases

   (1) Isolation treatment of early warning cases: Early warning cases of avian influenza in human should undergo immediate isolation treatment until avian influenza in human is excluded.
   (2) Epidemiological investigation and close contact tracing of early warning cases: the disease prevention and control agency carries out epidemiological investigation on early warning cases of avian influenza in human immediately after receiving the report of these cases. At the same time, the close contact of these cases is tracked and registered, self-isolation and daily temperature measurement are carried out, and the local disease prevention and control center is notified in time in case of fever and respiratory symptoms.

(3) Sample collection and detection.
   (a) Types of specimens: serum, blood clots, nasopharyngeal swabs (or throat swabs), throat swabs, tracheal aspirates, faeces (or anal swabs), urine and autopsy specimen. If conditions are limited, at least three specimens including nasopharyngeal swabs (or pharyngeal swabs), feces (or anal swabs) and serum should be collected. Autopsy of early warning cases of death and examination of samples [8].
   (b) Sampling of early warning cases of avian influenza in human: Collection of pharyngeal and nasal swabs or gargle of patients 1 ~ 3 days after onset, serum in acute phase within 7 days after onset and autopsy lung tissue and trachea secretions of death cases for virus isolation, detection of viral nucleic acids, and serum antibodies. If positive results appear, they shall be reported and dealt with immediately according to the relevant requirements of the National Health and Health Commission. If the test results are negative and avian influenza in human cannot be ruled out clinically, serum samples on week 2–4 post to onset shall be collected from patients. If the antibodies are still negative, this disease can be excluded.

   Collection, preservation, transport, and test of specimen are carried out in accordance with the requirements of the Technical Programme for Laboratory Testing of Avian Influenza.

5. Final diagnosis and exclusion of cases

   Once the early warning case is diagnosed as a suspected or confirmed case of avian influenza in human, the prevention and treatment work shall be carried out in accordance with the requirements of Emergency Plan for Highly Pathogenic Avian Influenza in Human issued by the National Health Commission.

15.3 Epidemic Report

China's infectious disease epidemic has a history of more than 50 years since its initiation in the 1950s. Since the promulgation and implementation of the Law of the People's Republic of China on the Prevention and Control of Infectious Diseases in 1989, reporting of infectious diseases in China has been arranged into the track of legal management. According to the Law of the People's Republic of China on the Prevention and Control of Infectious Diseases amended and promulgated on August 28th, 2004, avian influenza in human is a category B infectious disease, but it is prevented and controlled as category A infectious disease. It should be reported timely when patients diagnosed with or suspected of avian influenza are found [9].

(i) Reporting System for Avian Influenza in human
   1. Reporters Health care institutions, disease prevention and control institutions, and their medical personnel, quarantine personnel, disease control personnel, as well as individual practitioners and network manager in computerized disease management systems at all levels and of all kinds.

      When discovering confirmed or suspected cases of avian influenza in human, the responsible reporter fills in the Infectious Disease Report Card, and immediately reports the epidemic situation to the disease prevention and control authority at local county (district) through the computer network. No unit or individual may conceal, delay, falsely report the information or instruct others to do so.

(ii) Requirements on reporting [10]
   1. Health care facilities at all levels
      (1) First visit responsibility system must be implemented. When consulting or treating confirmed or suspected patients of avian influenza in human, medical practitioner should immediately report the information to the designated department of the hospital, regardless of whether the patient has a local household registration.
      (2) When the confirmed or suspected patient is cured and discharged or dies, the diagnosis and outcome of the patient are to be reported to the local disease prevention and control authority with simultaneous direct report via Internet, and the original report card is revised with a new outcome report.
      (3) Report of transference of confirmed or suspected patients with avian influenza in human. When confirmed cases or suspected patients with avian influenza in human are transferred to hospital, the Infectious Disease Report Card is transferred with the patient, and the medical and health care institution that receives the patient transferred is notified. In the network direct reporting system, the patient information reported by the transfer unit is accepted and confirmed. If the medical and health care institution to which the patient is transferred has no access to the internet, the patient's information should be handled by disease prevention and control center in local county (district).

2. Centers for Disease Control and Prevention

For centers for disease prevention and control at all levels, please log in to the website of http://211.167.248.17:8080 to enter the National Disease Surveillance Case Report System, and examine step by step the confirmed or suspected cases of avian influenza in human.

After completing the epidemiological investigation, the disease prevention and control agencies at county level will report Avian influenza in human Case Questionnaire directly online.

(iii) Reporting process and time deadline [11–13]

1. Upon receipt of visiting patients with confirmed or suspected avian influenza in human, the physician must report the epidemic by telephone or fax and network within 2 h.
2. Upon receipt of the epidemic report, the disease prevention and control authority at county level shall report the epidemic to the higher level of disease prevention and control authority and the health administration department at the same level within 2 h.

(iv) Types of epidemic reports

1. The first report of case. For the first report of confirmed or suspected case of avian influenza in human, the Infectious Disease Report Card should be sent to the local disease prevention and control agency as soon as possible.

   The first report of the case falls into the category of original report in the network direct reporting system, which requires the network direct reporting personnel to report in time and quickly; if the input is found incorrect, it should be revised in time. The information of the report card is involved in the statistics, only when the report card is reported from the provincial level to the country, and the Infectious Disease Report Card can be revised thereafter.
2. Correction report of the case. A dynamic correction is performed for the diagnosis of reported cases of confirmed or suspected avian influenza in human, including the conversion from suspected cases to confirmed cases, the exclusion of suspected cases, the conversion of confirmed cases to suspected cases, and the exclusion of confirmed cases. The correction card of Infectious Disease Report Card should be filled in and submitted on time.

   In case of the conversion from a suspected case to a confirmed one, the name of the disease shall be changed directly to "avian influenza in human" when revised. If a suspected case is excluded, the name of the disease shall be changed directly to "other diseases" when revised. In case of the conversion from a confirmed disease to the suspected one, the name of the disease shall be changed directly to "suspected case" when revised. If a suspected case is excluded, the name of the disease shall be changed directly to "other diseases" or "xx infectious diseases" when revised.
3. Outcome report. When a confirmed case or suspected case of avian influenza is cured, discharged, transferred to hospital or dies, an outcome report must be prepared and an outcome card of the Infectious Disease Report Card must be submitted. In the outcome card of the submitted Infectious Disease Report Card, the "discharge date" or "death date and date of receipt of death card" should be filled in.
4. Trans-regional epidemic reporting. The disease prevention and control authority shall promptly notify the local disease prevention and control authority by telephone timely after investigation and verification, and at the same time, send the copy of Infectious Disease Report Card and Questionnaire of Avian Influenza in Human Case to the disease prevention and control agencies by fax or computer network direct reporting system in order to disinfect the epidemic points, check and manage the close contacts.
5. Daily report and "zero case" reporting system. During epidemics of avian influenza in human, confirmed cases of avian influenza in human, onset in patients with suspected disease, outcomes, and so on within the past 24 h are summarized before 10 a.m. every day according to the request of the Ministry of Health, and reported by telephone or fax to the local disease prevention and control authority, including "zero" cases. Even if no cases occur, reporting should be continued.

   If confirmed or suspected patients with avian influenza in human are found to have left the current administrative area, the disease prevention and control agency in the current administrative area shall immediately report them to the health administration authority at the same level, and at the same time notify the disease prevention and control agency at the same level and the relevant transportation, railway, and civil aviation departments along the way.

(v) Completion of Disease Report Card

Use the current "Infectious Disease Report Card," including the disease card, correction card (corrected diagnosis), death card (outcome card), to fill in the name of the disease suspected or confirmed in the disease column.

(vi) Notification and publication of the epidemic situation of avian influenza in human

According to the situation of avian influenza in human, the National Health Commission shall promptly inform the relevant departments under the State Council and the health administrative authorities of provinces, autonomous regions, and municipalities directly under the Central Government, as well as the competent health departments of the military. The health administrative departments of provinces, autonomous regions, and municipalities directly under the Central Government where the avian influenza in human epidemic occurs shall promptly inform the health administrative departments of neighboring provinces, autonomous regions, and municipalities directly under the Central Government of the epidemic situation.

The administrative authorities of public health of provinces, autonomous regions, and municipalities directly under the Central Government receiving the notification shall promptly notify the medical and health institutions in their respective jurisdictions and do a good job of prevention and control.

The National Health Commission shall promptly and truthfully publish the epidemic situation to the public, and the health administrative authorities of provinces, autonomous regions, and municipalities directly under the Central Government shall promptly and truthfully publish the epidemic situation in their respective administrative areas.

15.4 Source Control

The source of infection refers to people or animals with the growth and reproduction of pathogens in their bodies, that can expel pathogens, including patients with infectious disease, pathogen carriers, and infected animals. So far, there is still no sufficient confirmation of human-to-human transmission of avian influenza. Therefore, the main source of infection of avian influenza is domestic poultries suffering the disease or carrying avian influenza virus, such as chickens, ducks, and geese, especially chickens. In addition, wild birds play an important role in the natural transmission of avian influenza, and the migration of migratory birds brings uncertainty to the control of avian influenza. Therefore, the countermeasures for the source of infection mainly include the control and management of epidemics of avian influenza in animals and in human, aiming at the prevention of new transmission.

I. Measures for patients with avian influenza

Avian influenza in human is a category B infectious disease but is managed as a category A infectious disease. Once the epidemic occurs, the principle of early detection, early reporting, early isolation, early treatment, and timely integrated measures must be followed to control the transmission and spread of the epidemic.

(i) Early detection

It is necessary to make use of all kinds of publicity tools to popularize the knowledge of prevention and control of avian influenza in human and improve the ability of public identification, improve health care organizations at all levels and raise the awareness of medical personnel on avian influenza in human. The first visit responsibility system should be implemented. Special observation rooms should be provided immediately for isolation of patients whenever suspected cases are found. Clinically diagnosed cases should be transferred to designated hospitals for hospitalization isolation and treatment. The quality of outpatient and emergency department should be improved to prevent misdiagnosis and missed diagnosis.

Health and medical institutions at all levels should pay close attention to the people seeing a doctor. When patients with fever accompanied by respiratory symptoms seek medical treatment, especially when patients present imaging manifestations of pneumonia, they should be inquired of possible contact history and presence of similar symptoms in surrounding populations such as their family members and colleagues. Special attention should be paid to the investigation on epidemiology and medical history of patients.

(ii) Early reporting

Early reporting can help us to grasp the epidemic situation in time, in order to facilitate the rapid adoption of epidemic prevention measures. When a patient suffering pneumonia with unknown etiology or suspected of avian influenza in human is found in the fever clinic or clinic of fever and respiratory diseases, a designated hospital or by other medical personnel, disease prevention and control authority within the jurisdiction shall be informed of the epidemic situation in accordance with the relevant provisions of the "Law of the People's Republic of China on the Prevention and Control of Infectious Diseases."

(iii) Early isolation

Early isolation should be emphasized for suspected or clinically diagnosed cases of avian influenza in human, so as to avoid long-distance transference. The purpose of early isolation is to prevent the spread of pathogens, facilitate management and disinfection, and make patients with avian influenza receive treatment timely.

II. Control of avian influenza in animals

When there is an avian influenza epidemic in animal, it is necessary to take corresponding control measures in the epidemic areas in accordance with the "Animal Epidemic Prevention Law of the People's Republic of China." The epidemic situation must be put out on the epidemic spot, the spread of the epidemic situation and its spread to human beings must be blocked, and if necessary the trading of live poultry must be prohibited and live poultry market must be closed.

15.5 Management of Contacts

Since 1997, there have been outbreaks of avian influenza in human in China. Breeders who come into contact with sick and dead poultry and those who rescue and care for patients, or live with or have direct contact with patients may be infected with avian influenza. In order to better identify and deal with the close contacts of avian influenza in human, timely and scientific medical observation and management shall be conducted for the contacts in order to prevent and control the spread of avian influenza in human among populations, and the criteria and treatment principles for close contacts of avian influenza should be formulated [14, 15].

I. Determination of close contacts
  (i) Close contacts of sick and dead poultry include [16].
    1. Those who raise, sell, slaughter, and process sick and dead poultry.
    2. Those who catch and handle sick and dead poultry, but fail to take protective measures in accordance with corresponding regulations.
    3. Other related personnel with direct contact with dead poultries and their excreta or secretions.
  (ii) Close contacts with suspected or confirmed cases of avian influenza in human.

II. Principles of treatment
  (i) The period of medical observation shall be 7 days, and the activities of subjects under medical observation shall not be restricted during the observation period, but the scope of activities of the observed subjects shall be within the scope of epidemic areas of avian influenza in animals.
  (ii) During the observation period, health personnel designated by the local health administration department shall test the body temperature of the close contacts once a day to understand their physical health condition, fill in the "Registration Form for Medical Observation of Close Contacts of Avian Influenza" and report it to the county-level disease prevention and control institutions daily according to the "Statistical Daily Report of Medical Observation of Close Contacts of Avian Influenza." Then disease control agencies at all levels make the daily summary according to the "Daily Statistical Summary Table of Medical Observation of Close Contacts of Avian Influenza" and report to the higher-level center for disease control and prevention and the health administrative department at the same level.
  (iii) Epidemiological investigation should be carried out in cases of abnormal clinical manifestations (body temperature over 38 °C with symptoms such as cough or sore throat).
  (iv) In case of human-to-human transmission of avian influenza, close contacts should be isolated for medical observation.

15.6 Division of Epidemic Areas

In controlling the source of infectious disease, it is very important to determine the epidemic point and divide the epidemic area. Only by correctly judging the epidemic point and the epidemic area can the measures adopted play their roles and the epidemic situation be controlled. On-site epidemiological investigation is the main method to determine the epidemic point and the epidemic area, and we can understand the source of the patient's infection and the range of possible spread through investigation.

I. Epidemiological survey
  (i) Purpose of investigation

    To verify diagnosis and investigate possible sources of infection, transmission routes, and their influencing factors.

  (ii) Subjects under investigation

    Confirmed and suspected cases of avian influenza in human, close contacts of cases, close contacts of dead animals of avian influenza, relevant basic information on the occurrence of avian influenza.

  (iii) Contents of investigation

    Birds where the avian influenza epidemic occurred and their incidence, epidemiological investigation of avian influenza in human cases, follow-up investigation of close contacts.

  (iv) Methods of investigation

    Investigation should be conducted by trained staff of disease prevention and control agencies; epidemiological investigations should be carried out quickly after avian influenza epidemic reports are made.

II. Identification of Avian Influenza Epidemic Point and Division of Epidemic Areas
  (i) Formation of epidemic focus of avian influenza

    The range that the source of infection and the pathogens it discharges can spread to is called epidemic focus. Avian influenza is a common infectious disease of human and poultry, so there are two kinds of focus, one is formed by poultry disease and the other is formed by human disease. The former is centered on sick poultry farms, and the scope of possible contamination of poultry and their excrement is usually within 3 km of sick and dead poultry. The latter is limited to the place where the patient lives and works and other places where the patient moves around during the illness [17].

(ii) Division of avian influenza epidemic areas

For the determination of epidemic spots, the epidemiological professionals of the disease prevention and control agencies should usually provide detailed investigation results, which should be determined by relevant experts. The delineation of epidemic areas should be determined in full compliance with relevant legal provisions and after serious discussion, on a basis of the division of epidemic spots and with the support of the health administration department. In accordance with the relevant provisions of the Law of the People's Republic of China on the Prevention and Control of Infectious Diseases, local governments at or above the county level shall report to the higher-level local government for approval before declaring this area such as a township, a street, a community or even a city as an epidemic area. The government shall arrange for professionals to implement health quarantine on personnel, materials, and vehicles entering and leaving the epidemic area.

III. Sanitary treatment of avian influenza focus

The main measures of sanitary treatment in avian influenza focus are disinfection. Disinfection should be carried out timely and effectively after the outbreak, and strict disinfection measures should be taken for the objects that must be disinfected. The disinfection measures for animal epidemics and avian influenza in human epidemics shall be distinguished. See the guidelines of the "Disinfection Technical Specification" for the medical equipment required for disinfection [18].

(i) Animal avian influenza outbreaks occurred only

It is necessary to carry out final disinfection on dead poultry and slaughtered poultry, poultry houses, and poultry excrement; to disinfect the articles that may be contaminated by diseases and dead birds in designated animal epidemic areas; to disinfect drinking water in designated animal epidemic areas; disinfection can be omitted for mobile water bodies and larger water bodies with difficulties in disinfecting, but strict management should be performed; disinfection should be performed for surfaces of objects that may be contaminated in designated animal epidemic areas when exceeding the blockade line; and air in poultry houses should be disinfected if necessary.

(ii) Avian influenza in human outbreaks occurred

Strengthen guidance on the disinfection on the epidemic spot and in the epidemic areas and evaluation of disinfection effects; disinfect patients' excreta, patients' living and working places, articles they have been in contact with and other articles that may be contaminated; and disinfect patients' possible contamination during diagnosis and treatment in accordance with the requirements applicable to intestinal and respiratory infectious diseases.

15.7 Immunization Prevention

Immunization prevention is a major measure to control the spread of infectious diseases. The fight against avian influenza in human, like that against other infectious diseases, ultimately depends on extensive vaccination of susceptible people to produce specific immunity to avian influenza. Immune prevention, including artificial automatic immunity and artificial passive immunity, lies in the development and application of vaccines. According to the infectious source of avian influenza and the susceptible population, the development of avian influenza vaccine includes the development and application of avian influenza both in human and in poultry [19, 20]. So far, China has successfully developed and popularized poultry vaccines, while vaccines for avian influenza in human have obtained preliminary results in the study. Although there is no vaccine for avian influenza in human at present, influenza vaccine for susceptible people can reduce the possibility of influenza virus infection and pneumonia, and reduce the chance of genetic recombination in human body between avian influenza virus and human influenza virus.

15.8 Prevention and Control of Nosocomial Infection

In accordance with the requirements of the management and technical documents "Technical Plan for Disinfection of Avian Influenza in Human, Nosocomial Infection Control and Personal Protection" issued by the National Health Commission, comprehensive protective measures should be taken to control nosocomial infection [21].

I. Basic protective techniques

According to the standard prevention principle, target measures should be taken based on the transmission route of avian influenza, so as to assess the risk of infection based on medical staff's contact with patients and take hierarchical protection measures.

The meaning of standard prevention is that all patients are considered potentially infectious and must be isolated. Regardless of whether there is obvious blood or contact with incomplete skin and mucous membranes, protective measures must be provided for those who contact the patient or their body fluids and excreta. Two-way protection should be emphasized, not only to prevent diseases from being transmitted from patients to medical personnel, but also to prevent diseases from being transmitted from medical personnel to patients.

The specific measures of standard prevention are to wear gloves when contacting substances such as blood, body fluids, secretions, excreta, and contaminated articles and wash hands immediately after removing gloves. Once one has been in contact with substances such as blood, body fluids, secretions, excreta, and contaminated articles, he/she should wash hands immediately. Medical staff shall wear disposable surgical masks or medical protective masks, protective glasses or masks, isolation clothing or aprons when their work clothes, faces, and eyes may be spattered with blood, body fluids, secretions, etc. Special attention should be paid to all sharp instruments to prevent stab wounds. Correct disinfection measures shall be taken for medical devices and appliances after use by patients.

II. Techniques for controlling nosocomial infection of avian influenza in human

Principle of patient isolation: Medical observation cases, suspected cases, clinically diagnosed and confirmed cases of avian influenza in human should be isolated in hospital as soon as possible. The confirmed cases can be placed in the same room, and the rest should be isolated in single rooms. Patients should be restricted to only move in the ward. In principle, no visit and no escort should be permitted. The diagnosis and treatment activities related to patients should be carried out in the ward as far as possible. The isolation measures of the hospital are as follows [22, 23].

(i) Areas for medical observation cases, suspected cases, and clinically diagnosed cases of avian influenza in human.

1. Independent areas are provided and separated from other areas without crossing, with a certain distance maintained.
2. They are divided into clean areas, semi-contaminated areas, and contaminated areas. The divisions are obvious without crossover and have obvious signs. Clean areas include duty rooms for medical staff, consultation rooms, changing rooms, bathrooms, warehouses, etc.; semi-contaminated areas include treatment rooms, medical staff's offices, disinfection rooms, and protective equipment replacement rooms; contaminated areas include wards, ward corridors and dirty clothes, and dirt temporary storage. Buffer zones and separate barriers are provided between clean and semi-contaminated areas, semi-contaminated areas and contaminated areas.
3. Keep the ward well ventilated.
4. The waste produced in the ward is put into the double yellow garbage bag as the infectious waste, and the damaged waste is put into the sharp box. Other medical items must be sterilized prior to their removal out of the ward.
5. One room is provided for one patient, with a toilet in the room.
6. Patients should wear medical protective masks and are forbidden to leave the ward or to visit each other.
7. In principle, there should be no escort and no visits. If visits are required, the visitors must strictly comply with the regulations and take personal protection measures.

(ii) Areas for confirmed patients with avian influenza.

1. Hospitals that have established negative pressure wards can adopt room isolation measures. Specific requirements for room isolation include:
   (1) Orient the airflow from office area → corridor → buffer room → isolation ward.
   (2) The isolation ward is a polluted area. A buffer room is set up between the corridor outside the isolation ward and the ward, and the protective equipment is placed in the buffer room.
   (3) Before entering the isolation ward, the medical staff changes the protective equipment in the buffer room; when leaving the isolation ward, he/she changes the protective equipment in the buffer room and perform hand hygiene operations.
   (4) The patient's diagnosis and treatment, nursing work and patient's life activities are completed in the hospital room.
   (5) Isolation signs should be provided in the isolation ward, and personnel access should be restricted, and the entering and leaving of anyone should be registered.
2. For hospitals without negative pressure wards, the following isolation measures should be taken:
   (1) Separate districts are provided, which are isolated from other wards and provided with obvious signs.
   (2) The layout is reasonable, divided into clean area, semi-contaminated area, and contami-

nated area. The three areas have no intersection.

(3) Special channels for medical staff and patients are set up in the ward.

(4) The area is well ventilated to ensure oriented airflow from clean area→ semi-contaminated area → contaminated area.

(5) The waste produced in the ward is put into the double yellow garbage bag as the infectious waste, and the damaged waste is put into the sharp box. Other medical items must be sterilized prior to their removal out of the ward.

(6) Patients shall wear medical masks and shall not leave the ward.

(7) Severe patients should be admitted to an intensive care unit or a ward with conditions for monitoring and rescue, and other patients are not allowed in this ward.

(8) In principle, there should be no escort and no visits, and the patient's critical condition should be made known by the medical staff to the family in time. If visits are required, the visitors must strictly comply with the regulations and take personal protection measures.

III. Guidelines for protection of personnel exposed to avian influenza in human

(i) Protection principles

All personnel exposed definitely or potentially to sick or dead poultry or avian influenza patients should take corresponding protective measures, including the following principles:

1. Protective measures should be taken to prevent respiratory, digestive, and contact transmission of avian influenza.
2. Medical masks should be worn to prevent respiratory transmission by anyone entering areas contaminated or potentially contaminated by the source of infection.
3. Protective measures should be adopted when contacting patients, suspected patients, sick and dead poultry in the epidemic area, and other sources of infection and their body fluids, secretions, and excrement. Protective measures should also be taken by anyone contacting items contaminated by the source of infection.
4. Measures should be taken to prevent the transmission of human avian influenza from patients to medical staff and from medical staff to patients.
5. The methods of basic protection, strengthened protection, and strict protection should be adopted according to the degree of hazard exposure.

(ii) Protection methods

1. Basic protection

(1) Applicable to: all medical staff engaged in the diagnosis and treatment of the hospital, and those who may come into contact with sick poultry or patients.

(2) Protective equipment: work clothes, work pants, work shoes, work caps, and medical protective masks.

2. Strengthened protection

(1) Applicable to: persons entering the observation room or inpatient area, persons entering the epidemic area, and other persons contacting the source of infection such as sick or dead poultry, and patients, as well as their body fluids, secretions, excreta, and contaminated articles.

(2) Protective equipment: isolation clothing, medical protective masks, caps, medical gloves or rubber gloves, and if necessary, used protective glasses, face shields, or shoe covers.

3. Strict protection

(1) Applicable to: persons slaughtering sick poultry, and persons performing invasive operations or autopsies on patients with avian influenza.

(2) Protective equipment: addition of positive pressure masks or full-scale respiratory protectors on the basis of enhanced protection.

(iii) Order of replacement of protective articles

Determine the changing sequence of the protective equipment according to the specific situation of the protective equipment, and the order of changing the protective equipment is based on the principle of convenient replacement of the protective equipment. After the work is over, the order of changing protective equipment is in principle to remove heavier and bulkier items first, and then remove the protective equipment for the most critical protective parts such as respiratory tract and eyes. For common protective clothing, protective equipment can generally be worn and taken off in relevant order.

IV. Management of patients with avian influenza.

(i) The confirmed or suspected patient shall enter the ward according to the prescribed route.

(ii) The patient's clothing shall be changed before entering the ward. After centralized disinfection of personal belongings and changed clothes, they shall be stored in a designated place for unified custody by the hospital.

(iii) Patients are strictly prohibited from going out during hospitalization. Their activities should be restricted to the hospital room, and all diagnosis and treatment activities should be completed as far as possible in this ward.
(iv) Strict visiting system should be implemented, and no escort and no visitation are permitted. If visits are required under special circumstances, the visitor should enter according to the specified time, along the specified route, and take strict protective measures before entry.
(v) Personal hygiene management of patients shall be strengthened.
(vi) The patient shall wear a mask when it is permitted based on his/her condition during the hospitalization.
(vii) The patient must take a bath when discharged or transferred. The patient can leave the ward only after changing clothes.
(viii) When the patient dies, the corpse should be treated in time. The treatment method: use 3000 mg/L chlorine disinfectant or 0.5% peracetic acid cotton balls or gauze to fill all open passages of the corpse, including mouth, nose, ears, and anus. The corpse shall be wrapped in double layers of cloth, put into a double-layer corpse bag, and sent directly to the designated place by a special vehicle for cremation.
(ix) The personal belongings used by the patient during hospitalization cannot be taken home with the patient or family member until they are disinfected.

15.9 Health Education and Health Promotion

Health education and health promotion are one of the most powerful weapons to prevent and control avian influenza. Through health education and promotion, strengthen government responsibility, mobilize social participation, educate people to establish health awareness and develop healthy behavior, promote healthy lifestyle, eliminate social panic, and instability, thereby creating a good atmosphere for preventing and controlling avian influenza in human. At the same time, everyone should do their best to cooperate actively in the implementation of the prevention and control measures taken by the relevant departments in order to reduce or eliminate the risk factors for the spread of avian influenza in human and implement prevention and control measures, through activities of health education and health promotion for preventing and controlling avian influenza in human.

(i) Important means to raise the public's knowledge level in preventing and controlling avian influenza

Various forms of health education activities have promoted the popularization of knowledge on the prevention and control of avian influenza in Shenzhen, met the requirements of various populations, and played a role of wide coverage. They have enabled all citizens to master the scientific knowledge of preventing influenza or avian influenza in human, and enhanced awareness of prevention and self-protection.

(ii) One of the most basic working methods in the prevention and control of avian influenza

The prevention and control of avian influenza is a complex social systematic engineering that requires energetic policy support, broad social collaboration, and comprehensive community actions, which are all the core of health promotion. Through health education and promotion, we can put prevention and control of avian influenza in human on the agenda of governments at all levels, departments and leaders at all levels, so that they can formulate policies and regulations on finances, publicity, education, and others in a timely manner, assume public health responsibilities, and promote extensive coordination and active cooperation in the society.

(iii) An effective way to develop healthy behaviors and lifestyles

The core issue of health education and promotion is to urge individuals or populations to change their unhealthy behaviors and lifestyles. We know that many bad behaviors and lifestyles are not just personal responsibilities, but also closely related to social customs, cultural traditions, economic conditions, living environment, etc. Therefore, changing behaviors and lifestyles is an arduous and complex process. The desired results can only be achieved by carrying out health education and promotion activities in a planned, organized, and systematic way.

(iv) The minimum investment and maximum benefit in prevention and control measures for avian influenza in human

The spread and epidemics of avian influenza in human are closely related to people's unhealthy hygiene behavior and lifestyle. Health education is to advocate a healthy lifestyle, change people's bad lifestyle and behavior, reduce the risk induced by their own activities, which is a business of great profit with little investment. For the prevention and control of avian influenza, health education is also the most effective measure with the least investment.

(v) Effective means of maintaining social stability and socioeconomic development

The spread and epidemics of avian influenza in human have disrupted people's normal order of life.

Some are afraid to eat poultry meat and processed poultry foods, some are afraid to use down products, some become indoorsy, and even postpone or give up their business trip opportunities, and some farmers suspend the chicken business. All these show that people's normal order of work and life is disrupted to some extent by avian influenza in human.

The epidemic of avian influenza in human will also undermine social cooperation, and even political and macroeconomic stability. At present, the world is increasingly concerned about the possibility of avian influenza pandemic and its adverse effects on mankind and the world economic and financial system. If the epidemic situation is serious, its impact on the world economy will also be serious, manifesting mainly the implementation of import and export restrictions, which will cause chaos in global trade and transportation, and may also lead to temporary and serious capital flows reduction. The biggest impact is likely to happen in countries with emerging market.

Because of this, through health education and promotion, the correct knowledge of prevention and treatment of avian influenza in human can be spread to the public, which can not only reduce the outbreak and epidemic of avian influenza in human, but also eliminate social panic in time during the epidemic of avian influenza in human. This plays a positive role in maintaining social stability and economic development.

15.10 Supervision and Law Enforcement

It is important to work, supervise, and enforce the law of human avian flu. In accordance with the relevant requirements of the "Law of the People's Republic of China on the Prevention and Treatment of Infectious Diseases" and the "Regulations on Emergency Response to Public Health Emergencies," enforcement work shall be carried out in a timely manner under the leadership of the health administration authorities [24].

I. Purpose and responsibilities
   (i) Take effective measures in conjunction with relevant departments to quickly control and eradicate the epidemics of avian influenza in human.
   (ii) Infectious disease supervisors shall supervise and cooperate with disease prevention and control personnel in the prevention and control of avian influenza in human.
   (iii) Infectious disease supervisors shall inspect relevant departments' implementation of the controlling measures for avian influenza in human, and impose administrative penalties on violators of laws and regulations related to infectious diseases.
   (iv) The health supervision agency shall supervise and inspect the following matters and supervise law enforcement on them:
      1. Epidemic reports from medical and health institutions and disease prevention and control institutions.
      2. Isolation, disinfection, protection, and treatment of medical waste, which are performed by medical institutions and detention stations (stations).
      3. Disinfection of public places.
      4. Medical observation of close contacts and environmental disinfection of epidemic points.
      5. The quality of disinfection products and protective equipment manufactured or being used.
      6. Carry out other supervision and inspection work in accordance with the law.

II. Supervise the preparations for law enforcement
   (i) The following documents must be available: " Report Registration Form for Avian Influenza in Human," " Case Investigation Form for Avian Influenza in Human," "On-site Inspection Record" and "Inquiry Record," "Notice of Preservation of Evidence," " Registration Form for Preservation of Evidence," "Sampling Record Form," "Health Administrative Control Decision," "Health Supervision Opinions," "Order Correction Notice," "Service Return Receipt" and "Seal," and so on.
   (ii) Supplies for on-site investigation and processing

      Protective equipment: work clothes, isolation gowns, masks, eye protection, gloves, water boots, etc.

      Forensic tools: cameras, tape recorders, cameras, etc.

      Reference: infectious disease diagnostic standards and treatment principles, relevant laws and regulations, standards and other relevant professional technical reference materials.

III. Supervision and law enforcement content
   (i) Health supervision of epidemic report.
      1. Ensure that reports of avian influenza in human meet the following requirements.
         (1) A control system for the epidemic situation of avian influenza in human shall be formulated in areas under its jurisdiction, and qualified professionals of preventive medicine shall be designated to manage reports of infectious diseases.
         (2) Disease prevention and control institutions at all levels, medical institutions within their jurisdiction, and disease prevention and control institutions at higher levels

operate the "National Disease Surveillance Case Report System" in a networked manner, which provides a special report on outbreaks of avian influenza in human, timely reports epidemic information within a specified time limit, and realizes a network of epidemic report information.

(3) Regularly and irregularly publish information on epidemics of avian influenza in human, and publish epidemic notifications every month during the epidemics. Report the analysis of the epidemic situation to the health administration in a timely manner.

(4) The epidemic report and analysis materials shall be complete, accurate, and timely. The high level of analysis has guiding significance for the prevention and control of avian influenza in human.

(5) The investigation plan should be available for missing reports of avian influenza in human in medical institutions in the jurisdiction, and shall be organized and implemented.

2. The infectious disease report of medical institutions in the supervision area shall meet the following requirements

(1) The epidemic situation management system of the institute shall be formulated, and the qualified professional and technical personnel shall be responsible for the management of infectious disease reports.

(2) The National Disease Surveillance Case Report System is networked with disease prevention and control institutions to report the epidemic situation of infectious pneumonia induced by avian influenza in human in a timely manner within the prescribed time limit, so as to realize the network of information on the epidemic situation.

(3) Timely notify the district disease prevention and control agency and the health administration department of the sudden outbreak of avian influenza in human.

(4) The epidemic report information should be complete, accurate, and timely.

3. Regular supervision, management and inspection of reports of avian influenza in human

Carry out supervision and inspection 1–2 time(s) every year from May to June or from November to December, or cooperate with superior authorities to arrange uniformly or carry out sudden supervision and inspection according to requirement. The objects of examination shall be general hospitals and hospitals of infectious disease within the jurisdiction. It is mainly to supervise the time limit, procedure, and quality of report filling implemented by relevant medical institutions and responsible persons in reporting avian influenza in human, and to bulletin the results of supervision and inspection [25].

(1) Whether an epidemic reporting system has been developed and implemented. Whether someone is responsible for the epidemic report.

(2) Randomly check the original records such as outpatient logs, medical records and prescriptions, and check with the infectious disease registration book and Infectious Disease Report Card submitted to the disease control institution. Check whether there is any missing report of epidemic situation.

(3) Check whether the main business departments of the outpatient clinic have the outpatient log, Infectious Disease Report Card, and infectious disease registry settings and registration, and whether the registration items are complete and accurate. Timely bulletin sudden and important epidemics. Check whether the Infectious Disease Report Card is reported in time according to the legal time limit.

4. Supervision and management of epidemic reports and notifications of relevant departments

(1) Check whether the disease prevention and control agencies of railways, transportation, civil aviation, factories (fields), and mines report the response to the epidemic situation to the disease prevention and control agencies designated by the health administration department of the local government in accordance with relevant provisions.

(2) Check whether the military medical and health institution reports outbreaks of avian influenza in human to the local disease prevention and control agency when diagnosing and treating local patients.

(ii) Health supervision of pre-screening and triage of avian influenza in human

1. Check whether the medical institution has established a pre-screening and triage system

for avian influenza in human. Check whether a fever clinic has been set up in a general hospital at or above level II to be specifically responsible for the triage of human avian flu in the medical institution, and organize and manage the preliminary examination and triage of avian influenza in human in the medical institution. Inspected whether the medical institutions without fever clinics have set up triage points for transmission of the disease.

2. Check whether the doctors in each department of medical institutions comply with the provisions on pre-detection of avian influenza in human in the process of consulting patients, whether a patient with confirmed or suspected avian influenza as revealed in pre-screening is referred to the fever clinic or the triage point in the department of infectious diseases for treatment, with necessary disinfection measures taken at the reception point. Check whether medical institutions strengthen the preliminary examination and triage of avian influenza in human in accordance with the requirements of the local health administration departments, after receiving the early warning information of avian influenza in human issued by the Ministry of Public Health and the people's governments of provinces, autonomous regions, and municipalities directly under the Central Government. When necessary, establish a relatively independent pre-inspection office for avian influenza in human.
3. Check whether medical institutions take measures to isolate patients with confirmed or suspected avian influenza according to law or adopt measures to control its spread, and perform medical observation or take other necessary preventive measures for the escorts and other close contacts of the patients according to regulations.

(iii) Hygienic supervision of isolation for avian influenza in human

Check whether the health care institution has established relatively independent fever clinics, isolation and observation rooms, or designated hospitals for treatment of avian influenza in human to set up special negative pressure wards.

1. The fever (emergency) clinic shall comply with the following guidelines for isolation work [9]
   (1) Set up an independent district separated from other outpatient and emergency departments and provided with obvious signs. There should be backup consultation rooms during the disinfection of the clinic.
   (2) Be well ventilated with qualified disinfection facilities.
   (3) There should be waiting areas, consulting rooms, treatment rooms, laboratory, radiological examination room (or mobile X-ray machine), special inspection rooms, and radiological inspection rooms. There should be separate toilets.
2. The isolation observation room shall comply with the following guidelines for isolation work
   (1) It shall be clearly marked with independent zoning.
   (2) It shall be divided into clean area, semi-contaminated area, and contaminated area, without any intersection among them.
   (3) There shall be a separation between the medical staff's office and the observation room without any cross-connection, and they are kept as far apart as possible.
   (4) The patient who is hospitalized in the observation room shall be kept in one room for each person. The patient shall wear a mask and shall not leave the room. Contact between patients shall be strictly prohibited.
   (5) Actively make differential diagnosis, and exclude upper respiratory infection, influenza, bacterial or fungal pneumonia, and so on. Quarantine observation is required for all patients whose diagnosis remains temporarily unknown or when the possibility of avian influenza in human cannot be ruled out.
3. Patients with confirmed or suspected avian influenza shall comply with the following guidelines for isolation work
   (1) Well ventilated, independently divided, isolated from other wards (including between patients and suspected patients) with clear labels.
   (2) It shall be divided into clean area, semi-contaminated area, and contaminated area, without any intersection among them.
   (3) The medical staff's office and the ward shall be separated without any intersection and kept as far apart as possible.
   (4) The suspected patient shall be kept in one room for each person. The patient shall wear a mask and shall not leave the room.

Contact between patients is strictly prohibited. Indoor conditions for washing, gargling, and excreting shall be provided.

(5) Critically ill patients shall be admitted to intensive care negative pressure wards or wards with conditions for monitoring and rescue, and intensive care wards for patients with avian influenza or wards with conditions for monitoring and rescue shall not admit other conventional patients.

(6) Strict visiting system should be established, and no escort or visit should be permitted. If there is a critically ill patient and there is any other circumstance under which visit is required, the visitor must take personal protection measures strictly according to the requirements of this guideline.

(7) There should be a particular person at the entrance and exit of the ward to check whether the persons entering and leaving meet the requirements of this guideline.

(iv) Supervision of health protection against avian influenza in human

Supervise whether the protection of medical personnel involved in the diagnosis and treatment of avian influenza in human conforms to the following principles:

1. Medical institutions shall strengthen the training of medical personnel on protection knowledge, correctly master the use of protective articles, and ensure the protective effect. Medical practitioners should wear protective items correctly according to the principle of grading protection.
2. Medical practitioners entering fever (emergency) clinic, isolation observation room, and isolation ward shall properly wear and remove protective articles according to the classification of clean area, semi-contaminated area, and contaminated area, and pay special attention to the hygiene and protection of respiratory tract, oral cavity, nasal cavity, mucosa, and eyes.
3. The disposable protective clothing used by medical practitioners shall meet the national standards of the People's Republic of China, and the protective masks used shall be disposable arched medical protective masks conforming to the national standards of the People's Republic of China or protective masks conforming to the standards of N95 and FFP2. The protective mask should be replaced after use for 4 h.
4. Hands should be cleaned and disinfected strictly according to procedures. Gloves must be worn by any person contacting patients or their blood, body fluids, secretions, excrement, and items contaminated by them (e.g., masks and oxygen pipes). After the treatment, gloves should be replaced and hands are cleaned and disinfected immediately.
5. Protective clothing (or isolation clothing), rubber gloves, protective glasses, protective masks, shoe covers, and other protective equipment must be worn when handling medical waste in fever (emergency) clinics, isolation observation rooms, and isolation wards.
6. In order to prevent needle injury and infection of medical personnel, medical institutions should be equipped with medical needle destruction devices to handle post-use needles or use self-destruction syringes in the treatment rooms of fever (emergency) clinic, isolation observation room, and isolation ward.
7. Medical institutions shall rationally arrange the work of medical staff to avoid overfatigue, care about the health of medical staff, and monitor the body temperature and respiratory symptoms of medical staff.

(v) Hygienic supervision on disinfection activities against avian influenza in human in medical institutions [26].

1. Disinfection scope: fever (emergency) clinic (including designated special laboratory and radiological examination room), isolation observation room, and special ward. If no particular laboratory or radiological examination room is designated, disinfection of the laboratory, and radiological examination room shall be strengthened.
2. Disinfection method: supervise whether air disinfection, ground and surface disinfection, disinfection of other items, and terminal disinfection are carried out in accordance with relevant requirements.

(vi) Sanitary supervision of disposal of medical wastes in medical institutions

Supervise whether the sewage disposal of medical institutions in the process of diagnosis and treatment of pneumonia of avian influenza in human meets the following requirements [27]:

1. The household garbage of the patient should be packed in double-layer garbage bags and disinfected in time to avoid contamination.

2. The isolation clothes, masks, hats, gloves, shoe covers, and other wastes shall be sorted, sterilized, and disposed in a timely manner after use, and the storage containers shall be covered to avoid contamination.
3. Dose of drugs for sewage treatment during the period of epidemic of avian influenza in human can be increased appropriately to make the total residual chlorine meet the required standards.

(vii) Sanitary supervision and management of disinfection products

Supervise the supply, usage safety, and disinfection effect of disinfection products related to the prevention and control of avian influenza in human and ensure they meet the following requirements:

1. Strictly manage and standardize the production and use of disinfection equipment and disinfectants used to prevent avian influenza in human.
2. Strengthen the sanitary supervision of disinfection products related to avian influenza in human. For supervision of disinfection products, disinfection equipment, disposable medical and sanitary products related to the prevention of avian influenza in human, special supervision and random inspection shall be conducted to ensure safe use and disinfection effect. Production and sale of disinfection products that have not obtained a sanitary license shall be prohibited. We must severely crack down on the illegal use of low-quality materials to produce disinfection products.
3. Health administrative departments at or above the provincial level shall promptly announce to the public the catalogue of disinfection products that have obtained valid sanitation licenses.

(viii) Cooperate with relevant departments to carry out on-site epidemiological investigations

After receiving the report of avian influenza in human, the health supervision agency shall promptly cooperate with the disease prevention and control agency to organize audit for epidemics and epidemiological investigations, grasp the epidemic rule of acute infectious disease outbreaks, identify the source, transmission route, and the scope of the epidemic, clarify epidemic factors, and provide scientific basis for formulating timely plans to control outbreak of epidemics.

(ix) Sanitary supervision of epidemic control measures

1. Supervise the isolation of patients with law enforcement: Issue the "Health Administrative Control Decision" for patients with confirmed or suspected avian influenza who refuse to be isolated or withdraw from isolation before the expiry of the isolation period. If necessary, the public security department can assist the medical institute to adopt mandatory isolation measures.
2. Cooperate with disease control institutions to conduct epidemiological investigation on people contacting closely the confirmed or suspected patients in accordance with relevant regulations, and adopt centralized or decentralized isolation measures for medical observation according to the actualities. When necessary, take preventive medicine or preventive injection measures and issue " Opinion on Health Supervision" and "Health Administrative Control Decision."
3. The supervising disease control agency shall implement necessary sanitization and preventive measures, such as disinfection, on the places and articles that may be contaminated by pathogens, and issue the "Opinion on Health Supervision" or the "Health Administration Control Decision" or "Notice of Ordered Correction."
4. In the event of outbreaks and epidemics of avian influenza, the governmental department can be requested to implement emergency measures if necessary including limitation and stopping of gatherings, shutdown of factories, businesses and schools, and cutoff of sources of drinking water of public health that might be contaminated by pathogen of infectious diseases, according to Article 25 of "Laws on Prevention and Control of Infectious Diseases of the People's Republic of China."
5. Inspect the implementation of control measures taken by medical care institutions and disease prevention and control institutions for patients with infectious diseases and the places, articles, and people in close contact with them. Sanitary penalties shall be imposed on acts violating the law on the prevention and control of infectious diseases. The institutes and individuals responsible for the transmission and spread of the avian influenza in human shall be punished accordingly.

IV. Administrative penalty
   (i) Content of administrative penalty [24].
      1. The administrative department of public health of the people's government at or above the county level shall order a corrections within a time limit, circulate a notice of criticism, and give a warning; give punishment to persons in charge and other persons directly responsible including demotion, dismissal or expelling according to law, and revoke the certificates of the relevant responsible persons according to law; with criminal responsibility investigated according to law in case of a crime committed, if any institution for disease control and prevention violates the provisions of the Law of the People's Republic of China on the Prevention and Control of Infectious Diseases and has one of the following situations: (1) Failing to perform duties in monitoring avian influenza in human in accordance with the law; (2) Failing to perform duties in reporting and notifying epidemics of avian influenza in human in accordance with the law, or concealing, falsely reporting, or delaying the reporting of epidemic situation of infectious diseases; (3) Failing to actively collect information on epidemic situation of the avian influenza in human, or failing to analyze, investigate and verify the epidemic situation information and epidemic report of infectious diseases in a timely manner; (4) failing to implement measures specified in this law in a timely manner according to duties when an epidemic situation of avian influenza in human is discovered; (5) Intentionally disclosing personal privacy-related information and data concerning patients with avian influenza, carriers of pathogen, suspected patients with infectious disease, and close contacts.
      2. If a medical institution violates the provisions of the Law of the People's Republic of China on the Prevention and Treatment of Infectious Diseases and falls under any of the following circumstances, the administrative department of public health under the people's government at or above the county level shall order it to make corrections, circulate a notice of criticism, and give it a warning. If an infectious disease has been transmitted or spread or other serious consequences have been caused, the persons in charge, and other persons directly responsible shall be punished with the punishment of demotion, dismissal from office or dismissal according to law, and the practice certificates of the persons concerned may be revoked according to law. If the case constitutes a crime, criminal responsibility shall be investigated according to law.

15.11 Quarantine

Since the avian influenza virus H5N1 caused many deaths in Hong Kong in 1997, avian influenza in human has become a newly discovered infectious disease that has attracted worldwide attention. Due to the migration of migratory birds, the epidemic spread quickly. Cases of avian influenza in human have occurred successively in areas with high poultry density such as Southeast Asia and China. In order to prevent and control avian influenza, all countries have strengthened quarantine measures. The main measures are quarantine of poultry from epidemic areas and medical observation and detention of patients with fever. According to the "Law of the People's Republic of China on the Prevention and Control of Infectious Diseases," avian influenza in human, like SARS, is a category B infectious disease managed as category A infectious disease and meets the conditions of the "Domestic Traffic Quarantine Regulations." To this end, the State Administration of Quality Supervision, Inspection and Quarantine issued the "Emergency Notice on Strengthening the Health and Quarantine Work for Prevention and Control of Avian influenza in Human at Ports." The "Notice" requires all ports to strictly implement eight port disease prevention systems: entry–exit health declaration system, entry–exit body temperature testing system, medical inspection system, patient control system, ventilation and disinfection system, epidemic report system, self-protection system, and publicity education system.

I. Frontier health and quarantine

   In order to prevent the spread of avian influenza into or out of China, international navigable ports, airports, land borders, and international rivers import and export ports shall implement quarantine on incoming and outgoing personnel, vehicles, poultry, and their products.
   (i) Passengers must declare health.
      1. Entry personnel and transportation staff should carefully fill in the Entry Quarantine Declaration Card, especially stating clearly the contact address and telephone number in China, so as to make contact when necessary. When a suspected case is found in a vehicle, all passengers and transport staff are required to provide identification, detailed address, and contact information for the journey within 7 days.
      2. The inspection and quarantine agency shall strengthen the on-site sanitation and quarantine (mainly temperature test), medical observation and medical inquiry of the entry and exit personnel, and promptly take controlling measures and report in time when suspected patients are found.
   (ii) Handling of suspected cases, clinically diagnosed cases, and their close contacts.
      1. If entry and exit personnel are found to have the following conditions at the port: high fever

(>39 °C), accompanied by respiratory symptoms such as dry cough, shortness of breath, or dyspnea with close contact with a patient with avian influenza within 1 week before the onset of illness or recent visits to poultry, influenza-affected areas, it is necessary to declare to the port inspection and quarantine agency, which shall immediately take necessary measures for suspicious cases, and immediately contact the local health administration department. People with the above symptoms will be transferred by 120 negative pressure ambulance to the local designated hospital for diagnosis and treatment. Those with the above symptoms observed after arriving at their destination should be diagnosed and treated on the spot in time, and the patients should explain the recent travel history to the doctor; travelers with the above symptoms are recommended to discontinue their voyage in order to get the diagnosis and treatment in time.

2. If passengers or staff with the above symptoms are found on planes, ships, trains, cars, and other transportation vehicles crossing the border, the vehicle manager should report to the port of destination, and the inspection and quarantine agency should contact immediately the local health authority. After the vehicle arrives, people with the above symptoms will be immediately escorted by a special 120 negative pressure ambulance and transferred to the local designated hospital for diagnosis and treatment. For other passengers and transportation employees, the inspection and quarantine agency shall issue a "Entry Health Advice" and disinfect the transportation means.
3. Ports, wharfs, airports, railway stations, and long-distance bus stations shall be provided with detention stations to retain infected persons or suspected persons who are coming from or intending to take transportation means.

II. Domestic traffic quarantine

(i) Health declaration and health quarantine.

1. Inspection stations shall be set up in railway stations, long-distance bus stations, and passenger terminals of airports, where people entering and leaving the local areas are required to make health declaration and registration, and medical examinations are carried out, including main test of temperature. People with a temperature of more than 38 °C are prohibited from taking transportation means and sent to the detention station for isolation and medical observation.
2. Strengthen sanitation inspections on the transportation vehicles and the materials they carry in and out of the local area, and implement strict sanitation treatments such as disinfection if any contaminated or potentially contaminated items are found.

(ii) Handling of suspected cases, clinically diagnosed cases, and their close contacts.

1. If fever is detected, the medical staff of the inspection station will make medical examination and epidemiological history inquiry according to the "Diagnosis and Treatment Plan for Avian Influenza in Human." If it is considered in preliminary judgment as a defined case of "unexplained pneumonia," local health administration department should be contacted immediately and persons with the above symptoms should be transported by special vehicles to the local designated hospital for diagnosis and treatment.
2. If a case of avian influenza or pneumonia of unknown etiology is found on a train, automobile, aircraft, or ship, the person in charge of the transportation shall immediately notify the railway, transport, or civil aviation department of the nearest city ahead and make the necessary preparations. At the same time, measures such as isolation and ventilation shall be taken immediately on the means of transport, investigation, and registration shall be conducted for passengers in the same cabin or carriage where the patient is in and other people who have close contact with the patient, and all stations along the way shall be notified to contact relevant departments to make preparations. Carry out epidemiological investigations and necessary medical examinations for passengers who get off the train and have close contact with patients.
3. If a patient with confirmed or suspected avian influenza is found during the voyage, the transportation means shall be terminally disinfected immediately after response measures are adopted for the patient.
4. The staff on the transportation means shall conscientiously perform their duties, assist in the searching, and take quarantine, ventilation and necessary disinfection measures, and immediately conduct the investigation and registration of close contacts, when the relevant CDC informs them to assist in the investigation and search for patients and suspected patients that need to be tracked down.
5. When an epidemic of avian influenza is identified on a transportation means in someone having passed traffic quarantine, the health administrative department of the province, autonomous

region, or municipality directly under the Central Government where the epidemics occur shall promptly report it to their counterparts in regions related to the epidemics.
6. When necessary, the health administrative department announces to the public the means of transportation that the patient has taken, and requires close contacts to go to the local quarantine office or medical institute for medical observation.

The prevention and control of avian influenza in humans is an eternal task for mankind.

Only by innovation and exploration can we remain invincible. We need to further sum up experience, and constantly perfect the working mechanism of integrated prevention and control, innovate working methods, increase investment, and raise the level of basic public health services, and combine the prevention and treatment of infectious diseases in key areas and key crowd, with prevention and control of the major epidemic, so as to guard people's health and make new contributions to a well-off society in an all-round way [28]. We should uphold the principle of grand health and grand hygiene, promote a new pattern of government-led work, departmental coordination, social participation, combination of special groups and mass prevention and control, actively participate in international public health governance and prevention and control of infectious diseases, and increase China's influence in major global disease prevention and control. We look forward to promoting exchanges and cooperation between Chinese health personnel and experts from around the world, integrating technologies and strategies in prevention and control of major infectious diseases into our public health services, and further enhancing our disease prevention and control capacity. By establishing an academic platform for avian influenza in human, we can face the problems with better and perfected strategies, thereby making a stride in the journey toward the goal of "healthy China" [29, 30].

References

1. State Council. Law of prevention and control of infectious diseases, People's Republic of China on, June 29, 2013.
2. Chen Q, Jin M, Chen H. Research progress of vaccines for avian influenza. Chin J Bioeng. 2004;04:34–8.
3. Li L. Epidemiological progress. Beijing: Beijing Medical University Press; 2002.
4. Ministry of Health. Emergency plan for human infection with highly pathogenic avian influenza on May 26, 2006.
5. Ministry of Health. Technical guidelines for preventing from and controlling epidemics of avian influenza in human. February 4, 2004.
6. Ministry of Health. Monitoring program for unexplained pneumonia. August 4, 2004.
7. Ministry of Health. Rules for treatment of patients with acute respiratory fever December 29, 2004.
8. Ministry of Health. Technical plan for laboratory detection of avian influenza. September 13, 2004
9. Ministry of Health. Management standard for reporting infectious disease information. October 29, 2015.
10. Ministry of Health. Administrative plan for reporting avian influenza in human. Chin Commu Med. 2004;010(001):5–8.
11. Ministry of Health. Emergency Regulations Regarding Emergency Public Health Incidents (January 18, 2011).
12. Ministry of Health. Management measures for public health emergencies and report of infectious disease monitoring information November 2003.
13. Ministry of Health. Notification on the revision of the management measures for public health emergencies and report of infectious disease monitoring information. August 22nd 2006.
14. Ministry of Health. Guiding principles for set-up of fever outpatient (emergency) department in medical institutions (run-in) May 2003.
15. Ministry of Health. Guidelines for protecting personnel with occupational exposure to avian influenza. February 27, 2004.
16. Ministry of Health. Criteria for determining close contacts of avian influenza and the administrative principle. February 27, 2004.
17. Ministry of Health. Epidemiological investigation plan for avian influenza in human. J Prev Med Inf. 2006;22(3):273–6.
18. Ministry of Health. Technology plan for disinfection of avian influenza. Chin Rural Med. 2004;03:74–5.
19. Zhang Y, Yu C. Types avian influenza vaccines and their advantages/disadvantages. Technol Inf Anim Husb Vet Sci 2006;(3):13–6.
20. Wang L, Li K. Research progress on immunogenicity of avian influenza virus and its vaccine. Prog Microbiol Immunol. 2006;34(2):54–7.
21. Yang H, Yi B. Modern disinfection science in hospital. Beijing: People's Military Medical Press; 2013.
22. Ministry of Health. Administrative measures for pre-examination and triage of infectious diseases in medical institutions. February 28, 2005.
23. Ministry of Health. Administrative measures for nosocomial infection. July 6, 2006.
24. Ministry of Health. Health administrative punishment procedures. June 19, 1997.
25. Ministry of Health. Implementation plan for monitoring avian influenza in human. Chin Rural Med. 2004;11(3):7–8.
26. Ministry of Health. Management measures for disinfection. December 26, 2017.
27. Ministry of Health. Administrative Regulations on Medical Wastes. 2011-1-8.16 Ministry of health, measures for the management of medical waste in medical and health institutions, October 15, 2003.
28. Hou Y. Controlling strategies and effects of major emerging infectious diseases. Electron J Emerg Infect Dis. 2019;4(3):129–32.
29. Li X, Yu X, Yu M, et al. Control of avian influenza in human in Guiyang City from 2009 to 2018 and strategy analysis. J Appl Prev Med. 2019;4(3):129–32.
30. Li L. Attentative analysis of prevention and control of avian influenza in human. Diet Health. 2018;5(29):256–7.

Prognosis

16

Gui-lin Yang, Dong-na Su, and Chen Qiu

Compared with SARS, human avian influenza can evolve more abruptly into hypoxemia, ARDS, shock, multiple organ failure, and other complications quickly, and most of the patients die of severe respiratory or circulatory failure. According to the analysis of available clinical data, age, sex, underlying diseases, peripheral white blood cells, lymphocyte and platelet counts, changes in T lymphocyte subsets, pulmonary lesion area, arterial blood gas, complications, different treatment measures, hospitalization time, and virus subtypes are all factors affecting the prognosis. The relevant evidence needs to be further confirmed by a large-scale worldwide epidemiological survey.

16.1 Prognosis and Outcome

I. Global fatality rate of human avian influenza

As of March 29th, 2007, cases of H5N1 avian influenza in human have been found in 12 countries around the world. Among them, 285 confirmed cases were reported in total with 170 deaths and a mortality of 59.7%. If the confirmed cases of H5N1 avian influenza in human in Hong Kong, China from 1997 to 2003 are included, there are 305 confirmed cases with 177 deaths and an overall mortality of 58.0%, which is far higher than that of SARS globally (10.9%) published by the WHO. As of March 2nd, 2018, a total of 1,567 laboratory-confirmed cases of human infected with H7N9 avian influenza have been reported globally through the reporting channel specified by International Health Regulations since 2013, including 615 deaths with a cumulative mortality of 39.2%.

II. Mortality of avian influenza in human in China

From 1997 to 2003, 23 cases of avian influenza in human in total were found in Hong Kong, China, of which there were 20 cases of H5N1 highly pathogenic human avian influenza and 3 cases of H9N2. A total of 7 cases were dead and they were all infected with H5N1, with a mortality of 35%, which was lower than the global average level [1]. As of June 30th, 2019, 52 cases of H5N1 avian influenza in human have been reported in China's mainland including 33 deaths with a mortality of 63.5%, which is slightly higher than the average level in the world. As of June 30th, 2019, a total of 1401 H7N9 cases have been reported in China including 562 deaths and a mortality of 40.1%. From March 30th to May 20th, 2013, 103 confirmed cases of human infected with H7N9 avian influenza were reported together with their onset time and confirmed time in China's mainland including 36 deaths with a mortality of 34.9%. From 2013 to 2018, 259 and 8 confirmed cases of human infected with H7N9 and H5N6 avian influenza were found in Guangdong Province of China, with a mortality of 38.6% and 62.5%, respectively [2]. As of January 2017, a total of 21 cases of human infected with H9N2 avian influenza has been reported in China's mainland including 1 death with a mortality of 4.8%.

III. Outcome

H5N1 and H7N9 avian influenza in human may cause various complications. Pneumothorax, acute lung injury

The original version of the chapter has been revised. A correction to this chapter can be found at https://doi.org/10.1007/978-981-16-1429-3_17

G.-l. Yang
Department of Infectious Diseases, Shenzhen People's Hospital (The Second Clinical Medical College, Jinan University, The First Affiliated Hospital, Southern University of Science and Technology), Shenzhen, Guangdong, China

D.-n. Su
Department of Infectious Diseases, Shenzhen People's Hospital, The Second Clinical Medical College of Jinan University, The First Affiliated Hospital of Southern University of Science and Technology, Shenzhen, Guangdong, China

C. Qiu (✉)
Department of Respiratory Diseases, Shenzhen People's Hospital, The Second Clinical Medical College of Jinan University, The First Affiliated Hospital of Southern University of Science and Technology, Shenzhen, Guangdong, China

C. Qiu et al. (eds.), *Avian Influenza in Human*, https://doi.org/10.1007/978-981-16-1429-3_16

(ALI), ARDS, secondary bacterial infection, fungal infection, pleural effusion, pleurisy, liver function damage, renal function damage, cardiac insufficiency, DIC, and others may occur in acute phase of the influenza. The main reason is that H5N1 and H7N9 avian influenza viruses cause systemic inflammatory response syndrome (SIRS) after the body is infected, thus leading to multiple organ dysfunction syndrome (MODS) [3]. For children infected with avian influenza who take aspirin during the onset, Reye syndrome mainly characterized by acute encephalopathy and fatty degeneration of hepatocytes may be induced. Osteoporosis, femoral head necrosis, mediastinal emphysema, and stress disorder related to human avian influenza may occur during the convalescent period. In addition, pulmonary fibrosis, an important pathological outcome of severely damaged lungs, can reduce lung compliance and lung volume, presenting restrictive, and diffuse ventilatory disorder. Pulmonary fibrosis also occurred in the course of the first patient in Shenzhen City, China infected with H5N1 human avian influenza who was successfully rescued by us. The lesions were not completely absorbed by the time of discharge, and pulmonary fibrosis was gradually absorbed and improved during long-term follow-up.

16.2 Factors Affecting Prognosis

Human avian influenza is an infectious disease that has not still been fully recognized. Based on the analysis of existing clinical data, factors affecting prognosis may include subtypes of avian influenza virus infected, age, sex, course of disease, underlying diseases, changes in hemogram and T lymphocyte subsets, pulmonary lesion area, arterial blood gas, complications, and treatment. As there are no results of large-scale worldwide epidemiological survey for further analysis of the multiple factors of death, further analysis and conclusion are still needed for the factors affecting the prognosis of human avian influenza.

I. Subtypes of avian influenza virus infecting human

The prognosis of patients infected with avian influenza is related to the subtypes of viruses. Most of the patients infected with subtype H9N2, H7N7, H7N2, and H7N3 have a good prognosis while those with highly pathogenic avian influenza in human such as H5N1, H7N9, and H5N6 are characterized by high rate of severe case and high mortality.

II. Age

According to statistical results of H5N1 human avian influenza cases in Hong Kong from 1997 to 2003, there were 12 cases under 18 among which 2 cases died, with a mortality of 16.7%. Both children died of multiple organ failure (MOF), and one of them died of Reye syndrome. There were 8 adult cases aged between 19 and 60 among which 5 cases died, with a mortality of 62.5%, showing a significant difference compared with the mortality in children ($P < 0.05$). However, the mortality rate of cases under 15 in Thailand is 89%, higher than that of adults. Based on the analysis of clinical data in China, it was found that the onset age of H5N1 human avian influenza patients amassed between 20 and 40. There were 15 cases in total, among which 10 cases died, with a mortality of 66.7%. There were 5 cases who were children under 10 years. Among them, 2 cases died, with a mortality of 40%. There were 3 cases above the age of 40 years among which 2 cases died, with a mortality of 66.7%. In light of the above results, the effect of age on prognosis is still uncertain and needs further study. Among the 30 confirmed cases of human infected with H7N9 avian influenza in Hangzhou, China in 2013, there were 23 males (Male:female = 3.29:1) and an age of 35–86 (M = 62) years [4]. The subtypes H7N9 and H5N6 of human infection with avian influenza viruses occurred in both men and women in Guangdong Province from 2013 to 2018. Among them, the cases with H7N9 were more common in men, accounting for 65.6% (170/259), and the cases with H5N6 subtype were more common in female, accounting for 62.5% (5/8). The minimum age of H7N9 cases was 0.8, the maximum age was 88.0, and the median age was 56.0. The minimum age of H5N6 cases was 4.0, the maximum age was 58.0, and the median age was 28.5 [2].

III. Gender

There were 41 cases infected with H5N1 avian influenza in China mainland and Hong Kong, including 17 male cases and 24 female cases. The sex ratio was 0.708. Of the only 20 cases in Hong Kong, China, the prognosis of female patients was slightly better than that of male patients; statistics on Chinese data showed a mortality of 66.7% (6/10) in males and of 64.3% (9/14) in females. There was no significant difference between them ($P > 0.751$). Among the 103 confirmed cases with H7N9 avian influenza in China, more were male [69.6% (87/125)] and those aged over 50 [72.8% (91/125)]. The cases were distributed in 10 provinces (municipalities directly under the central government) in China. The total number of reported cases in Zhejiang Province, Jiangsu Province and Shanghai (municipalities directly under the central government) accounted for 81.5% of the total cases. It is suggested that men, middle-aged and elderly people are the main populations susceptible to human infection with H7N9 avian influenza viruses, and the southeastern coast of China is the key area with human avian influenza monitored [5]. In Guangdong Province, H7N9 cases from 2013 to 2018 were mostly male, accounting for 65.6% (170/259); more female cases were observed for subtype H5N6, accounting for 62.5% (5/8) [2].

IV. Underlying diseases

The presence or absence of underlying diseases is an important factor affecting the prognosis of human avian influenza. Through researches, Chen Qi et al. [5] found that being elderly (over 60) combined with underlying diseases was the main risk factor for death caused by human avian influenza, OR = 8.075. This is also an important feature of H5N1 and H7N9 human avian influenza. For elderly patients, with the growth of age, their organ function gradually declines, accompanied by chronic diseases, especially combined with hypertension, cardiovascular and cerebrovascular disease, emphysema, chronic liver disease, and diabetes, which predispose them to multiple organ complications and lead to death [6].

V. Changes in the total number of white blood cells, lymphocytes, and platelets.

(1) The relationship between the total number of white blood cells and prognosis.

The total number of white blood cells of patients with human avian influenza is generally decreased to different degrees, which is closely related to the severity of the disease. The total number of white blood cells decreased significantly in both severe and critical patients [7, 8]. According to literature, 11 of the 18 patients with human avian influenza in Hong Kong, China showed a significant decrease in their peripheral white blood cells (WBC). Among patients in Vietnam and Thailand with avian influenza [9], the degree of leucopenia was significantly correlated with the severity of the disease and death of the patients. The average WBC was 3.70×10^9/L in the death group, and 6.0×10^9/L in the survival group. Therefore, strengthening the monitoring of the total number of white blood cells in patients with avian influenza is helpful to judge the disease progression and prognosis of patients with avian influenza.

(2) The relationship between the total number of lymphocytes and prognosis.

In most of the patients with avian influenza, the absolute value of lymphocyte count in peripheral blood decreased gradually, and there were cell morphological changes. Peripheral blood lymphocytes decreased significantly in severe patients, and the reduction of peripheral blood lymphocytes was significantly correlated with the severity of the disease [10]. At present, some studies suggest that changes in the absolute value of peripheral blood lymphocytes in newly diagnosed patients with avian influenza may be more significant in diagnosis than that of white blood cells.

(3) The relationship between total platelet count and prognosis.

For most patients with avian influenza, the peripheral total platelet was normal in their early onset. However, the total platelet count was decreased in some serious patients. Thailand's study found that the decrease of platelet count on admission was related to the increased risk of death. The average platelet count in the death group was 145×10^9/L and that in the survival group was 243×10^9/L. A small number of severe patients showed platelet elevation in the late stage of the disease due to secondary bacterial infection. Duration and bacterial infection are positively correlated.

According to literature reports, among the 15 cases of human avian influenza in Vietnam and Thailand, the count of 53.3% patients' peripheral blood platelet is less than 100×10^9/L at the time of admission, and the mortality rate of patients with a significantly lower platelet count at admission has increased significantly.

VI. Changes in T lymphocyte subsets and cytokines

For human avian influenza, the changes rule of T lymphocyte subsets is different from that of SARS. SARS patients may have a significant decrease in the absolute counts of $CD3^+$, $CD4^+$, and $CD8^+$ T lymphocytes during the course of the disease while patients with avian influenza mainly show a significant decrease in the $CD4^+$ T lymphocyte count, and the $CD8^+$ T lymphocyte count does not change significantly, so the $CD4^+/CD8^+$ ratio decreases. Observation of clinical cases of avian influenza in human [11] showed that the count of $CD4^+$ T lymphocytes significantly decreased with the progression of the disease, and the more severe the disease, the lower the count. According to the reports, the extent of damage of human avian influenza T lymphocytes is significantly related to the severity of the disease. That is, the T lymphocyte subsets of patients with severe human avian influenza have decreased significantly compared with mild cases, and the number of deaths has decreased more significantly. In addition, the reduction of T lymphocytes in human avian influenza patients is a reversible change, and gradually returns to normal levels as the disease improves. Unlike ordinary influenza, the recovery of the absolute number of lymphocytes and the ratio of $CD4^+/CD8^+$ often indicate the improvement of the disease. Therefore, changes in the absolute counts and proportions of T lymphocyte subsets of human avian influenza patients have important influence and predictive value on the prognosis of patients. The dynamic changes of lymphocyte count and $CD4^+/CD8^+$ ratio may be prognostic indicators of avian influenza inhuman. In addition, plasma cytokines such as TNF-α, IL-6, and IL-8 were significantly higher and lasted longer in the deaths than in the survivors, whose level of cytokines returned roughly to normal level during the recovery period [12]. The level of cytokines had a close relationship with acute lung injury.

VII. Complications

The main cause of death was the multiple organ failure (MOF) caused by avian influenza virus after infecting human beings, so the presence of multiple organ function impairments during the course of disease indicated a poor prognosis [13, 14]. The biochemical markers indicative of different organ damage also became important predictors of prognosis. LDH was an important indicator of cardiomyocyte damage and an important predictor of the prognosis of human avian influenza. A persisting high level of LDH often indicated a poor prognosis for the patient. When hepatic impairment happened, ALT and TBIL might be abnormal; when renal insufficiency occurred, BUN and Cr increased obviously. Under severe stress, endocrine metabolism became disordered, and blood glucose and blood lipids became abnormal. It is generally believed that the presence of multiple obvious abnormalities in the above biochemical parameters in patients with avian influenza patients indicated a poor prognosis.

References

1. Liang Z, He D, Weng W, et al. Review and implications of controlling avian influenza in human in Hong Kong, China. Chin J Tuberc Respir Dis. 2004;27(4):253–8.
2. Yang Y, Tan X, Ye M, et al. Epidemiological and clinical characteristics analysis of human infected with H7N9 and H5N6 avian influenza viruses in Guangdong Province, 2013–2018. Int J Virol. 2019;26(6):375–8.
3. Li C. A review of WHO risk assessment of influenza pandemic and response strategies. China Pharm Aff. 2006;20(6):370–4.
4. Xie L, Ding H, Sun Z, et al. Distribution and characteristics of cases of human infected with H7N9 avian influenza viruses in Hangzhou in 2013 and analysis of their exposure sources. Chin J Epidemiol. 2013;34(9):944–5.
5. Yan T, Xiao D, Wang B, et al. Epidemiological characteristics of 130 cases of H7N9 avian influenza in human in mainland China. Chin J Dis Control Prev. 2013;17(8):651–4.
6. Wan D, Kang X, Bai W, et al. Clinical characteristics and prognostic analysis of 20 cases of human infected with H7N9 avian influenza viruses. Chin J Tuberc Respir Dis. 2019;42(10):750–4.
7. Bi Y, Chen Q, Wang Q, Gao GF. Genesis, evolution and prevalence of H5N6 avian influenza viruses in China. Cell Host Microbe. 2016;20(6):810–21.
8. Luo R, Zhu Y, Xu Z, et al. The first case of H6N1 human avian influenza pneumonia reported in mainland China. Chin J Pediatr. 2006;44(5):342–5.
9. Zhao X, Jia N. Clinical observation of 22 cases with avian influenza in human in Vietnam. J China Jpn Friendship Hosp. 2004;18(6):369–70.
10. Zhang W, Wen L, Lu M, et al. Analysis of clinical characteristics of the first case of highly pathogenic H5N1 avian influenza in human in Jiangxi Province. Chine J Tuberc Respir Dis. 2006;29(5):300–6.
11. Peiris JS, Yu WC, Leung CW, et al. Re-emergence of fatal human influenza A subtype H5N1 disease. Lancet. 2004;363(9409):617–9.
12. Kandasamy M, Furlong K, Perez JT, et al. Suppression of cytotoxic T cell functions and decreased levels of tissue resident memory T cell during H5N1 infection. J Virol. 2020;94(9):e00057–20.
13. Yang L, Zhu W, Li X. Genesis and dissemination of highly pathogenic H5N6 avian influenza viruses. J Virol. 2017;91(5):JVI.02199-16.
14. Tran TH, Nguyen TL, Nguyen TD, et al. Avian influenza A (H5N1) in 10 patients in Vietnam. N Eng I J Med. 2004;350(12):1179–88.

Correction to: Avian Influenza in Human

Correction to: C. Qiu et al. (eds.), *Avian Influenza in Human,* https:// doi.org/10.1007/978-981-16-1429-3

The book has been inadvertently published with errors in chapters 1, 2, 3, 4, 5 and 16

In chapter 1, the below corrections have been updated

On page 1, the previous text "....strain of avian viruses in southern China...." has been changed to "...strain of avian influenza viruses in southern China..." and also "China mainland" to "China's mainland"

On page 4, the previous text "...stimulate CD8+T cells..." has been changed to "...stimulate $CD8^{+}T$ cells..."

In chapter 2, the below corrections have been updated

On page 9, "Mainland China" to "China's mainland"

On page 10, the previous text "(including Turkey,..." has been changed to "(including turkey,..."

In chapter 3, the below corrections have been updated

On page 19, the previous text "...performed by KatZJM et al." has been changed to "...performed by Kat ZJM et al."

On page 22, the previous text "The influenza virus is an..." has been changed to "The avian influenza virus is an..." and also the previous text "...commonly used for influenza virus..." has been changed to "commonly used for avian influenza virus..."

On page 27, the previous text "...outcome inhuman disease..." has been changed to "...outcome in human disease..." and also the previous text "...influenzaAH7N9..." has been changed to "...influenza A H7N9..."

In chapter 4, the below corrections have been updated

On page 31, the previous text CD4+T, CD8+T has been changed to CD4/CD8, and also the previous text $CD4^{+}T$, $CD8^{+}T$ has been changed to $CD4^{+}/CD8^{+}T$ cells

On page 34, the previous text "(Reye's Syndrome..." has been changed to "(Reye's syndrome..."

On page 36, Fig 4.4 and Fig 4.5 have been swapped

On page 37, the previous text "CD3, CD4, CD15, CD8, CD20, CD68" has been changed to "$CD3^{+}T$ cells, $CD4^{+}T$ cells, $CD15^{+}T$ cells, $CD8^{+}T$ cells, $CD20^{+}T$ cells, $CD68^{+}T$ cells"

On page 38, in legend of Fig 4.11, the previous text "The CD8..." has been changed to "The $CD8^{+}T$ cells..."

On page 39, the legend of Fig 4.19 has been changed to "In situ expression in pulmonary tissues in human infected with H7N9 avian influenza; positive signals are in blue, with stronger staining in nucleus than in the plasma, in situ hybridization ×400"

In chapter 5, the below corrections have been updated

On page 41, the previous text "...$CD4^{+}/CD8^{+}$ ratio..." has been changed to "...$CD4^{+}/CD8^{+}T$ cells..."

On page 44, in Table 5.1, the previous text H2N7 has been changed to H7N7

In chapter 16, the below corrections have been updated

On page 187 "China mainland" to "China's mainland"

The updated versions of the chapters can be found at
https://doi.org/10.1007/978-981-16-1429-3_1;
https://doi.org/10.1007/978-981-16-1429-3_2;
https://doi.org/10.1007/978-981-16-1429-3_3;
https://doi.org/10.1007/978-981-16-1429-3_4;
https://doi.org/10.1007/978-981-16-1429-3_5;
https://doi.org/10.1007/978-981-16-1429-3_16.

C. Qiu et al. (eds.), *Avian Influenza in Human*, https://doi.org/10.1007/978-981-16-1429-3_17

In chapters 1, 2, 6, 7, 15, 16, the affiliation of author Chen Qu has been changed from "Department of Respiratory and Critical Medicine, Shenzhen People's Hospital (The Second Clinical Medical College, Jinan University, The First Affiliated Hospital, Southern University of Science and Technology), Shenzhen, Guangdong, China" to "Department of Respiratory Diseases, Shenzhen People's Hospital, The Second Clinical Medical College of Jinan University, The First Affiliated Hospital of Southern University of Science and Technology, Shenzhen, Guangdong, China".

In chapters 4, 6, 7, the affiliation of author Shi-pin Wu has been changed from "Department of Infectious Diseases, Shenzhen People's Hospital (The Second Clinical Medical College, Jinan University, The First Affiliated Hospital, Southern University of Science and Technology), Shenzhen, Guangdong, China" to "Department of Infectious Diseases, Shenzhen People's Hospital, The Second Clinical Medical College of Jinan University, The First Affiliated Hospital of Southern University of Science and Technology, Shenzhen, Guangdong, China".

In chapters 8, 14, the affiliation of author, Jin-ping Wu has been changed from "Department of Radiology, Third People's Hospital of Changzhou City, Changzhou, Jiangsu, China" to "Department of Radiology, Third People's Hospital of Changzhou, Changzhou, Jiangsu, China".

In chapter 14, the affiliation of author Wei Huang has been changed from "Bacteriology and Antibacterial Resistance Surveillance Laboratory, Shenzhen Institute of Respiratory Diseases, Shenzhen People's Hospital (The Second Clinical Medical College, Jinan University, The First Affiliated Hospital, Southern University of Science and Technology), Shenzhen, Guangdong, China" to "Bacteriology & Antibacterial Resistance Surveillance Laboratory, Shenzhen Institute of Respiratory Diseases, Shenzhen People's Hospital, The Second Clinical Medical College of Jinan University, The First Affiliated Hospital of Southern University of Science and Technology, Shenzhen, Guangdong, China".

In chapter 4, the affiliation of author Xiao-hua Le has been changed from "Department of Pathology, Shenzhen Third People's Hospital, Shenzhen, Guangdong, China" to " Department of Pathology, The Third People's Hospital of Shenzhen, Shenzhen, Guangdong, China".

In chapter 5, the affiliation of author Wan-shui Shan has been changed from "Department of Clinical Laboratory, Shenzhen Third People's Hospital, Shenzhen, Guangdong, China" to "Department of Clinical Laboratory, The Third People's Hospital of Shenzhen, Shenzhen, Guangdong, China".

In chapters 10, 12, the affiliation of author Fei shi has been changed from "Emergency Department, Institute of Shenzhen Respiratory Diseases, Shenzhen People's Hospital (The First Affiliated Hospital of Southern University of Science and Technology, The Second Clinical Medical College of Jinan University), Shenzhen, Guangdong, China" to "Emergency Department, Institute of Shenzhen Respiratory Diseases, Shenzhen People's Hospital, The Second Clinical Medical College of Jinan University, The First Affiliated Hospital of Southern University of Science and Technology, Shenzhen, Guangdong, China".

In chapters 6, 16, the affiliation of author Dong-na Su has been changed from "Department of Infectious Diseases, Shenzhen People's Hospital (The Second Clinical Medical College, Jinan University, The First Affiliated Hospital, Southern University of Science and Technology), Shenzhen, Guangdong, China" to "Department of Infectious Diseases, Shenzhen People's Hospital, The Second Clinical Medical College of Jinan University, The First Affiliated Hospital of Southern University of Science and Technology, Shenzhen, Guangdong, China".

In chapters 2, 7, 13, the affiliation of author Dong-na Su has been changed from "Shenzhen Institute of Respiratory Diseases, Shenzhen People's Hospital (The Second Clinical Medical College, Jinan University; The First Affiliated Hospital, Southern University of Science and Technology), Shenzhen, Guangdong, China" to "Shen zhen Institute of Respiratory Diseases, Shenzhen People's Hospital, The Second Clinical Medical College of Jinan University, The First Affiliated Hospital of Southern University of Science and Technology, Shenzhen, Guangdong, China".

MIX
Papier aus verantwortungsvollen Quellen
Paper from responsible sources
FSC® C105338

If you have any concerns about our products,
you can contact us on
ProductSafety@springernature.com

In case Publisher is established outside the EU,
the EU authorized representative is:
Springer Nature Customer Service Center GmbH
Europaplatz 3, 69115 Heidelberg, Germany

Printed by Libri Plureos GmbH
in Hamburg, Germany